Battling Smallpox before Vaccination

Clio Medica

STUDIES IN THE HISTORY OF MEDICINE AND HEALTH

VOLUME 105

The titles published in this series are listed at *brill.com/clio*

Battling Smallpox before Vaccination

Inoculation in Eighteenth-Century Germany

By

Jennifer D. Penschow

BRILL

LEIDEN | BOSTON

Cover illustration: Allegorical image from Graeco-Roman mythology: the god of medicine, Aesculapius, forces death to retreat. Drawing attributed to Jacques-Charles Bordier du Bignon (1774–1826). Source: Wellcome Collection; V0007559. Public Domain Mark.

Library of Congress Cataloging-in-Publication Data

Names: Penschow, Jennifer D., author.
Title: Battling smallpox before vaccination : inoculation in eighteenth-century Germany / by Jennifer D. Penschow.
Description: Leiden ; Boston : Brill, [2022] | Series: Clio medica, 0045-7183 ; Volume105 | Includes bibliographical references and index.
Identifiers: LCCN 2021047207 (print) | LCCN 2021047208 (ebook) | ISBN 9789004465138 (hardback) | ISBN 9789004465374 (ebook)
Subjects: LCSH: Smallpox–Vaccination–Germany. | Smallpox–Germany–18th century.
Classification: LCC RA644.S6 P46 2022 (print) | LCC RA644.S6 (ebook) | DDC 614.5/210943–dc23/eng/20211103
LC record available at https://lccn.loc.gov/2021047207
LC ebook record available at https://lccn.loc.gov/2021047208

Typeface for the Latin, Greek, and Cyrillic scripts: "Brill". See and download: brill.com/brill-typeface.

ISSN 0045-7183
ISBN 978-90-04-46513-8 (hardback)
ISBN 978-90-04-46537-4 (e-book)

This book is printed on acid-free paper and produced in a sustainable manner.

Difficulties must inspire courage rather than crush it, in order to advance such a beneficial deed for mankind. Even if they cannot be overcome, compassion demands that the effort be made.

FRIEDRICH II (the Great), King of Prussia, 1778

Contents

Author's Note and Acknowledgements

German spelling in the eighteenth century was quite flexible and sometimes differed from modern spelling. Some of the more common differences were the addition of an 'h' after a 't' (*Theil* rather than the modern *Teil*), an omitted or an added 'e' in many words (*gegebne* rather than the modern *gegebene*; *gelehret* rather than *gelehrt*), the addition of a 'c' before 'k' in some instances (such as in *Gedancken*, now spelled *Gedanken*), and the interchangeable use of 'c' and 'k' before a vowel (*Carl* or *Karl*; *inoculation* or *inokulation*). Words such as the modern *medizinischen* were spelled with 'c' (*medicinischen*), and 'ei' in modern usage was 'ey' in certain contexts (*vorbey* rather than the modern *vorbei*).

All of the translations are my own, unless otherwise stated.

I wish to thank, firstly, my husband Reinhold for his encouragement, companionship, and for sharing his enduring interest in his German homeland. I also thank Jacqueline Gratton for our engaging discussions, Michael Bennett for his historical insights and for checking the manuscript, and Elizabeth Freeman for helpful advice. I am grateful to the University of Tasmania for the provision of research materials, particularly the librarians, and to the reading room staff at the *Historisches Gebäude* at the *Niedersächsische Staats- und Universitätsbibliothek Göttingen*, the *Universitätsbibliothek Kiel*, the *Bibliothek J.C. Senckenburg* at the University of Frankfurt am Main, and the *Universität Rostock Bereichsbibliothek 2*, for assistance in providing source material. I thank, too, the archivists at the *Stadtarchiv Göttingen* and the *Hessische Hauptstaatsarchiv* for their searches.

Figures

Illustrations

Maps

Table

Abbreviations

ADB	*Allgemeine deutsche Bibliothek*
AFS	*Auszüge aus den besten französischen periodischen, medicinischen, chirurgischen, und pharmaceutischen Schriften*
AGM	*Archiv für Geschichte der Medizin*
ALZ	*Allgemeine Literatur-Zeitung*
Apx	Appendix
ASZ	*Aerztliche sachverständige Zeitung*
BA	*Braunschweigisches Anzeigen*
BMN	*Bunzlauische Monatsschrift zum Nutzen und Vergnügen*
BMS	*Berlinische Monatsschrift*
BRM	*Braunschweigisches Magazin*
BSA	*Berlinische Sammlungen zur Beförderung der Arzneywissenschaft*
CM	*Clio Medica*
DM	*Deutsches Museum*
DMS	*Deutsche Monatsschrift*
DVG	*Deutsche Vierteljahrsschrift für öffentliche Gesundheitspflege*
FAE	*Fränkische Acta Erudita et Curiosa*
FGN	*Fortgesetzte neue Genealogish-historische Nachrichten*
GA	*Göttingische Anzeigen von gelehrten Sachen*
GB	*Gelehrte Beyträge zu den Braunschweigischen Anzeigen*
HAM	*Hamburgisches Magazin, oder gesammelte Schriften aus der Naturforschung und den angenehmen Wissenschaften überhaupt*
HB	*Hannoverische Beyträge zum Nutzen und Vergnügen*
HM	*Hannoverisches Magazin*
HUN	*Hamburgische freye Urtheile und Nachrichten zum Aufnehmen der Wissenschaften und Historie überhaupt*
JAW	(*Hufeland's*) *Journal der practischen Arzneykunde und Wundarzneykunst*
JCH	*Journal of Contemporary History*
JD	*Journal von und für Deutschland*
JE	*Journal der Erfindungen, Theorien und Widersprüche in der Natur und Arzneiwissenschaft*
JHM	*Journal of the History of Medicine and Allied Sciences*
JP	*Journal für Prediger*
JRS	*Journal of the Royal Society*
LI	*Leipziger Intelligenzblatt*
LM	*Lausitzisches Magazin, oder Sammlung verschiedener Abhandlungen*
MCZ	(*Hartenkeil's*) *Medicinisch-chirurgische Zeitung*

MF	*Gemeinnütziges Magazin für die Freunde der nützlichen und schönen Wissenschaften und Künste*
MM	*Monatsschrift von und für Mecklenburg*
NB	*Niederrheinisch-westfälische Blätter*
NMI	*Neue Miscellaneen historischen, politischen, moralischen, auch sonst verschiedenen Inhalts*
NS	*Nützliche Sammlungen*
NZT	*National Zeitung der Teutschen*
PA	*Physikalisch-Oekonomische Auszüge aus den neuesten und besten Schriften, die zur Naturlehre, Haushaltungskunst, Policei, Kameral-, auch andern damit verwandten Wissenschaften*
PAD	*Patriotisches Archiv für Deutschland*
PJ	*Philosophisches Journal für Moralität, Religion und Menschenwohl*
PT	*Philosophical Transactions of the Royal Society*
RA	*Kaiserlich priviligierter Reichs-Anzeiger*
RNS	*Das Reich der Natur und der Sitten*
SP	*Schlesische Provinzialblätter*
TM	*Der teutsche Merkur*
UCP	*University of California Publications in Modern Philology*
VSH	*Verhandlungen und Schriften der hamburgischen Gesellschaft zur Beförderung der Künste und nützlichen Gewerbe*
WM	*Westphälisches Magazin zur Geographie, Historie und Statistik*
ZGH	*Zeitschrift für die gesamte Hygiene*
ZMG	*Zeitschrift für die gesamte innere Medizin und ihre Grenzgebiete*
ZMK	*Zahn-, Mund-, und Kieferheilkunde*

Abbreviations for the additional journals listed in Appendix 2 are shown at the beginning of that appendix.

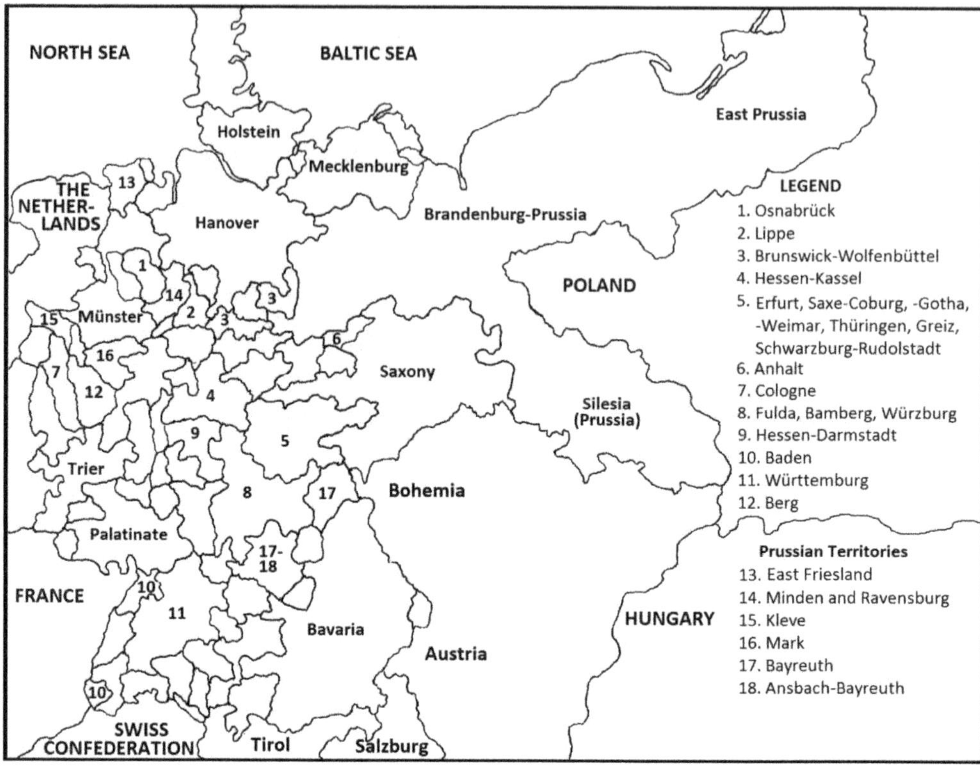

MAP 1 A disunited Germany and its neighbours, ca. 1791
© JENNIFER PENSCHOW

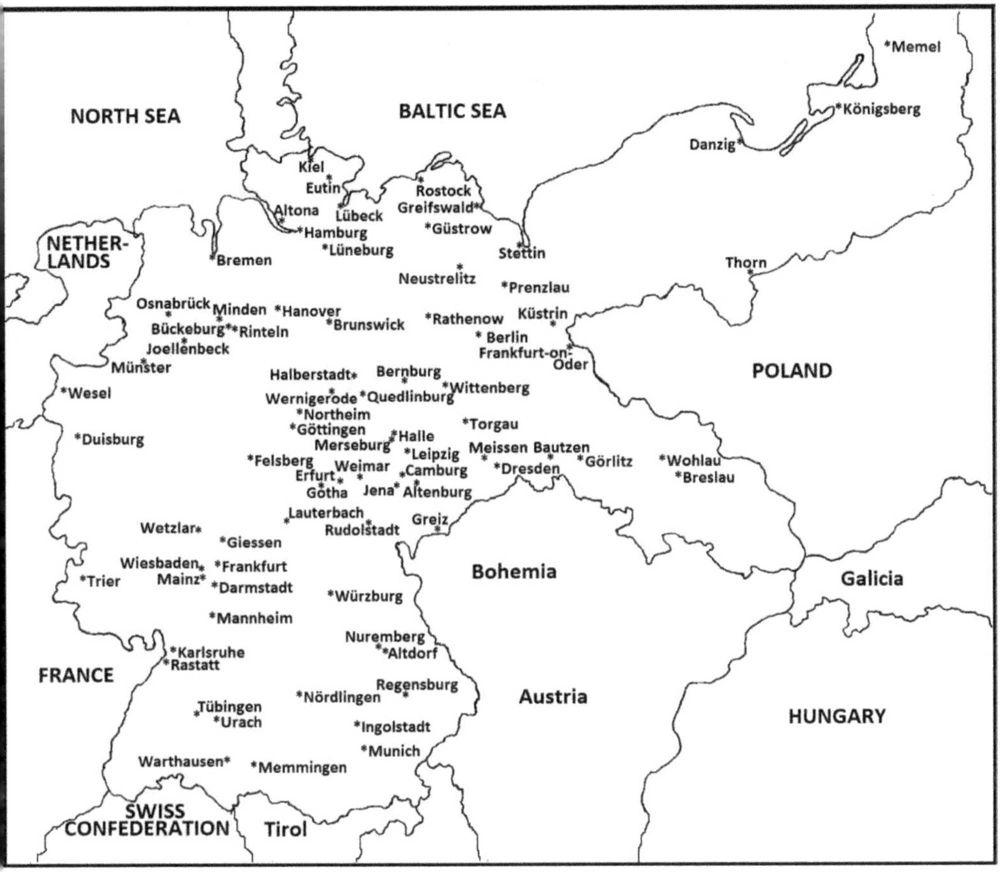

MAP 2 Cities and towns in Germany in the eighteenth century
© JENNIFER PENSCHOW

Introduction

Vaccination – the cornerstone of preventive medicine – has tragically become a victim of its own success in pushing back many of the infectious diseases that killed and maimed past generations. Now the very idea of vaccinating children seems to arouse greater fear among some parents than the afflictions that immunisation prevents. New pestilences, too, threaten to overwhelm us if newly-developed vaccines are shunned to the extent that 'herd immunity' cannot be achieved. Opponents of vaccination would perhaps reconsider their stance if they were to see their child suffer in this way:

> The face is monstrously swollen and horrifyingly disfigured, the eyes are unseeing, the nose is blocked, the swollen-closed gullet begs for water but cannot get it down; … the whole body from the scalp to the soles of the feet is pustules and pus; … the body and face are covered in a brown, or often black, crust interspersed with runnels of stinking pus, a rotting purulence that has sometimes corroded the flesh from the bones; … after ten or more days and nights of such torment, the mother and father sigh and wish that death will end the indescribable screaming, that heart-rending suffering of the sick one who has passed into putrefaction.[1]

That was a death from smallpox. All but 5 per cent of eighteenth-century Europeans were afflicted at some time in their lives by that disease caused by the *Variola major* virus, which commonly killed one in three or four victims in the most virulent of the epidemics that swept across the landscape every four to seven years.[2] Indeed, smallpox killed so many children that it was personified in Germany as the 'murdering angel' for mimicking the biblical *Würgeengel* sent by God to murder the first-born Egyptians.[3] Modern children and parents

1 Bernhard C. Faust, "An den Kongreß zu Rastadt über die Ausrottung der Blattern," *Deutsches Magazin* 16 (1798): 379–80.

2 N.A. Humphries, "English Vaccination and Small-Pox Statistics: with Special Reference to the Report of the Royal Commission, and to Recent Small-Pox Epidemics," *Journal of the Royal Statistical Society* 60 (1897): 523; Andreas-Holger Maehle, "Conflicting Attitudes Towards Inoculation in Enlightenment Germany," CM 29 (1995): 200.

3 Eberhard Wolff, "Der 'willkommene Würgeengel,' Verstehende Innenperspektive und 'genaue' Quellen-interpretation – am Beispiel des erwünschten Kindertods in den Anfangen der Pockenschutzimpfung," in *Neue Wege in der Seuchengeschichte,* ed. Martin Dinges

 | DOI:10.1163/9789004465374_002

can be eternally grateful to the Gloucestershire surgeon-scientist Edward Jenner for demonstrating that vaccination with cowpox prevented smallpox, providing the weapon that slashed the smallpox death-rate soon after its introduction in 1799 and paved the way for the eventual global eradication of the disease in 1978.[4]

This book is a social history of smallpox in Germany before the introduction of Jenner's cowpox vaccination. More specifically, it explores the encouragement and adoption, or indeed rejection, of a crude form of immunisation known as inoculation or variolation, which was first practised by western medical men in 1721. The 300th anniversary of the initiation of smallpox inoculation in Europe and North America, coinciding as it does with the optimistic rollout of vaccines to curb the Covid-19 pandemic that has caused so much global dislocation and death, seems an ideal time to reflect on the pre-vaccination era approaches to combating smallpox, particularly through the encouragement of inoculation in the face of widespread doubts about the morality and safety of the practice.

Inoculation, in its simplest form, involved merely scratching the skin with a needle and inserting infectious matter from a smallpox pustule, in the hope of producing mild symptoms that would protect against a potentially fatal future case of the disease.[5] The practice first came to the attention of western medical men through a number of different avenues that led back to the procedure used by Greek women in Constantinople (modern Istanbul) to protect their children from severe smallpox.[6] Descriptions of the method first began appearing in British and European journals during 1714–17, beginning with an article in the *Philosophical Transactions of the Royal Society* by the Greek doctor Emanuele Timoni, a graduate of Padua who was working in Constantinople.[7] According to Timoni, inoculation arrived in the city from Circassia and Georgia about forty years earlier and had been used successfully on thousands of people in the previous eight years without cause for concern. The procedure has also been traced to Armenia and Samarkand as well as parts of Africa, India, and the Ottoman Empire, while in China the preferred method, known

(Stuttgart: Steiner, 1995), 104–7; *Die heilige Schrift*, trans. S.G. Dom, part 3 (Berlin and Basel, 1782), 321.

4 Donald A. Henderson, *Smallpox: the Death of a Disease* (New York: Prometheus, 2009).

5 Michael J. Bennett, *War Against Smallpox. Edward Jenner and the Early Global Spread of Vaccination* (Cambridge: Cambridge University Press, 2020), 10–12, 18.

6 Genevieve Miller, *The Adoption of Inoculation for Smallpox in England and France* (Philadelphia: University of Pennsylvania Press, 1957), 56–7, 67–9, 72, 92, 173.

7 Miller, 55–9, 287–8.

as insufflation – blowing dried, powdered smallpox material up the nose – was already firmly documented in the sixteenth century.[8]

Western medical men began to inoculate in 1721 in Massachusetts, England, Anhalt-Bernburg (Germany), and Hungary in response to severe epidemic smallpox.[9] The most inoculations at that time were carried out in Boston at the urging of the Reverend Cotton Mather, a medical doctor and member of the Royal Society who had read Timoni's account of inoculation in a 1714 issue of the Society's journal. Noting the similiarity of the method to the childhood experience related by his slave Onesimus, a Guaramante from the region of modern southern Libya who bore the scar from inoculation on his arm, Mather's curiosity prompted him to make further inquiries among the local Africans and traders. Having learned that the procedure was quite common in parts of Africa, and was known to provide reliable protection against future smallpox, Mather was confident in pushing for inoculation when smallpox struck Boston in 1721.[10] Dr. Zabdiel Boylston, the only practitioner willing to make a start, initially inoculated his own children, and was so encouraged by the outcome that he offered his new-found expertise more widely. While the physician William Douglass issued a prescient warning of the potential spread of the contagion from inoculated individuals, Boylston kept inoculating while Mather continued to defend the practice against the opponents accusing supporters and practitioners of opposing the will of God. When the epidemic ended, Boylston's tally of inoculations in one year had reached 247.[11]

Inoculation was initiated in Britain in April 1721, a month before Boylston began his impressive effort, when Lady Mary Wortley Montagu called in Charles Maitland to inoculate her daughter. The method was quite familiar to both the child's mother and to Maitland, who was the embassy surgeon during Lord Montagu's term as the British Ambassador to the Ottoman Empire. On the occasion when Lady Montagu arranged for an old Greek woman to inoculate her young son in Adrianople in 1718, Maitland gained first-hand experience by intervening with his lancet to complete the procedure when the woman's rusty needle proved inadequate.[12] His successful inoculation of the Montagu's

8 Alicia Grant, *Globalisation of Variolation: the Overlooked Origins of Immunity for Smallpox in the 18th Century* (New Jersey: World Scientific, 2018), 261, 280; Arthur Boylston, "The Origins of Inoculation," *JRS* 105 (2012): 309–12, https://doi:10.1258/jrsm.2012.12k044 (accessed 13 February 2021); Bennett, *War*, 17–18.

9 Miller, *Adoption*, 67–8, 72, 92, 173.

10 Miller, 92–6; Boylston, "Origins," 309–10.

11 Ian Glynn and Jennifer Glynn, *The Life and Death of Smallpox* (London: Profile, 2004), 60–3.

12 Miller, *Adoption*, 68–72.

daughter in London three years later generated considerable interest among leading medical men while also capturing the attention of the scientifically-inclined Princess of Wales, Caroline of Ansbach, who was keen to follow Lady Montagu's example.[13] The royal interest led to an initial experiment on six adults undertaken by Royal Society medical men, and to a second involving six orphaned children, which was funded by the princess. The success of both trials paved the way for the inoculation in 1722 of two of Princess Caroline's daughters. Yet despite such an auspicious start, the practice became mired in controversy rather than being greeted with widespread enthusiasm, though aristocratic and elite parents tended to follow the royal lead rather than being dissuaded by the polemic.[14]

By the end of the 1720s inoculation had faded in Britain as well as in the few parts of Europe where it had been tried on small numbers of children.[15] Yet the procedure was soon making a comeback in North America, beginning in Boston where a smallpox outbreak in 1730 led to 2,000 inoculations among residents willing to defy a ban on the practice. A further 500 individuals were inoculated in Philadelphia in 1730–31, and more than 800 during a smallpox outbreak in Charleston in 1738, while hundreds more were reported in Barbados and St. Kitts.[16] News arriving in London of such high numbers of inoculations in North America and the Caribbean helped to bring about a recommencement of the practice in various parts of Britain struck by smallpox in the 1740s, and in 1744 approval was granted for the inoculation of children admitted to the London Foundling Hospital. The groundwork had well and truly been laid for a major resurgence in activity when severe smallpox struck London in 1751.[17] The procedure was making a comeback in Europe too, initiated by the Swiss physician Theodor Tronchin's inoculation of his son and other children in Amsterdam in 1748. Its further spread in Europe largely followed the smallpox epidemic that swept across the continent in the mid-1750s, with inoculations reported in many regions, though the activity was quite sporadic and usually involved very few candidates.[18]

---

13 Isobel Grundy, *Lady Mary Wortley Montagu* (Oxford: Oxford University Press, 1999), 211–2.

14 Miller, *Adoption*, 84–5, 96–7; Glynn and Glynn, *Smallpox*, 53–5, 64–7.

15 Neither the five inoculations in 1721 in Bernburg, nor the one in Eperjes, nor the other inoculations reported in Europe during the 1720s led to further inoculations at the time: Miller, 67–8, 173–8; Arnold C. Klebs, *Die Variolation im achtzehnten Jahrhundert: ein historischer Beitrag zur Immunitätsforschung* (Gießen: Töpelmann, 1914), 58–9.

16 Bennett, *War*, 55.

17 Bennett, 23, 34–6, 55, 63.

18 Klebs, *Variolation*, 36, 45, 48, 52–4, 56, 59.

Inoculation was hotly debated and widely rejected in European states during the subsequent decade, echoing the controversies that had surrounded its use in Boston and Britain in the 1720s.[19] The moral and ethical dilemma of inoculating a healthy child with a potentially deadly disease caused considerable disquiet, as did the perception that inoculation interfered in Providence. Nor could parents' fears that their child may die from inoculation be lightly dismissed, nor the problem of failed inoculations, nor the contagiousness of inoculated smallpox. The longstanding belief that smallpox was innate, inevitable, and indeed necessary as well as beneficial for purging the body of disease-causing contaminants was another major disincentive to the adoption of the practice. Those kinds of issues as well as local influences largely determined the popularity and longevity of inoculation in communities across Europe before the procedure was superseded circa 1800 by cowpox vaccination.[20]

In Germany, inoculation was tried on individuals and on small groups of candidates in several places during the 1720s, accompanied a surge of largely unrelated publications on the topic. Yet the interest soon waned to relative dormancy until influences from abroad brought about a reinvigoration in 1750.[21] The recommencement of inoculation procedures in Germany in 1755 initiated a continuous practice for the remainder of the eighteenth century that generated vigorous discussion in the print media.[22] This book explores the social and cultural influences that shaped the evolving approaches to curbing the high smallpox mortality in Germany at that time, including not only the encouragement and practice of inoculation but also strategies aimed toward convincing parents to modernise their home treatments for smallpox, and the eventual promotion of isolation measures to prevent the spread of the disease. With regard to inoculation, the extent to which the practice spread in German territories during the second half of the eighteenth century had much to do with regional differences in enthusiasm for Enlightenment-inspired ideas for

---

19 Antoinette S. Emch-Dériaz, "L'Inoculation Justifiée, or Was it?," *Eighteenth-Century Life* 7 (1982): 65–9; Arnold H. Rowbotham, "The 'Philosophes' and the Propaganda for Inoculation of Smallpox in France," UCP 18 (1935): 271–83.

20 Peter Skold, *The Two Faces of Smallpox, A Disease and its Prevention in Eighteenth and Nineteenth-Century Sweden* (Umea: Umea University Press, 1996), 268, 289–90, 344; Maehle, "Attitudes," 203–5, 215–6; Eberhard Wolff, *Einschneidende Maßnahmen: Pockenschutzimpfung und traditionale Gesellschaft im Württemberg des frühen 19. Jahrhunderts* (Stuttgart: Steiner, 1998), 106–8.

21 References listed in Apx 1 and Apx 2: Miller, *Adoption*, 67–8, 71–2, 84–5, 172–9.

22 Apx 2; Maehle, "Attitudes," 203–5; Wolfram Kaiser, "Impfärzte des 18. Jahrhunderts," ZMK 64 (1976): 387–95.

improvements in public health and disease prevention.[23] At that time, articles promoting inoculation were regularly published in the plethora of new kinds of journals that were a feature of the flourishing publishing scene linked to the expansion of the public sphere.[24] Such journals were being read by not only subscribers from the well-educated social echelon but also by an increasingly literate broader cross-section of society. Yet women and readers in rural areas had less access to the range of periodical publications available to men in the larger towns, who could read journals and newspapers at public libraries or reading societies, and at some cafés.[25] Other influences shaping the differing regional approaches to ameliorating the impact of smallpox emanated from the fragmentation of the German 'fatherland' into hundreds of free cities and sovereign states of vastly differing sizes and complexities. The many universities, sponsored mainly by princes ruling the larger states, had an important influence on high-level decision-making by shaping the ideas of the graduates recruited by the multitude of local and territorial governments requiring large numbers of well-educated officials.[26] Some of the university-educated men (women were excluded from university courses), including many poets and writers, formed an influential intelligentsia with a shared objective of achieving enlightened social change.[27] Those men were among the social commentators, academics, doctors, and other Germans who came to regard inoculation as not only the hallmark of the new disease prevention approach of the so-called medical Enlightenment, but also as an emancipation from the notion that man's destiny was determined by God.[28] Lutheran pastors, too, were among the university-educated groups that largely subscribed to the new ideas and were keen to encourage enlightened social change.[29]

---

23 Ute Frevert, *Krankheit als politisches Problem, 1770–1880* (Göttingen: Vandenhoek & Ruprecht, 1984), 49–53; 108–9; Mary Lindemann, "'*Aufklärung*' and the Health of the People; '*Volksschriften*' and Medical Advice in Braunschweig-Wolfenbüttel, 1756–1803," in *Das Volk als Objekt obrigkeitlichen Handelns,* ed. Rudolf Vierhaus (Tübingen: Niemeyer, 1992), 108–9.

24 Eckhart Hellmuth and Wolfgang Piereth, "Germany, 1760–1815," in *Press, Politics, and the Public Sphere in Europe and North America, 1760–1820,* eds. Hannah Barker and Simon Burrows (Cambridge: Cambridge University Press, 2002), 70–6. See also Table 1 and Apx 2.

25 Ulrich Im Hof, *Das Europa der Aufklärung* (Munich: Beck, 1993), 106–7.

26 Peter Watson, *The German Genius* (London: Simon and Schuster, 2010), 51–4, 826; Tim C.W. Blanning, *The Culture of Power and the Power of Culture; Old-Regime Europe, 1660–1789* (Oxford: Oxford University Press, 2002), 205–6.

27 Blanning, 207–11; Hellmuth and Piereth, "Germany," 69–70.

28 Maehle, "Attitudes," 203–4; Wolff, *Maßahmen,* 23–4.

29 Lindemann, '*Aufklärung,*' 105–6; Anthony J. La Vopa, *Grace, Talent, and Merit. Poor Students, Clerical Careers, and Professional Ideology in Eighteenth-Century Germany* (Cambridge: Cambridge University Press, 1988), 337–8.

Around the turn of the twentieth century a number of German scholars marked the centenary of the adoption of Jenner's cowpox vaccination by examining the influence of the prior inoculation period as a forerunner to vaccination. Arnold Klebs concluded from his exploration of the origins of inoculation and of the medical men who facilitated the spread of the practice across Europe, that inoculation provided the great benefit of inspiring an unprecedented level of sharply-focused research into smallpox, which considerably increased medical knowledge of the disease.[30] The general conclusion drawn by Gustav Behrend, Gotthold Mamlock, and Peter Kübler from their own respective studies was that inoculation was beneficial for familiarising parents with the insertion of smallpox matter into the skin to prevent severe smallpox, which aided the later public acceptance of the insertion of cowpox matter in the same way, for the same purpose.[31]

In a much more recent study focused on the Duchy of Württemburg, Eberhard Wolff too examined the influence of inoculation as a forerunner to cowpox vaccination. He showed that inoculation began in the territory in 1768, was adopted among the elite, and was not influenced by any actions of the prince. Yet he found that it was limited even among the upper social echelon by concerns about the contagion and the potential for a severe case of the inoculated disease, while the broader society generally rejected the procedure on the basis of misconceptions about smallpox or religiously-based prejudices.[32] Peter Albrecht showed that inoculation was generally unpopular in Brunswick-Wolfenbüttel at much the same time, even after the government publicised the successful inoculation of the crown-prince's first-born son and other elite children during 1767–68, and followed up with an ongoing offer of free inoculation and after-care for the poor.[33] Gotthold Mamlock showed that the Prussian public was similarly reluctant to accept inoculation, despite the attempts of

30 Klebs, *Variolation*, 63.

31 Gustav Behrend, "Ueber Variolation," *DMW* 20 (1896): 311–12; Peter Kübler, *Geschichte der Pocken und der Impfung* (Berlin: Hirschwald, 1901), 141; Gotthold L. Mamlock, "Friedrich der Grosse und die Einführung der Impfung in Berlin," *ASZ* 10 (1904): 38–41. Some of those pre-war publications as well as Moritz Pistor, "Geschichte der preussischen Medizinalverwaltung," *DVG* 40 (1908): 749–810, are invaluable for their extensive citations of eighteenth-century records that have since been lost.

32 Woff, *Maßnahmen*, 12, 104–8.

33 Peter Albrecht, "Von den vergeblichen Mühen, die Bevölkerung der Stadt Braunschweig von der Nützlichkeit des Impfens gegen Blattern zu überzeugen (1754–1787)," in *Gotts Verhengnis und seine Straffe – zur Geschichten der Seuche in der frühen Neuzeit*," ed. Petra Feuerstein-Herz (Wolfenbüttel: Herzog August Bibliothek, 2005), 128–32, 135–6.

the king, Friedrich II (the Great), to improve the inoculation expertise of Prussian medical men by arranging targeted training by British experts.[34]

Peter Albrecht and Andreas-Holger Maehle examined the German inoculation discourse, particularly the contentious religious and medical issues previously debated in Britain and France. While Albrecht focused on the conundrum confronting parents deciding whether or not to adopt inoculation, and on the arguments raised by doctors as well as by philosophers and theologians, Maehle turned his attention to the broader discourse. From various doctors' reports and publications, he notes quite low numbers of inoculations with a usual but not exclusive upper-class bias.[35] Maehle also points to the promotion of isolation measures in the 1790s, with or without inoculation, particularly Professor Johann Christian Wilhelm Juncker's initiatives that included the organisation of a society of doctors to work toward the eradication of smallpox. He places a strong focus on Juncker's invitations to several German philosophers to express their views on the ethics and morality of inoculation, and their responses, particularly whether those views accorded with pronouncements made by the erudite Immanuel Kant from Königsberg.[36] Juncker's inoculation-related activities were more of a central focus for Kurt Werner, Wolfram Kaiser, and Arina Völker from the medical faculty at the Martin-Luther University Halle-Wittenberg, Juncker's *alma mater*. As part of their studies of doctors who engaged in inoculation in Germany, those scholars paid particular attention to the influence of Juncker and other academics from their own faculty who encouraged inoculation, as well as to the Halle graduates who became known as inoculators.[37]

This book paints a broader picture of inoculation in Germany than the one that has already emerged, by examining which social and professional groups were encouraging inoculation, how those groups structured their various

34 Mamlock, "Einführung," 39–40; Gotthold L. Mamlock, *Friedrichs des Grossen Korrespondenz mit Aerzten* (Wiesbaden: Sändig, 1966), 24, 106–9.

35 Maehle "Attitudes," 200–209; Peter Albrecht, "Wie hältst Du es mit der Blatterninokulation? Eine 'Gretchenfrage' im 18. Jahrhundert," *Praxis Geschichte* 5 (1999): 58–60.

36 Maehle, 212–15; Andreas-Holger Maehle, "The Ethics of Prevention: German Philosophers of the Late Enlightenment on the Morality of Smallpox Inoculation," in *Coping with Sickness. Perspectives on Health-Care Past and Present*, eds. John Woodward and Robert Jütte (Sheffield: E.A.H.M.H., 1996), 94–104.

37 Wolfram Kaiser and Kurt Werner, "Die Anfänge der Pockenschutzimpfung in Halle und Umgebung," *ZGH* 19 (1973): 807, 809–11; Kaiser, "Impfärzte," 387–8, 392–5; Arina Völker, "Johann Christian Wilhelm Juncker (1761–1800) und die Dessauer Impfpropagisten," in *Johann Juncker (1679–1759) und seine Zeit*, eds. Wolfram Kaiser and Hans Hübner (Halle-Wittenberg: Martin Luther University, 1979), 86–90, 95; Arina Völker, "Einige Markierungspunkte aus der Geschichte der Pockenschutzimpfung," *ZMG* 45 (1990): 394–6.

approaches, what kind of responses they encountered in various communities, which other strategies were adopted or proposed to ameliorate the impact of smallpox, and what influences shaped the various approaches. It relies on published sources, owing to the relative scarcity of pertinent archival records. The *Stadtarchiv* in Göttingen (Hanover) produced no relevant records at all, even though inoculation was practised in the town for a considerable time,[38] yet vaccination in the years after 1800 was well-documented. Eberhard Wolff reported similarly that his perusal of various archives in Württemburg revealed little about smallpox prophylaxis until the nineteenth century when official cowpox vaccination initiatives were under way.[39] On the other hand, as Peter Albrecht showed in his study of government-supported inoculation in Brunswick-Wolfenbüttel, the archives in that region contain a rich store of material about inoculation. Many other, potentially relevant, archival records were lost during World War II and the subsequent occupation.

Published dissertations, statutes, letters, reports, books, articles, novels, reviews, and poetry, the main sources used here, are unfortunately unsuited to statistical analysis of whether inoculation reduced regional smallpox mortality to a measurable extent. On the other hand, some of the reports provide sufficient indications of local inoculation activity for rough assessments of that kind to be made if matching smallpox mortality data is available. More comprehensive demographic studies are hampered by not only the relative scarcity of archival records but also by a dearth of accurate smallpox mortality figures. Most surviving church registers fail to show a cause of death before 1764 when Prussia led the way with a new regulation requiring that information. Subsequent records from the remainder of the inoculation period usually list only the last observed symptom before death, with rarely a mention of smallpox or any other underlying disease.[40] As Walter Rödel points out in his demographic analysis of smallpox in Mainz in 1766–67, since no cause of death was recorded alongside the names of the many children who died, his calculations of smallpox mortality relied on a report of the disease in the area at the time and on age-related probability based on the knowledge that children were the primary victims of smallpox.[41]

38 Albrecht, "Mühen," 128–36; Apx 2: Klärich (1778), 209–22.

39 Wolff, *Maßnahmen*, 43–5.

40 Frevert, *Krankheit*, 25; Heinrich A. Gins, *Krankheit wider den Tod* (Stuttgart: Fischer, 1963), 67–8.

41 Walter G. Rödel, "Die Pocken in Mainz in Jahre 1766," *Medizinhistorisches Journal* 14 (1979): 55, 78–9.

The published sources used for this book all have particular strengths that collectively provide the material for painting a broad picture of the medical and social history of smallpox and inoculation in Germany in the eighteenth century. The seven volumes of Professor Johann Christian Wilhelm Juncker's so called 'archive' (1796–99) of his smallpox eradication campaign, which include reports published exactly as they were submitted to Juncker by pastors, doctors, and local officials across the length and breadth of Germany, are crucial sources that provide a range of important insights into local attitudes to smallpox and inoculation.[42] Multiple observations of similar attitudes among various social groups, by different commentators, lends a collective authenticity to the observations. Similarly, the considerable body of books and articles about inoculation used as source material, when assessed chronologically and collectively, shows the extent to which the topic was being discussed by doctors, churchmen, and other interested commentators at various times. Those kinds of sources also reveal the evolving ideas about smallpox that underpinned the gradual change in the commentary and the eventual recommendations for a new approach to prophylaxis. At a more individual level, some of the reports and articles by country pastors and others in close contact with their communities are important for revealing local attitudes toward smallpox that shaped much of the parental decision-making about inoculation. The obituaries and other laments in verse offer an emotional view of the impact of smallpox through their power to convey the agony and anguish of the illness for victims and their loved-ones. Other kinds of poetry and literature are valuable for their intrinsic ability to illustrate the cultural history of smallpox and the hope offered by inoculation, particularly for young women and mothers.

In the first chapter, the suffering and death that motivated the efforts to improve smallpox treatments and promote inoculation are underscored through poetic laments, while a variety of contemporary reports reveal the raft of deeply-entrenched myths and misconceptions that gave rise to much scepticism about the purported benefits of inoculation. Letters, statutes, reports, and journal articles, which are the main sources for chapter 2, reveal the intuitive inoculation-related intiatives of a number of princes, in addition to those examined previously, and the contribution of princes' wives and elite physicians as well as the rural nobility in encouraging the local adoption of inoculation. Academia comes into the spotlight in chapter 3 where dissertations, books, and articles by professors and their former students, backed up by contemporary histories of various universities, identify medical school professors who were encouraging the spread of inoculation by not only teaching

42 Johann C.W. Juncker, *Archiv der Aerzte und Seelsorger wider die Pockkenoth,* 7 vols. (Leipzig: Weygand, 1796–99).

the procedure to their students but also by providing other kinds of inspiration. This chapter shows that the University of Halle (Prussia) medical school, highlighted previously as a focal point from which inoculation practice spread around Germany, was neither alone nor indisputably the most influential of the twenty-eight German medical schools, in having such an impact. The work of the surgeons, a largely overlooked group of inoculators who rarely put pen to paper, are examined in this chapter too, through local reports of surgeons' activities.

Chapter 4 explores the discourse involving a broad cross-section of Germans who promoted inoculation in the print media, or indeed argued against it. From the articles published by the various journals that facilitated the discussion, it is evident that the editors of some provincial publications played an important role in giving 'average parents' the opportunity to engage in the discussion. With regard to the dissemination of the preferred viewpoints of the educated elite, the important issue emerges of potential 'censorship' occurring at the various stages of the publication process. The focus of chapter 5 is women's attitudes to inoculation, and men's attitudes to women making their own decisions on the matter, which are revealed largely through the works of enlightened poets who directed pertinent 'advice' in their verse. Such poetry brings into sharp focus the insecure future facing women disfigured by smallpox and the hurdles facing those who resisted the patriarchal dictates of the society of the time. Chapter 6 explores the challenges of curbing the impact of smallpox across the vast rural landscape where three-quarters of Germans lived and worked in agriculture. Reports by the occasional doctor and particularly by the country pastors provide much of the detail about attempts to assist country folk in dealing with smallpox, and the overall effectiveness of the various approaches adopted by not only the pastors themselves but also by governments and local landowners. Some rural inoculation initiatives explored in this chapter, when related to a set of regional smallpox mortality statistics published by Rolf Gehrmann, suggest that inoculation may have had a noticeable impact in lowering smallpox mortality in particular regions.[43] Inoculation in Germany has otherwise been generally regarded as either too unpopular, too limited, too poorly recorded, or too contagious to have had such a demonstrable positive influence.[44]

43 Rolf Gehrmann, "The impact of smallpox and vaccination in Northern Germany in the 18th and 19th centuries," *Przeszlość Demograficzna Polski* 36 (2014): 48–9.

44 Kübler, *Geschichte*, 139; Albrecht, "Mühen," 134–5; Wolff, Maßnahmen, 106–7; Maehle, "Attitudes," 209–10; Behrend, "Variolation," 310–11; Mary Lindemann, *Health and Healing in Eighteenth-Century Germany* (Baltimore and London: Johns Hopkins University Press, 1996), 332.

Chapter 7 moves on to the final phase in the evolution of doctors' and other commentators' opinions about inoculation: the increasing demands in the 1790s for a change of approach. These are revealed in the plethora of published proposals aimed toward the eradication of smallpox through containment and quarantine measures. By the time those proposals crystallised into two campaigns for smallpox eradication, which were both actively fund-raising from the mid-1790s, the question demanding an answer was the reason behind the growing perception that the eradication of smallpox was actually achievable without any improvements or additions to the tools that had long been at hand.

Works primarily about inoculation that were published in Germany during the eighteenth century are listed in two appendices: Appendix 1 shows dissertations; Appendix 2 lists journal articles, books, and reviews. Sources listed in the appendices are cited in footnotes as: Apx 1 or Apx 2: the author or an abbreviated title if the work is anonymous, the journal (if relevant to the discussion), the year of publication (in brackets), and the page number(s). An abbreviated title is added if the author published more than one listed work in that year.

CHAPTER 1

Realities, Myths, and Perceptions

The spectre of smallpox was ever-present in eighteenth-century society. Faces marred by the characteristic disfigured features or pitted scars were in every crowd and social gathering, and children blighted by pustules were a common sight whenever smallpox was on the march. Diminished families and grieving mourners going to and from the all-too-frequent funerals for the smallpox dead at such times issued sobering reminders of the destructive capacity of the disease. Yet the impact of smallpox was far worse than statistics suggesting that it caused 10–20 per cent of of all deaths.[1] Such figures fail to consider the many survivors left so weak that they died after the sickness had passed, or the countless victims left crippled, blind, or disfigured.[2] A more realistic view of the impact of smallpox is revealed by the concerted efforts to curb the disease and by the heartfelt laments for victims than by the understated mortality figures. Although inoculation inspired initial optimism that the suffering and deaths could be reduced, such hopes were soon quashed by public resistance to the practice, based to some extent on myths and misconceptions about smallpox that denied the very concept of prophylaxis.[3] While the smallpox suffering continued, so did the laments.

1 Reality and Mythology of Smallpox

'Smallpox poetry' bewailing the destructive effects of severe smallpox on its tragic victims provides us with vivid reminders of the ability of smallpox to kill and to maim, as do inspirational poetic accounts of determined efforts to end the suffering and deaths. Another value of 'smallpox poetry,' pointed out

1 Bernhard C. Faust, "Versuch über die Pflicht der Menschen, jeden Blatternkranken der Gesunden abzusondern; und dadurch zugleich in Städten und Ländern und in Europa die Ausrottung der Blatternpest zu bewirken," *PJ* 4 (1794): 49; Donald R. Hopkins, *The Greatest Killer: Smallpox in History* (Chicago: University of Chicago Press, 2002), 75.

2 Deafness, blindness, closed nostrils, disfigured jaws, tooth loss, and crippled, wasted limbs were among the lasting effects of smallpox: Carl A.W. Berends, *Handbuch der praktischen Arzneiwissenschaft* (Vienna: Hapkul, 1830), 45–6. One in eight or nine survivors died from after-effects of smallpox, and one in ten was disfigured or weakened: Faust, 49–53.

3 Christoph W. Hufeland, "Neue Aussicht zur Vertilgung der Blattern," *TM* 4 (1786): 167–81, 253–63; Apx 2: Heinsius (1780), 89–90, 96.

 | DOI:10.1163/9789004465374_003

by David Shuttleton, is the recruitment of the reader's imagination to consider the victim's ordeal.[4] Just two lines from a 'burial poem' is indeed sufficient for the squeamish mind to recoil at the unimaginable torment endured by a woman whose death was attributed to the pain of giving birth while suffering from fatal smallpox:

Ist gleich der Schmerzen groß, wenn Schmerzen sich verbinden,	The agony is great when pains are joined together,
Wenn Pocken und Geburt mit sich vergattet sind.[5]	When smallpox and childbirth pair with one-another.

Others watched in horror as their children succumbed to the sickness. One such excruciating ordeal that caused great distress to the boy's parents was described at length by the Hamburg senator Barthold Heinrich Brockes, in his poignant farewell to his fourteen year-old son Johann who endured a lingering death from smallpox in 1731.

Die Glut, die dich erhitzt, die Angst, die dich erfüllt,	The glowing fire that's heating you, the pervasive fear
Durch Schmerzen, welche dir das Blut so heftig pressen,	Arising from your pain and worsened by the pulsing blood,
Daß dein verwirrter Geist entstellet, flüchtig, wild,	That your muddled mind, distorted, wild and flighty,
Ohn alle Regel wirkt, ganz aussern Schranken schweift,	Now working without discipline, wanders unconfined,
Und (einem Uhrwerk gleich, das ohne sein Gewicht	And like a clock that's lost its weights
Mit lautem Rasseln rennt) auch ohnaufhörlich läuft,	Still runs, but rattling loudly with no time,
Erhitzt, erfüllt und presst auch mich.[6]	Heats, pervades, and pressures me, as well.

4 David E. Shuttleton, *Smallpox and the Literary Imagination, 1660–1820* (Cambridge: Cambridge University Press, 2007), 3, 6, 14, 51, 53.

5 "Begräbniß Carme," M. Francisco Wokenius, *Anleitung zur teutschen Poesie* (Leipzig: Cörner, 1715), 25.

6 Barthold H. Brockes, "Letzte Gedanken über einen kranken und sterbenden Sohn Johann Bernhard Brockes," in *Weichmann's Poesie der Nieder-Sachsen,* ed. J.P. Kohlen, vol. 6 (Hamburg: Herold, 1738), 265–6.

Brockes reveals elsewhere that one of his daughters died from smallpox some time before Johann's passing, and that he and his wife held great fears for six more of their children suffering from the illness, one of whom came close to death:[7]

Zumal der Aelteste, den wir in letzten Zügen,
Wol fünff mahl ausser Hoffnung liegen,
Und fast schon todt, gesehn.
Ja wär auch nicht an ihm ein Wunder fast geschehn,
Das unsrer ganzen Stadt bekandt,
So deckt auch ihn bereits des Grabes Sand.[8]

Then, seeing the eldest boy's laboured breaths,
About five times we lost all hope
As we saw him there, almost dead.
Yet, for him, a near-wonder came about,
That's known to folk all 'round our town
Aware of preparation of his burial ground.

Yet not all parents regarded their child's survival from severe smallpox as cause for celebration. The Schwarzburg-Rudolstadt *Stadt- and Landphysikus* Johann Gottfried Otto recalls his dismay when a mother admonished him for helping her son survive after smallpox destroyed the sight in one eye.[9] Such 'thoughts' of mothers whose children emerged from smallpox disfigured and disabled were considered in 1743 by Daniel Wilhelm Triller (Figure 3):[10]

Wie viel Kinder gegentheils schlugen durch das Gift der Seuchen,
So entsetzlich aus der Art, daß sie keinem Menschen gleichen,
Und nicht sehen, oder riechen; daß die Mutter selbst erschrickt,
Wenn sie gleichsam Wechselkinder, wie man sonst geglaubt, erblickt.

How many did the poison so badly misshape,
That all human appearance has gone from the face,
And they can't see or smell; leaving mothers appalled,
Upon seeing their changelings, as others will call them.

---

7 Barthold H. Brockes, "Selbstbiographie," *Zeitschrift des Vereines für hamburgische Geschichte* 2 (1847): 223.

8 Barthold H. Brockes, "Bei dem 1732sten Jahres-Wechsel," in *Barthold H. Brockes: Irdisches vergnügen in Gott* (Hamburg, Herold, 1740), 427.

9 Johann G. Otto, *Medicinische und chirurgische Bemerkungen* (Leipzig: Böhme, 1793), 69–70.

10 Triller was *Leibarzt* to the Crown-Prince of Nassau-Usingen at the time. He accepted a professorship at Wittenberg in 1747: Friedrich C.G. Hirsching, *Historisch-litterarisches Handbuch berühmter und denkwürdiger Personen welche im achtzehnten Jahrhundert gelebt haben* (Leipzig: Schwicker, 1810), 369, 371.

Viele wünschten sich vielmehr ihre Kinder zu begraben;	Many wish much more they could bury their children,
Als in solcher Ungestalt, sie noch neben sich zu haben.[11]	Than still have them, so badly disfigured, beside them.

Yet Triller's contemplation of the impact of smallpox, in this thanksgiving poem for that year, was focused largely on his recollection of his anguish at seeing his own five children suffer through the disease, and his joy at their survival relatively unscathed:

Dennoch, Herr, gefiel es dir, alle von des Todtes-Rachen,	Oh Lord, you granted that they'd all survive,
Und des Giftes Schädlichkeit, nebst der Blindheit, frey zu machen;	And not be disabled, nor would they be blind:
Jedes hat gesunde Glieder, sein gebildet Angesicht,	Each still has sound limbs and a face shaped quite right,
Nebst noch unverletzten Augen, als des Lebens Trost und Licht.[12]	And undamaged eyes for comfort and light.

Adults and adolescents suffered greatly from smallpox as well as children. Many young women who ended up with catastrophic disfigurement faced a future offering little else than spinsterhood and insecurity. Nor could betrothed or married women be sure that their men would not abandon them for a more alluring bride after seeing their chosen partners' "ideal of beauty turned into a loathsome lump of flesh," as Dr. Christoph Wilhelm Hufeland described cases of disastrous disfigurement.[13] Men harmed by smallpox found their future prospects dimmed, as well:

Mein mattes Haupt hängt nach der Seit,	My dull head hangs off to the side,
Und krümmt den Mund ob seinen Plagen,	And makes the mouth misshapen, oddly,
Der Fuß voll schwacher Müdigkeit	The feet are now so weak and tired

11 Daniel W. Triller, "Neujahrs-Gedicht auf das Jahr 1743," in *Daniel W. Triller: Poetischer Betrachtungen über verschiedene Natur-und Sittenlehre* (Hamburg: Herold, 1747), 210.

12 Triller, 210.

13 Hufeland, "Vertilgung," 169. Hufeland was a medical practitioner in Weimar at that early stage of his illustrious career. For more biographical details, see pp. 87–88.

Kann nicht den magern Leib mehr tragen.[14]	They cannot bear the wasted body.

Smallpox tended to be endemic in larger towns and to spread across the landscape every four to seven years claiming many young children born since the previous epidemic, who lacked immunity.[15] The initial symptom, heralding the beginning of four recognised stages of the smallpox disease, was a severe headache that began approximately six days after infection. In the next two to four days, the patient could experience headache, fever, lethargy, loss of appetite, sweating, pains, or nausea. Stage two (eruption), which lasted for about three days, began with the appearance of the pustules as red dots followed by their enlargement and the return of the fever. An eruption occurring about three days late accompanied by restlessness, waking up startled, convulsions, or twitching tended to presage confluent smallpox (Figure 1), known in Germany as *Kristalblattern*, which afflicted about one-third of patients and had a fatality rate of around 75 per cent.[16] During the third stage (suppuration), the pustules filled with white pus and grew to their maximum extent accompanied by the rotting flesh stench that was an unmistakable feature of smallpox. Less than one thousand discrete, whitish, 'good' pustules accompanied by mild symptoms presaged a high probability of survival, whereas confluent smallpox tended to be fatal when accompanied by extreme swelling of the surrounding tissues, intense pain, extreme lethargy, a raging thirst, a racing pulse, and a high fever causing hallucinations and convulsions. The rare kinds of 'bad' pustules – those filled with blood, known as *Blutblattern* (haemorrhagic smallpox), and flattened grey pustules referred to as *nabelförmige Blattern* (malignant smallpox) – presaged almost certain death.[17]

Patients who survived the stage three symptoms, which lasted for about three days, proceeded to the fourth and last stage (drying) that usually began on the ninth to eleventh day after the initial symptoms. During this stage, the skin shrivelled and scabs formed, then fell off in a massive exfoliation enabling

14 Hans Aßmann von Abschatz, "Die Blattern oder Kinder-Pocken," part 3 of *Hans Aßmann von Abschatz: Poetische Uebersetzungen und Gedichte* (Leipzig und Breslau: Bauch, 1708), 86.

15 Claudia Huerkamp, "The History of Smallpox Vaccination in Germany: a First Step in the Medicalization of the General Public," *JCH* 20 (1985): 618.

16 J.J. Schmidt, "Einige gemeinnützige Regeln, über das beste Verhalten des Landmanns bei grassirenden Pokken und Scharlachfiebern," *Neue MM* 6 (1797): 89–90.

17 Samuel G. Vogel, *Handbuch der practischen Arzneywissenschaft zum Gebrauche angehende Aerzte* (Vienna: Trattner, 1789), 21–9.

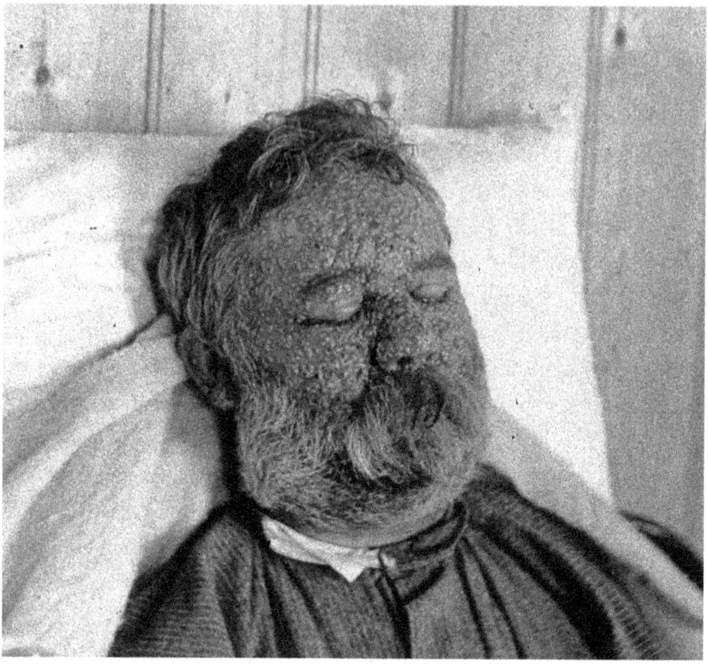

FIGURE 1 A patient with Confluent Smallpox, Gloucester Smallpox Epidemic, 1896
PHOTO BY H.C.F. WELLCOME COLLECTION: 590928I. PUBLIC DOMAIN MARK

the infection to be transmitted over long distances on letters, cloth, and other materials to which the scabs became attached.[18] Yet, even after the drying stage, death still stalked the patients left with corrosive ulcers that were difficult to heal and often turned gangrenous, as in the case of Senator Brockes's son, Johann:

Wie ihm, fast jährig ists, ein Zufall beyde Beine	About a year ago when both his legs, as it happened,
Bis auf die Knochen, ganz verbrannt;	Were full of gangrene right down to the bone;
Indem er dazumal ohne Aechzen und Geweine	He never groaned nor complained on seeing

18 Vogel, 29–30; Johann C.W. Juncker, *Archiv der Aerzte und Seelsorger wider die Pockkenoth*, vol. 5 (Leipzig: Weygand, 1798), 5; vol. 6, 49. The shedding of scabs, like autumn leaves, gave rise to the colloquial German term *Blattern* (leaves) for smallpox, which was used more commonly than the more formal *Pocken*.

Die nackten Sehnen sah, samt der entfleischten Knocken.[19]	The naked tendons and the bones in his ulcerated legs.

An ulcer caused by smallpox also caused the death (1777) of Elector Maximilian III Joseph, the Duke of Bavaria, when he seemed to have almost recovered from the disease. A royal physician even resorted to giving the elector a small image of the Virgin Mary to swallow in a desperate final attempt to save him after all the other medicines in his arsenal had failed.[20] That occasion underscores the helplessness of eighteenth-century medical men facing severe smallpox symptoms in their various manifestations. The vast range of products used to prevent and treat smallpox at that time were summarised in this way by Dr. J.O. Kleine in an article in a Hanover journal (1767):

> We know now, unfortunately, that no bleeding, no mineral or plant acids, nor soapy products, no 'mercury of life,' no perspiration-inducing antimony sulphide, purgative mixed with heart stimulants, bezoar products, copper sulphate, nor vomit-inducers, neither gold antimony sulphate, nor sweetened mercury, nor aloes, nor guajac sap, camphor, mercuric chloride, mineral mud, sulphur-antimony, salpeter, cinchona bark, nor tar-water, neither cooling substances, nor musk, nor bile, nor the stinking sap, can place us in safety from this disease, smallpox.[21]

The tar water and mercury compounds were thought to prevent smallpox, while various heavy-metals were used as emetics and purgatives, and concotions containing certain kinds of tree-bark given to reduce fever.[22] Over-administration of medicines was apparently common and caused much harm, judging by the eminent Professor Hufeland's warnings (1790s) that excessive use of emetics and purgatives tended to worsen the illness, and that generous dosages of opiates used for pain relief could be fatal, particularly in small children.[23]

Most patients treated by doctors after the 1750s were fortunate that cool conditions were then being recommended for smallpox, in a complete reversal

19 Brockes, "Letzte Gedanken," 267.

20 Thomas Christan, *Beiträge zur Geschichte und Behandlung der natürlichen Pocken* (Vienna: Obelen, 1781), 28.

21 Apx 2: Kleine (1767): 615–6.

22 Apx 2: Hensler, vol. 1 (1765), 14–15.

23 Christoph W. Hufeland, *Bemerkungen über die natürlichen und geimpften Blattern, verschiedene Kinderkrankheiten und sowohl medizinische als diatetische Behandlung der Kinder*, 3rd ed. (Berlin: Rottmann, 1798), 116–22, 225.

of the longstanding idea that patients should be 'heated up.'[24] The 'heating treatment' would have been abandoned much sooner if the distinguished British physician Thomas Sydenham's challenge (1662) to the traditional regimen were promptly accepted by his colleagues rather than being dismissed as a slight on their professional judgement. Only after the highly-esteemed Professor Hermann Boerhaave (1668–1738) from Leiden agreed that cooler conditions were preferable for smallpox patients, and some of his more prominent peers followed his lead, was the 'heating treatment' gradually abandoned by doctors more generally.[25] Yet the changed approach among the medical men made little difference to the vast majority of children suffering from smallpox who were 'heated up' by parents who knew no better or were reluctant to alter their traditional practices.[26] As Pastor Weniger from the Glogau region of Silesia (Prussia) reported in 1798:

> Here, the poor children suffering from smallpox are packed up in quilts, as it is believed they cannot be kept warm enough. The summer heat increased the children's torture. No wonder that here nearly every fourth child died![27]

Smallpox was such a common childhood affliction that medical help was rarely sought.[28] While some parents adopted treatments recommended by doctors or their pastor, others used traditional home remedies that in some cases involved superstitious practices.[29] According to the belief that 'like cured like,' based on similar shapes or colours, the appearance of the bread taken out of the oven took on a special significance at times of smallpox: a smooth loaf was thought to presage a smooth complexion after the illness had passed, and vice versa.[30] More active 'intervention' was to place a dish of steaming peas under the sick child's bed to expedite the eruption of the pustules, with

---

24 James Burges, *An Account of the Preparation and Management necessary to Inoculation* (London: Vaillant, 1754), 31; Apx 2: Tissot (1756), 88.

25 Thomas Sydenham, *The Whole Works of Dr. Thomas Sydenham,* trans. John Pechey, 10th ed. (London: Feales, 1734), 95–100; Peter Kübler, *Geschichte der Pocken und der Impfung* (Berlin: Hirschwald, 1901), 106–8.

26 Juncker, *Archiv*, 1:194; 3:126–7, 129, 131; 4:106; 5:229; 6:34, 50–1, 100, 131; 7:221.

27 Juncker, 4:104.

28 Juncker, 3:90; 4:69, 98; 5:109, 119, 4:143, 198; 5:34; 7:225.

29 Juncker, 3:92; 4:93; 5:3, 35; 6:35; 7:224; Christian A. Struve, *Miscellaneen für Freunde der Heilkunde* (Breslau: Korn, 1796), 73–4.

30 Mary Lindemann, *Health and Healing in Eighteenth-Century Germany* (Baltimore and London: Johns Hopkins University Press, 1996), 309; Oscar Hovorka and Adolf Kronfeld, *Vergleichende Volksmedizin: eine Darstellung volksmedizinischer Sitten und Gebräuche,*

the swelling of each pea representing a pustule, or to hang a small taper from a yellow wax plant high around a child's neck with the aim of preventing the formation of pustules inside the throat.[31] Another superstitious notion, rooted in the belief that the disease symptoms could be transferred to something else, motivated the action in a Prussian village in 1788, which was intended to cure a boy suffering from the after-effects of an incompetent inoculation. On that occasion, a cow-herder took the boy into the forest at sundown, dipped a nail from a black stallion's shoe into the pus in the boy's wound, and hammered it into a tree while uttering incantations. Any improvement in the boy's health would be attributed to the nail in the tree, enhancing the cow-herder's reputation as a 'healer.'[32] Another kind of approach relied on 'holy objects' or amulets of various kinds to ward off illness (Figure 2). In an area of Brandenburg, such amulets were created from pieces of paper bearing blessings or figures drawn by a miracle-worker or exorcist.[33] In other instances, 'healing' would be performed by an old woman known for 'talking the illness away.'[34] A different kind of 'magical' remedy captivated the people of Berlin in the 1780s, when the 'moon-doctor' attracted thousands of well-dressed citizens to his door for a 'cure' effected by moonlight, much to the amazement of the more enlightened residents.[35]

A more down-to-earth custom for dealing with smallpox, which was reported from many regions of Europe and other parts of the world, was the ritual of 'buying smallpox.'[36] In Germany the *Pockenkaufen* tradition was more common among farmers than townsfolk, owing to the seasonal nature of farm-work and the possibility of co-ordinating children's smallpox illness with a period of lighter workload. Although the ritual varied in some respects in different areas, the identification of a mild smallpox case in a village initiated the action, prompting a parent to take their child to 'purchase' scabs from the infected child. The custom in Hanover and Prussia required the sick child to count the scabs into the hand of the purchasing child in exchange for coins,

---

Anschauungen und Heilfaktoren, des Aberglaubens und der Zaubermedizin (Stuttgart: Strecker and Schröder, 1909), 746.

31 Juncker, *Archiv*, 5:128; Struve, *Miscellaneen*, 74.

32 Heinrich L. Fischer, *Beiträge zur Beantwortung der Frage, ob Aufklärung schon weit genug gediehen oder vollendet sey? Als Anhang zu dem Buch vom Aberglauben* (Hanover: Rischer, 1794), 134–5; Lindemann, *Health*, 310.

33 "Etwas zur Characteristik des Landmanns in der westphälischen Grafschaft Mark," *Neues WM* 3 (1792): 198.

34 Juncker, *Archiv*, 4:79; 5:35; 7:228; Apx 2: Piccard (1794), 668.

35 "Die Wallfahrt zum Monddoktor in Berlin," *BMS* 1 (1783): 379–82.

36 David Schultz, *An Account of Inoculation* (London: A. Linde, 1758), 65–6; James Kirkpatrick, *The Analysis of Inoculation* (London: Millan, Buckland, and Griffiths, 1754), 148–9.

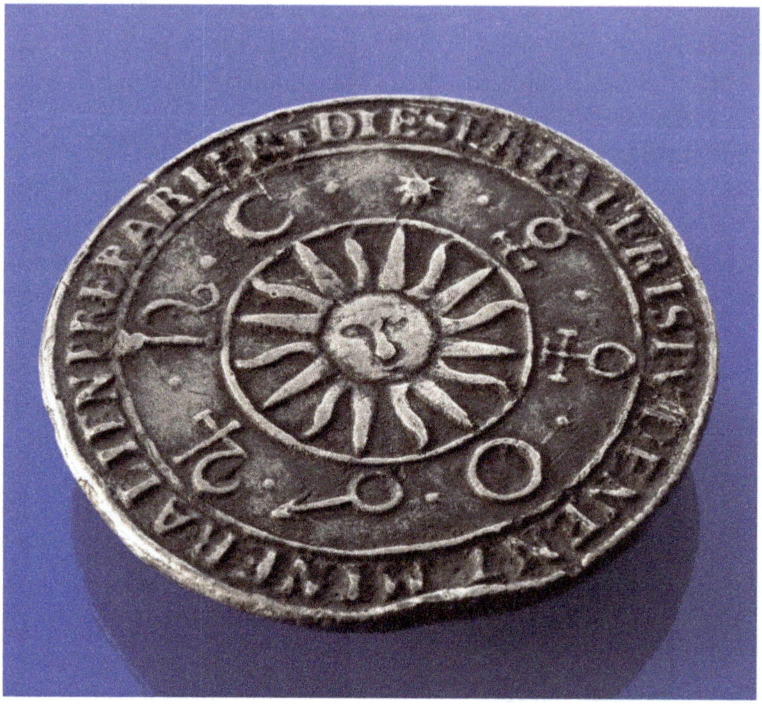

FIGURE 2 Eighteenth-century astrological amulet from Germany engraved with planetary symbols

supposedly ensuring that the recipient's pustules would not exceed the purchased number. A parent would then rub the scabs into the skin of their child's upper arm in the hope of producing a mild bout of smallpox.[37] Although *Pockenkaufen* was based on the same concept as inoculation, it posed the added danger of the purchasing child becoming infected by inhaling or ingesting the contagion from the donor or from other infected children in the donor's household. A general reluctance to admit to a child's death from 'bought smallpox' apparently helped to perpetuate the ritual's reputation for being quite safe.[38]

Smallpox and other contagious diseases that caused highly visible corruption of the flesh tended to inspire a variety of moral messages and metaphors rooted in Christian theology. Adult afflictions of that kind, such as leprosy and

37 G.F. Wehrs, "Vom Blatternkaufen unter den Landleuten, nebst einigen Anmerkungen über das Alter der Kinderpocken," *HM* 27 (1789): 453–4; Juncker, *Archiv*, 3:140–1; 4:111, 156; 6:28.

38 "Eine ungekünstelte Art der Blattermittheilung, unter den Landleuten," *Hildesheimisches Magazin* 41 (1789): 148; Apx 2: Klose (1786), 418.

syphilis, were deemed to be God's punishment for immoral behaviour, while the mainly childhood illness, smallpox, was placed in the broad category of diseases inflicted by God to punish mankind for the original sin.[39] In the public mind, however, smallpox tended to be regarded as God's punishment for worldly sins.[40] Hans Aßman von Abschatz's depiction of a nobleman severely afflicted with smallpox for his sin of vainglory, warning his extravagant peers that they will suffer the same fate, indicates that the notion of punishment by smallpox transcended social class:

Diß ist der Sünden Liberey,	This that I bear in all my limbs
Die ich an meinen Gliedern führe:	Is for the sin of ostentation:
Vielleicht kommt bald die Zeit herbey	Perhaps the time is imminent
Die Euch nach gleicher Art beziere,	For you to wear the same decoration.
Den stolz-gesinnten Hochmutt lege,	The arrogant pride will soon be replaced
Des Todes Bildnis in Euch präge.[41]	By the new imprint of death's portrait.

Religiously-inspired linkages between highly recognisable features of past smallpox and notions of divine punishment for sin gave rise to evocative poetic imagery implying that smallpox scars were taints of sinful behaviour, such as these few lines by Johann Christian Günther (1739):

Was soll das Unschlit-Licht, das auf der Canzel brennt?	Why does that tallow candle burn upon the pulpit?
Vielleicht, daß man dabey die Narben besser kennt,	Perhaps to show the scars more clearly,
Womit dich die Natur in Blattern zeichnen lassen,	As Nature sketched you, with taints of smallpox,
Um einmal deinen Kopff mit Hörnern einzulassen.[42]	That now reveal your head adorned with horns.

39 Christi Sumich, "'A Christian's Groans under the Body of Sin:' the Pox and the Pious Physician," *CM* 91 (2013): 139–41; William F. Hezel, *Die Bibel mit vollständig-erklärenden Anmerkungen*, part 4 (Lemgo: Meyer, 1783), 159; Leonis Strobel, *Geist der Wahrheit oder gesammelte Glaubens-und Sittenlehren*, part 1 (Freising: Mösmer, 1769), 178.

40 Juncker, *Archiv*, 3:127; 5:211–12; 6:130–1.

41 Abschatz, "Blattern," 86.

42 Johann C. Günther, "An einen guten Freund," in *Sammlung von Johann Christian Günther's Gedichten*, 2nd ed. (Breslau and Leipzig: Hubert, 1739), 486.

German poets of the classical literary period were inclined to parody the religious notion of God inflicting smallpox as punishment, invoking malevolent deities from Graeco-Roman mythology as the punitive agents. In doing so, they held to the Olympian deities' well-known literary predilection for wielding supernatural powers to meddle in the affairs of mortals in order to gain some kind of personal advantage in their own power relationships, with callous disregard for their hapless victims. Depictions of jealous goddesses inflicting smallpox on beautiful women reflect the competition in the beauty contest that characterised upper-class female society, where some ladies may have wanted to destroy their beautiful rivals' appeal. Justus Wilhelm Zachariä invokes an unnamed weather-goddess spreading pestilential diseases in the warm south-wind, as his choice of malevolent divine agent:

Ueber die zitternde Stadt schaut sie verwüstend herunter,	Over the trembling town she looks down with destructive intent,
Mit der Medusa verderbenden Blick …	With her ruinous Medusa gaze …
Schönen von himmlichen Reiz sehn durch verwüstende Blattern	The most alluring beauties see ruinous smallpox
Ihr bezaubernde Schönheit verheert.[43]	Overwhelm their bewitching charms.

Venus was much more selective in her targets, according to an anonymous idyll from Saxony in which the goddess 'uses' smallpox to punish only the women whose behaviour displeases her.[44] The idyll revolves around the young shepherd Palemon's concerns about his girlfriend, who was ill with smallpox, after the rustic god Pan told him in a dream that Venus habitually transmitted the disease to beautiful young women for failing to tread the fine line between squandering their beauty with prudish behaviour and flaunting their looks by flirting. Palemon offers this advice to his beloved Henriette:

Der Venus Zorn ist nun gestillet,	The wrath of Venus is now suppressed,
O! reiz ihn nicht durch neue Sprödigkeit,	Don't excite it by hiding your charms,

43 Justus F.W. Zachariä, "Die Seuche," in *Justus F.W. Zachariä: Scherzhafte epische Poesien nebst einigen Oden und Liedern* (Brunswick and Hildesheim: Schröder, 1754), 385–6. Zachariä's south-wind deity is an allusion to the mysterious continent of Africa once thought to be the source of pestilential diseases in Europe. The Medusa gaze refers to the mythical multi-headed snake-like Gorgon, Medusa, whose blood was shed in the Libyan desert after she was slain by Perseus: Ovid, *Metamorphoses*, trans. A.D. Melville (Oxford: Oxford University Press, 1986), IV.17–24.

44 "Die Blattern. Eine Idylle," *Magazin der sächsischen Geschichte* 7 (1790): 302–3. The idyll was written in 1777.

Du weißt, sie ist mit Nachsucht angefüllet	You know that she is filled with vengeance,
Besänftge sie durch Unterwürfigkeit.[45]	Be also submissive, to keep her calm.

The gnome Uriel, the archangel for elemental earth, was another character endowed with the poetic power to inflict smallpox. In the following anonymous verse from Saxony (1759), the disease is once again depicted as a weapon used by divine agents to control the behaviour of mortals, particularly women:

Den einzigen Gefallen,	The only favour you can grant
Den bitt ich iezt von dir,	That I now ask of you,
Der uns Jünglingen allen	Is to me as important
So wichtig ist als mir:	As to all of our young group:
Laß deine schwarzen Blattern,	Arrange for your black smallpox,
Im fürchterlichem Heer,	In its ghastly masses,
Zu ** Antlitz flattern,	To flutter onto **'s face,
So höhnt sie niemand mehr.[46]	To stop her mocking someone else.

The trope of smallpox being inflicted by one or other classical deity faded with the changing direction of the literary movement to sensibility and romanticism. Yet the longstanding popular idea that God wielded smallpox as punishment for sin still resonated among the common folk as well as in some intellectual minds.[47] The elderly Professor Triller (1695–1782; Figure 3) from the medical faculty at the University of Wittenberg (Saxony) affirmed his own ideas on the matter (1766) in his lengthy poem, *Geprüfte Pockeninoculation* (An Evaluation of Smallpox Inoculation):

Doch dieser Grundsatz steht unüberwindlich fest,	This principle, indeed, is unassailable,
Weil er sich aus der Schrift, genau erwiesen lässt;	Since the proof is shown quite clearly in the Bible;
Gott schicht zur Züchtigung, aus seinem Zorn, die Seuchen,	Diseases are God's punishment, His way of venting rage,
Und lässt sie wiederum, aus seiner Huld, entweichen.	And then, from His grace, He lets them fade away.
Er schlägt und heilet uns, so wie es ihn gefällt:	He strikes us and heals us as and when He wants:

45 "Die Blattern," 304.
46 "An den Gnomen Uriel," *Lyrische Muse an der Saale* (Jena: Schill, 1759), 184.
47 Wolff, "Maßnahmen," 240–1.

Drum ist die Propfkunst wohl nicht aus der besten Welt.[48]	So inoculation's surely not the ideal thing for us.

In this 214-page poem, which is essentially a treatise in rhyming couplets, Triller explains his opposition to the crude form of immunisation known as inoculation that had proven its worth in ameliorating the severity of smallpox in individuals. While he based some of his arguments on medical cases and on common misconceptions about smallpox, he placed his main emphasis on man's audacity in engaging in inoculation and usurping God's exclusive prerogative to inflict smallpox.[49]

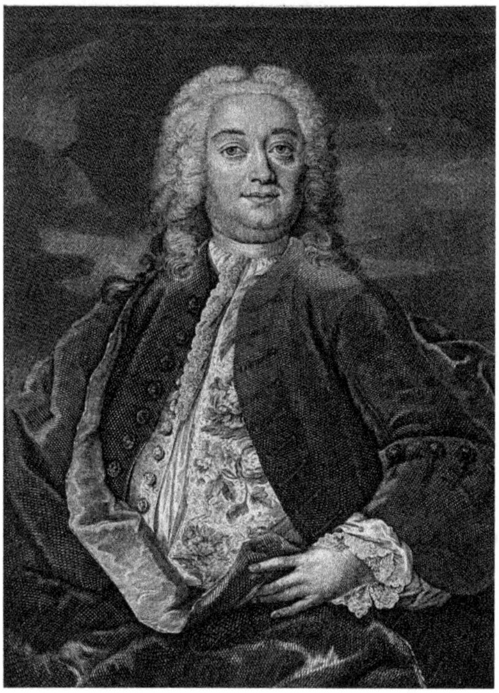

FIGURE 3
Daniel Wilhelm Triller. Line engraving by C. Fritsch, 1759, after F. Lippold
WELLCOME COLLECTION: 92621. PUBLIC DOMAIN MARK

48 Apx 2: Triller (1766), 12–13; see similar sentiments on pp. 14–15, 111, 135–6, 147, and elsewhere in the poem.

49 Triller's footnotes referencing the Bible and scholarly literature in several languages, and his pertinent comments occupy approximately half the 214 pages of the poem. The eminent physician Paul Gottlieb Werlhof from the Royal Hanover Court, and Dr. Johann Gottfried von Hahn from Breslau both regarded Triller as the most learned scholar of Medicine and Philology of their time: "Geschichte von den Herrn Daniel Wilhelm Triller," *Beyträge zur Historie der Gelartheit, worinnen die Geschichte der Gelehrten unserer Zeiten beschrieben worden* (Hamburg: Geißler, 1748), 154.

2 Inoculation Offers a New Approach

The spread of inoculation to Germany in the 1720s occurred largely due to influences emanating from Britain after the Prince and Princess of Wales's daughters, Amelia and Caroline, came through the procedure in 1722. The sisters' Hanover-based eldest brother Frederick Lewis was so impressed that he sought permission to have himself inoculated, which the king granted in the knowledge that the London trials to test the safety and efficacy of the procedure were just as successful as the inoculation of his granddaughters.[50] The highly-publicised experiment involving three women and three men from among the condemned prisoners at Newgate, who were given a king's pardon for their participation, was conducted in August 1721 by Royal Society doctors led by Sir Hans Sloane. After the candidates inoculated by Charles Maitland had recovered from their smallpox, Sloane and his colleague Johann Georg Steigerthal, King George I's physician, seized the opportunity to answer the crucial question – whether the procedure offered protection against future smallpox. They obtained their answer by paying one of the inoculated female former-prisoners to nurse and lay with a child suffering from smallpox, concluding from her failure to contract the disease that her inoculation was indeed protective.[51] Steigerthal reported the Newgate trial in a German surgical journal, while an invited witness from Königsberg (East Prussia), Dr. Matthias Ernst Boretius, alerted his countrymen not only to the successful trial but also to inoculation more generally.[52]

More experiments were carried out in Hanover to prepare for the inoculation of eighteen-year-old Prince Frederick Lewis. Between February and June 1723 the prince's surgeon Johann Ernst Wreden inoculated five children and one adult, in conjunction with physicians from the Royal Hanover Court who joined him in closely observing and recording the progress of the disease.[53]

---

50 Hans Sloane, "An Account of Inoculation," *PT* 49 (1755), 517–9; Genevieve Miller, *The Adoption of Inoculation for Smallpox in England and France* (Philadelphia: University of Pennsylvania Press, 1957), 176.

51 Charles Maitland, *Account of the Inoculation of the Small Pox* (London: Peele, 1723), 19–21, 25. The one female prisoner who had smallpox matter put up her nose instead of being inoculated was unwell but failed to come down with smallpox: Sloane, 517.

52 Apx 2: Steigerthal (1722); Boretius (1722), (1723), 204–12.

53 Apx 2: Wreden (1723, 1724). Wreden provides a more complete description in a later publication: Johann E. Wreden, *An Essay on the Inoculation of Smallpox. To which are added, some Examples of Persons Inoculated with Good Success at Hanover* (London: Jackson, 1729), 30–2, 34–42.

While the inoculated individuals all survived, one child passed the infection to two companions, causing the death of one and the near-death of the other.[54] Fatalities in similar circumstances in England also confirmed that inoculated smallpox was not only transmissible but lost its characteristic mildness when passed on through contagion.[55] On the other hand, the mildness of the smallpox ensuing from the vast majority of inoculations offered considerable encouragement to expand the practice, with the 1–2 per cent fatality rate regarded as generally acceptable in light of the much higher mortality from naturally-acquired smallpox.[56]

While the German experiments were very limited and received little publicity, medical men in Britain with an intense interest in inoculation continued to collect, examine, and publish relevant data. Their close scrutiny of the symptoms and course of inoculated and of naturally-acquired smallpox resulted in the publication of comparisons, with close attention to detail. Cumulative observations of that kind enabled conclusions to be drawn about the best age for inoculation, a season when smallpox seemed less virulent, and other important factors such as the dangers of inoculating during pregnancy and during teething in young children.[57] The new parameters set sensible limits when inoculation practice increased in Britain during 1751–52 and commenced in many European states in the mid-1750s in response to virulent epidemic smallpox, after a period when both the disease and inoculation were in relative abeyance.[58]

The inoculation procedures in use in Europe at the time included not only those translated from English but also the methods of the Swiss doctors Jean-Antoine Butini from Geneva and Samuel-August Tissot from Lausanne, which were available in French.[59] However, the methods of the British medical men tended to be quite complex owing to significant changes to the original procedure transmitted from Turkey. One important innovation was the

54 Wreden, 32–3, 43.

55 Kirkpatrick, *Analysis*, 100–01, 286–7; Schultz, *Account*, 30–31.

56 Kirkpatrick, 106–13; Schultz, 106–10.

57 Schultz, 7–8, 21–2, 26–7. Spring and autumn were regarded as the best times for inoculation, and 2 to 12 years the best age: Samuel Sharp, *Treatise on the Operations of Surgery*, 4th ed. (London, 1743), 225; Burges, *Account*, 15–16.

58 Michael J. Bennett, *War Against Smallpox. Edward Jenner and the Early Global Spread of Vaccination* (Cambridge: Cambridge University Press, 2020), 34–6; Klebs, *Variolation*, 36, 45, 48, 52–4, 56, 59.

59 Jean-Antoine Butini, *Traité de la vérole, communiquée par l'inoculation* (Paris: Hérissant, 1752); Samuel-Auguste Tissot, *L'inoculation justifiée, ou dissertation pratique et apologétique sur cette méthode* (Lausanne: Bosquet, 1754).

pre-inoculation 'preparation' for candidates with 'high' or 'energised' constitutions that were believed to predispose to more virulent smallpox. In order to correct the 'condition,' those candidates were subjected to a three-to-six week regimen of bleeding, purging, and dietary restrictions intended to ameliorate the inoculated smallpox symptoms and aid recovery.[60] Dr. Henry Bracken from Lancaster opposed such 'preparation' procedures, arguing (1760) that "preparation of the body for inoculation is an absurdity ... brought about by the self-interest of doctors ... requiring a patient's visits to be extended." He also pointed out the dangers of dehydration caused by harsh preparation regimens. The high-profile Dr. Angelo Gatti in Paris similarly referred to the "uselessness and danger" of preparation (1767).[61]

Doctors in Germany had the choice of either following the more stringent regimens of the British medical men or using the European methods with limited 'preparation,' such as those described by Butini and Tissot. The Göttingen professor Johann Georg Röderer adopted the British approach, as Dr. Philipp Gabriel Hensler indicated some years after assisting with Röderer's inoculations in 1762 as part of his doctoral studies, admitting that prolonged administration of the professor's 'secret medicine' robbed their candidates of energy. Dr. Elias Henschel from Breslau (Prussia) was much more critical of Röderer, blaming the harsh 'preparation' for the failure of a number of the professor's procedures in 1758 that sparked adverse publicity when five sisters he inoculated contracted smallpox later, harming the reputation of the practice.[62] The folly of debilitating 'preparations' so outraged the Wittenberg professor, Triller, that he even paused his staunch opposition to inoculation for a moment to offer grudging praise for the simple Turkish procedure:

Man pflegt die Kinder nicht vorher zu präpariren,	Preparation of the children is not their usual habit,
Braucht keiner Arzeney, den Unrath abzuführen,	They don't give them purgatives, nor do they make them vomit,
Stöhrt auch durch Hunger, nicht die Ordnung der Diät,	And they don't let them hunger, nor change their usual food,
Da doch die Pfropfung selbst dort, wohl von statten geht.	So inoculation there proceeds in just the way it should.

60 Burges, *Account*, 9–11, 19–22; Kirkpatrick, *Analysis*, 233–7; Thomas Frewen, *The Practice and Theory of Inoculation* (London: Austen, 1749), 17–20; Sharp, *Treatise*, 224–5.

61 Apx 2: Bracken (1760), 448; Angelo Gatti, *Nouvelles réflexions sur la practique de l'inoculation* (Brussels: Musier, 1767), 48.

62 Apx 2: Henschel (1795), 50–1.

Nun diesen Völkern ist hierinnen Recht zu geben,	Now these folk, with their practice, seem to do things right,
Sie schwächen nicht zuvor, der Kinder frisches Leben,	Yet we're inclined to weaken the children's fresh, young life,
So daß dann die Natur, weil sie bereits zu matt,	So they have no natural strength left in their constitution,
Die Pfropfung auszustehen, zu wenig Kräffte hat.[63]	And they become too weak to withstand inoculation.

Since most inoculators had already moderated their 'preparation' regimens by 1766 when the poem was published, Triller's criticisms, though justified, were somewhat belated.

The use of incisions was another innovation that helped to transform the simple Turkish-style inoculation into a dangerous, cumbersome procedure that harmed many, dissuaded others, and was too costly for all but the wealthy.[64] Charles Maitland initiated the change by preferring a lancet-wound over the needle-prick he witnessed in Turkey; he reports inoculating the Newgate prisoners in 1721 using an "incision in both arms and the right leg."[65] Lady Montagu was so dismayed by the modified approach that she publicly criticised the infliction of such "gashes in the flesh," while the practitioners argued that the incision was beneficial in providing a larger outlet for the expulsion of the smallpox matter, and denounced the use of a small inoculum as insufficient to produce the disease.[66] German doctors discussing inoculation in the 1750s-60s agreed that an incision wound acting as a *fontanelle* was beneficial for assisting the expulsion of the smallpox material contaminating the blood.[67] Yet, as Triller explains, the change from the needle-prick to the incision was ill-conceived and caused much harm:

Bisweilen ist allda, sogar der Brand entstanden;	Sometimes, in those places, gangrene will appear;
Und denn ist die Gefahr des Lebens selbst, vorhanden,	Then life is under threat, with danger very near,
Daß mancher, der mit Glück, erst durch die Pocken kam,	So some who had good fortune to at first survive unharmed,

63 Apx 2: Triller (1766), 211–12.

64 Peter Razzell, *The Conquest of Smallpox: the Impact of Inoculation on Smallpox Mortality in Eighteenth-century Britain* (London: Caliban, 2003), 13–16.

65 Maitland, *Account*, 7, 21 (quote).

66 Isobel Grundy, *Lady Mary Wortley Montagu* (Oxford: Oxford University Press, 1999), 217–218 (quote); Frewen, *Practice*, 41; Kirkpatrick, *Analysis*, 162–4.

67 Apx 2: Hensler (1765), 1:35–42; Constantini (1757), 694; Kleine (1767), 612.

Noch durch den Schnitt am Arm ein traurig Ende nahm.[68]

Still reached a tragic end through the cut made in their arm.

The sight of poorly-healed inoculation incisions, and the disability and death from wounds that became infected turned Germans away from inoculation.[69] Yet incisions were indispensable for practitioners who adopted the convenient method developed in Britain, of placing pre-prepared, dried, smallpox-impregnated threads in shallow incisions, enabling the inoculator to dispense with the need for a suitable smallpox donor on each occasion.[70] Triller found fault with that innovation too:

Um diesen Ort, wo man die Fäden eingelegt,
Wird offt Geschwulst und Brand, mit grösser Pein erregt,
Sie zucken fürchterlich das Haupt und alle Glieder,
Ja fallen endlich auch bißweilen todt darnieder.[71]

Around that very place where the thread was laid,
An ulcer often forms, then gangrene, with dreadful pain,
Appalling jerking may ensue in limbs and with the head,
Eventually, those affected tend to fall down dead.

The Essex apothecary Robert Sutton's advertisement (1762) for inoculation "without an Incision, the most curious Eye cannot discern where the Operation is performed," marked the beginning of a widespread procedural change.[72] Sutton and his six sons, all surgeon-inoculators, were soon famous for the sheer numbers who attended their respective practices and emerged with an inoculation they barely noticed. Minimal 'preparation' and encouragement to stroll around in the fresh air after inoculation added to the favourable experience. The Suttons's success is reflected in the spread of their franchises, which by 1768 were located across Britain as well as in Paris, Jamaica, and Virginia.[73] Daniel Sutton's reported tally of 40,000 successful inoculations by 1768 with very few fatalities forced other doctors to concede that the Suttons's simple

68 Apx 2: Triller (1766), 57–8.

69 Apx 2: "Zu der Geschichte" (1770), 216, 233–5; Migula, "Noch etwas" (1787), 422–3; Thebesius (1788), 126–7.

70 Burges, *Account*, 22; Apx 2: Constantini (1757), 679.

71 Apx 2: Triller (1766), 199. For a description of a fatality caused by poorly-prepared inoculation incisions, see in Apx 2: "Zu der Geschichte" (1770), 233–6.

72 Razzell, *Conquest*, 17 (quote) -19.

73 Deborah C. Brunton, "Pox Britannica: Smallpox Inoculation in Britain, 1721–30" (PhD diss. University of Pennsylvania, 1990), 102–6.

skin-prick method and recuperation in the cool, fresh air was superior.[74] Dr. Angelo Gatti, consultant to the King of France, published his own simplified method in 1767, agreeing that the incision was one of the biggest problems with inoculation. The English doctor, Thomas Dimsdale, followed suit in 1768.[75] With the gradual spread of various less-invasive techniques in the 1770s, Germans were offered a more persuasive argument in favour of inoculation. Yet the procedure still posed quite a dilemma for parents. Many feared that their child may die from inoculation, seemingly unable to think in terms of the statistical reality that very many more children were killed by naturally-acquired smallpox than the number who died from inoculation.[76] In addition, a raft of myths, and misconceptions about smallpox that acted as a disincentive to inoculation needed to be overcome before much progress could be made in curbing the impact of the disease.

Beliefs about smallpox were still firmly rooted in the 'innate smallpox theory' proposed at the turn of the tenth century by the Arabic physician known as Rhazes (865–925), chief physician at the main hospital in Baghdad.[77] Rhazes's ideas about the origin of smallpox and the cause of its symptoms endured largely because they provided a logical explanation for the characteristics of the illnesss, as Dr. Elias Henschel from Breslau pointed out in 1796:

> We believed, because we were led astray by incorrect assumptions, that the child already received a fermentation agent in the womb, which would be activated either earlier or later to produce the illness. This fermentation agent would subsequently, by means of the illness, be expelled from the body, having cleansed the blood of all harmful constituents, so this illness can come only once in a lifetime … Smallpox was thus regarded as a natural and beneficial illness … the only ones who died either had too strong a fermentation, or received too much or too little of the agent in the womb.[78]

74 "The Opinion of his Majesty's Physicians and Surgeons, given Jan. 23, 1768, in regard to Messrs. Sutton's Practice of Inoculation, in Consequence of a Letter from Sir John Pringle," *Gentleman's Magazine*, 38 (1768): 74–5.

75 Gatti, *Nouvelles réflexions*, 73–8; Thomas Dimsdale, *Neue Methode für die Einpfropfung der Pocken, auch Anhang* (Zürich: Füssli, 1768), 31–2.

76 Lindemann, *Health*, 331–2; Apx 2: Sintenis (1790), 109–14; Vasmer (1795), 855–9.

77 Abú Becr Mohammed Ibn Zacaríyá al-Rází, *A Treatise on the Small-pox and Measles*, trans. William A. Greenhill (London, 1868); Kübler, *Geschichte*, 37–9.

78 Elias Henschel, *Von den Blattern und deren Ausrottung* (Breslau and Leipzig: Korn, 1796), 11–12.

The concept of innate smallpox initiating a fermentation, from which the reaction products caused skin eruptions that aided the expulsion of 'contaminants' involved in the fermentation process, was so closely aligned with common occurrences in nature that it was easily understood. Yet, unfortunately for many smallpox victims, that explanation for the disease process gave rise to misconceptions resulting in adverse consequences. The idea that residual smallpox and other 'contaminants' caused ill-health and premature death if they were not expelled, and that smallpox actually performed a necessary function in purging those 'contaminants,' prompted misguided attempts to accelerate and exacerbate the eruption, usually by means of the deadly 'heating treatment' in its various forms.[79] The seemingly logical assumption that an abundance of pustules was necessary to complete the 'purging process,' which the heating of the patient was supposed to assist, had the other far-reaching consequence of arousing widespread public scepticism about the benefits of the usually mild symptoms ensuing from inoculation.[80] The supposition that inoculated smallpox was too weak to generate the necessary 'purging power' gave rise to the gleeful predictions by inoculation opponents that inoculated individuals would suffer ill-health and premature death owing to the residual 'contaminants.' As a result, deaths of inoculated individuals often prompted jubilant proclamations that the inoculation was to blame, regardless of the actual cause of death or the time interval since the procedure.[81]

An additional disincentive to inoculation arising from the innate smallpox theory was the 'belly-button' ritual that misled parents into believing their child was protected from the disease. The custom of pushing out a newborn's belly-button, rubbing the skin with salt, and washing it clean to remove all traces of smallpox 'seeds' from the umbilical blood was thought to prevent the child from contracting smallpox.[82] Even though generations of children kept disproving that idea by suffering from the illness despite being subjected

79 Juncker, *Archiv*, 4:114–5; 5:136–7, 229–30; Apx 2: Büscher (1755), 749–50. Christian Gottlieb Weis interpreted the progression of mild smallpox symptoms to "foulness" through heating the patient, in terms of vegetables fermenting rapidly to rottenness in warm conditions, see in Apx 2: Weis (1773), 51–3.

80 Juncker, *Archiv*, 5:237; Büscher, 747–52; Anton von Haen and Ernst Platner, *Anton von Haen's kaiserlichen Leibarztes Heilungsmethode, in dem kaiserlichen Krankenhaus zu Wien*, vol. 5 (Leipzig: Weygand, 1782), 437–8.

81 Apx 2: Klose (1786), 413–4; Heinsius (1780), 134–5; Hirschel (1771), 657.

82 Ulrich C. Salchow, "Ein durch Versuch geprüftes und durch die Erfahrung bestätigtes Vorbauungsmittel wider die Pokken," *BSA* 9 (1777): 231–5. Prophet Ezekiel's suggestion, "why did you not rub yourself with salt?" (Ezekiel 16.4) was cited in 1798 as justification for the 'belly-button prophylactic:' Juncker, *Archiv*, 5:202.

to the ritual at birth, the belly-button washing was still being recommended in the 1790s as a safe 'new' protective measure against smallpox.[83] While one commentator openly called the ritual *charlatanerie,* a like-minded counterpart warned against debunking the myth so firmly that the cleansing ritual was abandoned, arguing that thorough washing of a newborn's abdomen was a beneficial hygienic measure.[84]

Another longstanding notion increasingly under challenge was the presumption of God's displeasure at mankind's inoculation practice, which was believed to usurp His prerogative to inflict smallpox as punishment.[85] The pious Professor Triller shared the view that God would seek vengeful retribution, envisaging this vivid scenario of divine wrath:

Von Gott und der Natur, weil sie zur Felde gehn,	Both God and Nature take the field eventually,
Und der Verwegenheit derselben widerstehn,	Opposing man's foolishness and his audacity,
Die gegen die Natur, die unverschämt empören,	In attacking unashamedly Nature's rightful borders,
Und sie mit Ungestüm, in ihrer Ordnung stöhren;	And violently interfering in her natural order,
So, daß sie endlich sich, mit Unmuth und Verdruß,	So that finally, in a rage and very much displeased,
Zu einer Kranckheit noch, gezwungen, lencken muß,	Nature was compelled to act and send out a disease
Die sie vielleicht, von selbst, noch lange nicht erreget,	That otherwise she'd perhaps keep in a state of pause,
Vielleicht auch wohl noch nie, den Grund dazu geleget.[86]	Possibly forever, if there's no sufficient cause.

Such religiously-based arguments from a seventy-one year-old scholar from Wittenberg, in the heart of Martin Luther territory, epitomise the clash between the conservative mindset and the more secular-oriented new ideas becoming entrenched in the Protestant universities and among the younger educated

83 Apx 2: Hufeland, *Bemerkungen* (1789), 33–4.

84 Johann S. Halle, *Fortgesetzte Magie, oder die Zauberkräfte der Natur* (Berlin: Pauli, 1793), 520; Wehrs, "Blatternkaufen," 463–4.

85 Juncker, *Archiv*, 3:22; Apx 2: Ehrhart (1789), 32–5.

86 Apx 2: Triller (1766), 107–8.

elite.[87] Triller's notion of a vengeful Nature spitefully inflicting a pestilence on an errant mankind was quite the converse of the new Enlightenment-inspired perception of Nature as a powerful ally in the maintenance of good health and in disease prevention.[88] To Dr. Rudolph Christian Opitz from Minden (Prussia), one of many adherents to the more enlightened view, inoculation was an intervention that "Nature promotes, common-sense advises, and religion allows." Along similar lines, the Rinteln (Schaumburg-Lippe) professor Ludwig Philipp Schröter saw "Nature and common sense" as the teachers inspiring the re-simplification of cumbersome inoculation methods.[89] Opitz and Schröter were among many commentators railing against the prejudices hindering the adoption of inoculation, some of which endured into the nineteenth century as a cause of resistance to cowpox vaccination. Only after vaccination showed that smallpox was indeed preventable was the broader public prepared to accept that the disease was neither inborn, nor inevitable, nor necessary, nor willed by God.[90]

3 Perceptions of a Benevolent 'Murdering Angel'

Parental opposition to inoculation was in many cases rooted in medical or religious preconceptions, or in parents' fear of unbearable guilt if their child were to die from the procedure.[91] Another, unspoken, reason for some parents' opposition to inoculation and to the later cowpox vaccination was apparently a desire to 'keep smallpox coming' as a way of thinning their numbers of children. Pastor Schwager (see Figure 16 on p. 179) from Joellenbeck (Minden-Ravensburg, Prussia) expressed the view that to some parents "the children are a burden … and if one dies they are pleased. Now they see that children do not die when they have inoculated smallpox."[92] He continued with the following explanation in his circular to his parishioners, "Is Inoculation a Duty, or Not?" (1784), of how he believed such parental attitudes may have developed:

---

87 Johann M. Stroup, *The Struggle for Identity in the Clerical Estate* (Leiden: Brill, 1984), 86–94.

88 Peter Watson, *The German Genius* (London: Simon and Schuster, 2010), 82–3; Ute Frevert, *Krankheit als politisches Problem 1770–1880* (Göttingen: Vandenhoek & Ruprecht, 1984), 32–3.

89 Apx 2: Opitz (1774), 109; Schröter (1773), 19.

90 Eberhard Wolff, *Einschneidende Maßnahmen: Pockenschutzimpfung und traditionale Gesellschaft im Württemberg des frühen 19. Jahrhunderts* (Stuttgart: Steiner, 1998), 239–41.

91 Apx 2: Sintenis (1790), 112–4; Vasmer (1795), 857–8.

92 Apx 2: Schwager, "Patriotische" (1786), 201, 215.

> The love in marriage is merely animal among very many married people; they marry because of sexual excitement, they come together out of lust, poverty was their wedding present, and a lack of means to feed themselves the first wellsprings of cold-heartedness. No wonder that the familiar love can never take root, that children who are not the result of a higher love but mere fruits of an animal need become a burden for you, and that you see their deaths as a benefit. Yes, you say, they are indeed well looked-after when dead, when they are with God; who would not wish them to be in Heaven?[93]

Many other pastors, doctors, and officials agreed that poverty was a common basis for parents' rejection of inoculation, or later (1804–20), of vaccination.[94]

A high-ranking Catholic official in Württemburg reported (1815) that the primary cause of rejection of vaccination was likely to have arisen from many parents' "secret wish for smallpox to claim some of their children, whose upkeep had become a burden."[95] In some cases smallpox was regarded as a kind of benevolent spirit that would take children to a better place, as the Swabian doctor J.E. Wetzlar indicated in his admonition to parents who rejected vaccination with such an outcome in mind (1807): "many of you parents with large numbers of children wish that some would die, so you welcome the *Blatternmann*, as you call it, to come for his share."[96] A similar personification of smallpox was reported at that time during an epidemic of the disease in Ansbach: "some families seemed to expect the welcome murdering angel to reduce the domestic burden of their number of children."[97]

Poverty-stricken parents were in some cases inclined to adopt a belief system that regarded death not as a threat but as a transitional phase between the here and the hereafter. Very real visions of a miserable life of hunger and deprivation on earth, alongside mental images of a blissful life in Heaven helped to consolidate that idea and enable parents to come to terms with their desire to reduce their family size. The word *Himmeln* (to send to Heaven) was even coined to accommodate the concept of an innocent child passing seamlessly

---

93 Schwager, 215–6. For further discussion of Schwager and his ministry, see ch. 6, pp. 179–80 below.

94 Eberhard Wolff, "Der 'willkommene Würgeengel,' Verstehende Innenperspektive und 'genaue' Quellen-interpretation – am Beispiel des erwünschten Kindertods in den Anfangen der Pockenschutzimpfung," in *Neue Wege in der Seuchengeschichte*, ed. Martin Dinges (Stuttgart: Steiner, 1995), 110–13.

95 Cited in Wolff, 110.

96 Cited in Frevert, *Krankheit*, 70.

97 Cited in Wolff, "Wurgeengel," 111.

from life on earth into life in Heaven.[98] Another common form of consolation for desperate parents with a sense of guilt about wishing for the death of one of their offspring was the notion that God wanted, and indeed expected, a share of their children, and that their babies would be better off among the angels' chorus.[99] Justus Möser, the high-profile Osnabrück jurist and social analyst, used clever satire to highlight the mindset that accepted children's deaths from smallpox as God's will, when inoculation could prevent such deaths (1783): "I support natural smallpox, which gets rid of the excess so effectively leaving a few in each household who have enough to eat, and God is in agreement because many angels are delivered."[100]

Some peasants struggling to support their families were inclined to regard smallpox as a test for selecting the strongest children able to provide the most help with the heavy burdens of farm-work.[101] Poor peasants in rural Livonia who deliberately exposed their children to smallpox admitted to thinking that "it is better if the child dies now, if it has to die, than if it first eats a lot of bread and then dies."[102] A similar attitude toward smallpox among the despairing rural poor in Prussia may explain the exceptionally high smallpox death-rate of 44 per cent in a group of poverty-stricken villages, in 1796. In that area, where 129 deaths were recorded from 292 smallpox cases, a local doctor noted that some parents failed to provide their sick children with anything to drink, despite the familiarity of the saying *aut bibendum aut moriendum* (either drink or die).[103] The high child mortality in those times seems to have given rise to a general acceptance of post-natal birth control, and to the notion of smallpox as a convenient way of alleviating the burdens of a large family without arousing suspicions of infanticide, a commonplace crime that was usually difficult to prove.[104]

---

98 Wolff, 115–6, 119–22; Kerstin Michalik, *Kindsmord. Soziale- und Rechtsgeschichte der Kindstötung im 18. und beginnenden 19. Jahrhundert, am Beispiel Preußen* (Pfaffenweiler: Centaurus, 1997), 35, 44.

99 Rolf Gehrmann, *Bevölkerungsgeschichte Norddeutschlands zwischen Aufklärung und Vormärz* (Berlin: Spitz, 2000), 293; Wolff, 110–12.

100 Apx 2: Möser (1783), 43.

101 Juncker, *Archiv*, 4:182; Wolff, "Würgeengel," 127–8.

102 Garlieb Merkel, *Die Letten in Liefland am Ende des philosophischen Jahrhunderts* (Leipzig: Gräff, 1800), 52–3. Livonia covered an area roughly corresponding to modern southern Estonia and northern Latvia.

103 Juncker, *Archiv*, 3:90, 123–4; 4:168 (quote), 182; 7:234.

104 Frevert, *Krankheit*, 70. Modern scholars have linked poverty with infanticide: Edward Shorter, "Die Grosse Umwalzung in der Mutter-Kind-Beziehung vom 18. bis zum 20. Jahrhundert," in *Zur Sozialgeschichte der Kindheit*, eds. Jochen Martin et al. (Munich: K.A. Freiburg,

According to a report from Ansbach-Bayreuth during the 1796–97 smallpox epidemic, the common folk regarded smallpox as a necessary evil, and their child's death as a benefit that not only spared the child from other plagues but also alleviated the cost of upbringing.[105] Local teachers' ideas cited in the report were likely to have reinforced such sentiments:

> Some among the teachers, out of fear and dread of excessive population increase and famine, would explain the smallpox horror as an apparent evil through which benevolent Nature would avert the seeming over-population of humans.[106]

Perceptions of the necessity of smallpox were also evident in comments by *Stadt- and Landphysikus* Bachmann from Brandenburg-Kulmbach, who noted (1796) that "most parents ... were inclined to regard smallpox as a necessary and unavoidable evil against the lives of their children, who would best be in Heaven with God."[107]

The perceived 'necessity' of smallpox, and the notion that children would be better off with God were clearly quite at odds with inoculation, vaccination, or any other form of smallpox prophylaxis. Professor Friedrich Benjamin Osiander from Göttingen argued that parents who cited religious reasons for opposing inoculation saw "a benefit in God occasionally taking a few of their children through smallpox, because in their opinion God had given them too many."[108] Pastor Lohe from Brand, in Ansbach-Bayreuth, wrote (1798) that the rejection of inoculation in his parish was in some cases because "parents are happy when God looked after their children, and may leave a single one behind."[109] Some apparently believed that God had every right to take smallpox-afflicted children, as suggested by the accusations of jeering inoculation opponents that a father "robbed our God of his child" by having his son

---

1986), 519–20; Michalik, *Kindsmord,* 44–5; Otto Ulbricht, *Kindsmord und Aufklärung in Deutschland* (Munich: Oldenbourg, 1990), 171–2; Wolff, "Würgeengel," 114–5, 130–1.

105 Juncker, *Archiv*, 3:123.

106 *Unter den Lehrern, es noch einige giebt, die aus Aengstlichkeit für übergrosse Menschen Vermehrung und Hungersnoth sich fürchten, und darum die Pokkennoth auch für ein scheinbares Uebel erklären möchten, durch welches die wohltätige Natur dem scheinbaren Ueberflußе an Menschen-Menge vorbeuge*: Juncker, 3:123–4; see 3:113–4 for a comment on such sentiments.

107 Juncker, 3:90.

108 Friedrich B. Osiander, *Lehrbuch der Hebammenkunst* (Göttingen: Rosenbusch, 1796), 602–4; Review of *Vorschläge zur Ausrottung der Kinderblattern und anderen ansteckenden Seuchen,* by Francesco M. Scuderi, *GA* 1 (1795): 283.

109 Juncker, *Archiv*, 7:234.

inoculated after losing a daughter to smallpox.[110] Pastor Schwager, who witnessed that outburst, had this to say some years later:

> Many parents regard their substantial number of children as a burden, and wish secretly that God would like to take some ... To them, every denigration of inoculation is welcome, and every sermon reminding them of the duty to preserve their children whenever possible is a barbed nail in the heart. These are the very ones who shout most loudly against inoculation.[111]

Overall, the stark reality of smallpox was suffering, death, and disability on the one side of the equation, and the promise of relief offered by inoculation, on the other. The raft of myths and misconceptions, leaving parents relying largely on futile treatments that often did more harm than good, rather than choosing inoculation, reflect the dichotomies in German society as the new ideas of the Enlightenment clashed with long-entrenched traditions resistant to change. On the other hand, the new humanitarian approach to suffering and death inspired many public-spirited protagonists to become involved in the effort to improve home-treatments for smallpox and to encourage inoculation, in the face of much public scepticism.

110 Apx 2: Schwager, "Patriotische" (1786), 207.
111 Apx 2: Schwager, "Diesmalige" (1790), 20–21.

CHAPTER 2

The Ruling Class and the Nobility

Smallpox cut a swathe through the ruling houses of Britain and Europe for centuries, causing dynastic shifts on many occasions. It even caused an armed conflict, the War of the Bavarian Succession, by killing the childless Elector Maximilian III Joseph of Bavaria in 1777, at age thirty-two, without an obvious successor. Smallpox precipitated the end of the Stuart reign in Britain too, by claiming Queen Anne's last heir, eleven-year-old Prince William, in 1700 after killing two of his sisters and several other close relatives during the previous fifty years.[1] The Hanoverian ascent following the queen's death in 1714 led to enduring royal support for inoculation initiated by the new Princess of Wales, Caroline of Ansbach, who had good reason to fear smallpox. Not only had the disease caused the tragic death of young Prince William that opened the path for her own family's elevation to British royal ranks, but smallpox had also killed her father Margrave Johann Friedrich of Brandenburg-Ansbach when Caroline was three years old. Smallpox claimed her stepfather too, eight years later, and caused grave concerns in 1721 that her eldest daughter Anna was about to meet the same fate.[2] Caroline's embrace of inoculation, highlighted by her public show of confidence in having her two younger daughters inoculated in 1722, helped to halt the carnage from smallpox in her own family by inspiring her eldest son and her grandchildren to follow suit. Other families in which the parents followed her example benefited as well.[3]

Compared to British royalty and aristocracy in the 1720s, German princes tended to be more curious about inoculation than enthusiastic, quickly losing interest after witnessing the occasional test.[4] They began to pay closer attention in the mid-1750s after the reinvigoration of inoculation, when deadly

1 Donald R. Hopkins, *The Greatest Killer: Smallpox in History* (Chicago: University of Chicago Press, 2002), 36–46, 56–8, 61–4; Evelyne Bechmann, *Die Frauen der Wittelsbacher: Ein Frauenbild von Mittelalter bis in die Gegenwart* (Norderstedt: BoD, 2014), 41.

2 Caroline's father died in 1686; her step-father Elector Johann Georg IV of Saxony died in 1694: Marieke Böth, *Erzählweisen des Selbst. Körperpraktiken in den Briefen Liselottes von der Pfalz (1652–1722)* (Böhlau, Cologne, 2015), 64. Hans Sloane, "An Account of Inoculation," *PT* 49 (1755): 517–8.

3 Hervé Bazin, *Vaccination: a History. From Lady Montagu to Genetic Engineering* (Esher, UK: John Libbey Eurotext, 2011), 31–2.

4 Genevieve Miller, *The Adoption of Inoculation for Smallpox in England and France* (Philadelphia: University of Pennsylvania Press, 1957), 67–8, 176–7; Apx 2: "Methode" (1726), 130–6.

 | DOI:10.1163/9789004465374_004

smallpox was once again spreading across Europe. While some princes acted quite promptly to have their children inoculated by their own *Leibarzt*, others were more inclined to either invite a specialist to carry out the procedure at their court, or take their children on a sometimes lengthy journey to a skilled practitioner.[5] The recognition by princes and ther officials that the amelioration of severe smallpox on a wide scale would not only benefit state finances but also boost a government's enlightened credentials led to initiatives aimed toward curbing the disease mortality.[6] Some officials advocated inoculation, which was being promoted at that time by a number of German pioneers of public health policymaking as well as by other influential inoculation advocates.[7]

1 Princes, and 'Travelling Inoculators'

When the pros and contras of inoculation became a point of public discussion during the smallpox epidemics of the mid-1750s, some princes and their officials were inclined to view inoculation as a humanitarian benefit that should be bestowed on the people.[8] For others, another tenet of Enlightenment ideology came to the fore: disquiet about compulsion.[9] By the time smallpox was claiming a new harvest of unfortunate victims in 1767–68, princes and their officials had abandoned the idea of compulsory inoculation in favour of strategies based on encouragement, though some local authorities continued to

5 Marie-Hélène Cotoni, *Correspondance de Frédéric II avec Luise-Dorothée de Saxe-Gotha (1740–1767)* (Oxford: Alden, 1999), 10; *Leipziger gelehrte Zeitung*, no. 7 (1757): 60ff; Élie-Catherine Fréron, "Arrivée d'un de Mrs. Sutton & d'un de ses beaux-frères à Paris," *L'année littéraire. Année 1771*, vol. 3 (Paris: Delalain, 1771), 193–5, 199–200.

6 Ute Frevert, *Krankheit als politisches Problem 1770–1880. Soziale Unterschichten in Preußen zwischen medizinischer Polizei und staatlicher Sozialversicherung* (Göttingen: Vandenhoek & Ruprecht, 1984), 24–5; Moritz Pistor, "Geschichte der preussischen Medizinalverwaltung," *DVG* 40 (1908): 780; Apx 2: Möhsen, part 2 (1775), 8–9.

7 Johann P. Süßmilch, *Die göttliche Ordnung in den Veränderungen des menschlichen Geschlechts, aus der Geburt, dem Tode und der Fortpflanzung desselben erwiesen,* 2nd ed., vol. 2 (Berlin: Buchhandlung der Realschule, 1762), 440–3; Johann C. Scherf, *Archiv der medizinischen Polizey und die gemeinnützigen Arzneikunde*, vol. 2 (Leipzig: Weygand, 1783), 215–41; Apx 2: Justi (1755), 169–71; Weinland (1770), 12–15.

8 Apx 2: de Redern (1765), 81–2.

9 Pistor, "Geschichte," 781; Peter Albrecht, "Von den vergeblichen Mühen, die Bevölkerung der Stadt Braunschweig von der Nützlichkeit des Impfens gegen Blattern zu überzeugen (1754–1787)," in *Gotts Verhengnis und seine Straffe – zur Geschichten der Seuche in der frühen Neuzeit,*" ed. Petra Feuerstein-Herz (Wolfenbüttel: Herzog August Bibliothek, 2005), 128.

inoculate children in orphanages and work-houses.[10] The usual first step taken by European princes keen to expand inoculation was to have the procedure carried out on their own children or grandchildren, and to ensure that a good outcome was publicised so that the people were aware of their sovereign's example.[11] Such was the case in 1756 when the Duke of Orléans called in one of the champions of inoculation, Theodor Tronchin, to carry out the procedure on his children, causing great jubilation in Paris, and turning inoculation into a fashion.[12]

Count Heinrich XI of Obergreiz was arguably the first German prince to have his children inoculated, when in 1757 he called upon his *Leibarzt* Johann Gottlob Sturm to inoculate two of his sons, named Heinrich XIV and Heinrich XV according to family tradition.[13] In nearby Saxe-Gotha in the following year, Duke Friedrich III's younger son August was inoculated by the duke's Swiss *Leibarzt* Johann Caspar Sulzer, who prepared for the occasion by carrying out the procedure on twenty-six children, including his own.[14] While there is no evidence of any broader emulation of the princely initiatives in Obergreiz and Saxe-Gotha, the inoculation of Prince-Elector Friedrich Christian's children in nearby Saxony in 1763 attracted considerable attention among the elite. According to the children's mother Electress Maria Antonia, her example in having her children inoculated saved the lives of "about a thousand children whose parents followed my example."[15] A similar response was noted in neighbouring Anhalt-Dessau after the Anglophile Duke Leopold III Friedrich Franz and his wife Luise Henriette had themselves inoculated soon after their marriage in 1768, setting an example that reportedly inspired "the majority of the upper-class and others to follow."[16]

While princes may have had good access to skilled practitioners to inoculate their children at their respective courts, a shortage of expertise in many regions during the 1750s-60s caused difficulties for other parents keen to adopt the procedure. Justifiably believing that the newer British inoculation methods were superior, elite parents were inclined to seek out one of the inoculation

10 Apx 2: "Etwas von" (1769), 347; Lichtenstein (1787), 399–400; "Werkhaus" (1788), 164–7.
11 Apx 2: Weinland (1770), 126–31.
12 Arnold H. Rowbotham, "The 'Philosophes' and the Propaganda for Inoculation of Smallpox in France," *UCP* 18 (1935): 268.
13 *Leipziger gelehrte Zeitung*, no. 7 (1757): 60ff.
14 Charles-Marie de la Condamine, *Histoire de l'inoculation de la petite vérole* (Amsterdam: Typographic Society, 1773), 267.
15 *Correspondance de Frédéric II, roi de Prusse*, eds. Johann D.E. Preuss and Adolph von Menzel, vol. 9 (Berlin: Decker, 1854), 47.
16 Apx 2: Weinland (1770), 141.

specialists from Britain aiming to capitalise on the relative dearth of local expertise. Johann Wolfgang von Goethe remarked on the opportunistic 'inoculation business,' in his reminiscences:

> among us, inoculation was still viewed as very problematical ... German doctors were hesitant about using a procedure that seemed to pre-empt nature. Consequently, speculating Englishmen came over to the Continent and, for a considerable fee, inoculated the children of persons they found to be well-to-do and unprejudiced.[17]

The first wave of such British practitioners came to Germany during 1754–55. A London newspaper's Berlin correspondent reported on 17 January 1755 that "Dr. Geseke, an eminent physician of this city, has begun to introduce the inoculation of smallpox, in which he has proven very successful." Mr. Middleton began practising in Hamburg at much the same time.[18] The Scottish doctor, George Motherby, joined the subsequent wave inspired by the increasing confidence in inoculation following the Suttons's technical improvements.[19] His arrival in Prussia in 1770 was announced officially: "With the permission of His Majesty the King, Mr. G. Motherby, a medical doctor from England, has come to inoculate smallpox using the latest and best method ... in the royal Prussian lands." Motherby focused his activities on the Danzig-Königsberg region of East Prussia, receiving high praise from a father amazed that the doctor was able to inoculate his daughter without the girl even noticing because he distracted her so effectively with a small toy.[20]

A number of doctors trained by the pre-eminent Sutton family of inoculation specialists from Essex were offering welcome British expertise to the European elite more generally at that time. Daniel Sutton's father-in-law Simeon Worlock was practising in Paris in the 1770s, and a brother-in-law, Dr. Andrew Hewit, established a successful practice in The Hague in 1768 with a

---

17 *Goethe's Werke,* vol. 24, *Aus meinem Leben, Dichtung und Wahrheit* (Stuttgart and Tübingen: Cotta, 1839), 51–2.

18 *London Gazette,* no. 94, January 28 - February 1, 1755 (quote); Charles-Marie de la Condamine, *Seconde mémoire sur l'inoculation de la petite vérole* (Geneva: Du Villard, 1759), 33.

19 "Vorbericht," *Stuttgarter Allgemeines Magazin* 1 (1767): 4–5; *Augspurgisches Extra-Blätel,* no. 174 (Augsburg), July 23, 1767, 3.

20 William Ebstein, "Georg und William Motherby und ihren Beziehungen zur Variolation (Königsberg)," *AGM* 4 (1911): 37 (quote); Review of *Von der vorzüglichen Geschichtlichkeit des herrn Georg Motherby, bey der Einpfropfung der Pocken, ertheilet aus eigner Erfahrung an seinem Kinde sichere Nachricht,* by Friedrich S. Bock, *TM*, no. 12 (1775): 283–5.

Sutton-trained colleague Dr. Alexander Sutherland.[21] Hewit's high reputation led to invitations to inoculate at princely courts, sometimes necessitating considerable travel. Following such a journey to the Crown-Prince of Brunswick-Wolfenbüttel's court in 1770, Hewit carried out a number of inoculations at the Duke of Holstein-Oldenburg's residence in northern Germany, and at the Danish Royal Court in Copenhagen. Many other elite parents from far and wide took their children to Hewit in The Hague for inoculation appointments.[22] The Hessen-Kassel minister, Count von Oeynhausen, made the trip in 1768, as did the Margrave of Nassau-Weilburg (Rhine-Lahn region) and his wife, who used their public announcement of the successful inoculation of their three children as an opportunity to entreat other parents to follow their example.[23] Yet emulation was not so easy considering the ongoing scarcity of skilled inoculators in many regions.

Dr. William Baylies (see Figure 6 on p. 65) was another of the British inoculators helping to fill the gaps in expertise in Europe. After fleeing from Bath to France in 1766 during a property dispute, he worked as a 'travelling inoculator' until the early 1770s, using a *Poste Restante* address in Metz as his point of contact.[24] Although he visited the occasional high-profile client in more distant towns, such as the Prince of Thurn and Taxis in Regensburg (Bavaria) and Count von Stadion in Warthausen (southern Württemburg), most of his clients were invited to take their children at a particular time for a group inoculation in Metz or in one of several other towns not too far away: Spa, Strasburg, Mannheim, Worms, or Frankfurt.[25] Indeed, Goethe's much-cited remark about 'speculating' English inoculators may have been modelled on Baylies, whose inoculation activities in the Frankfurt region coincided with the period in autumn 1768 when Goethe was living at his parents' home in Frankfurt being cared for by his mother during a long illness.[26]

Goethe's suggestion that German doctors were disinclined to inoculate is borne out to some extent by the experiences of one of Baylies's clients, Baron

---

21 Michael J. Bennett, "Curing and Inoculating Smallpox: the Career of Simeon Worlock in Paris, Brittany, and Saint-Domingue in the 1770s," *French History and Civilization* 7 (2017): 29–30; Fréron, "Arrivée," 193–5.

22 "Inoculation," *Journal Oeconomique, ou mémoires, notes et avis. Année 1770* (July 1770): 321–2; Fréron, "Arrivée," 193–4, 199–200.

23 Fréron, 193; *Augspurgische Ordinarii Postzeitung von Staats-politischen und andern Neuigkeiten* (Augsburg), April 4, 1768, 2.

24 "Letter to the editor," *The Gentleman's Magazine* 25 (1846): 592–3; A. Seitz, "Etwas vom Impfen aus dem Jahre 1768," *AGM* 2 (1909): 421.

25 Seitz, 420–1; Apx 2: "Zu der Geschichte" (1770), 211.

26 Goethe, *Dichtung*, 51–2; Dorothea Hölscher-Lohmeyer, *Johann Wolfgang von Goethe* (Munich: Beck, 2007), 19.

von Botzheim from Wachenheim, near Worms (Palatinate). The baron finally had his children inoculated, though not by Baylies, a full seven years after Baylies failed to turn up in Mannheim at the arranged time in 1768, and failed to make a suggested later visit to Worms.[27] The ongoing scarcity of skilled inoculators in southern Germany is underscored by the inoculation in 1803 of young Friedrich Eser in Hürbel (southern Württemburg) after three of his siblings died from smallpox. The Count of Stadion's *Leibarzt* Jakob Christian von Bourdon, who lived nearby, offered to carry out the procedure, claiming that he had obtained the necessary instruments and medicines from England. He then proceeded to inflict deep incisions on the hapless three-year-old child, using a discredited method dating from the 1720s.[28]

Baylies halted his activities as a 'travelling inoculator' and settled in Dresden during the early 1770s, perhaps enticed by the lucrative prospect of inoculating princely children following the marriage in 1769 of nineteen-year-old Elector Friedrich August. However, the Elector invited Dr. Johann Friedrich Probst from Bautzen to inoculate himself and other family members, while his uncle Carl Christian, the deposed Duke of Courland who resided at the Dresden court, chose his own *Leibarzt* Montanus to inoculate his baby daughter.[29] Baylies's expertise nonetheless attracted elite clients from farther afield, such as Baron Friedrich Wilhelm von Arnim-Boizenburg. The baron travelled from Berlin to Dresden with his son in early-1774 so they could both be inoculated by the British specialist; the practice was in disrepute in Berlin at that time, as it had been ever since the deaths in 1765 of several high-profile clients inoculated by high-ranking practitioners.[30]

In the small south-western territory of Baden in the 1760s, inoculation was not such a rarity as in many other regions. Margrave Carl Friedrich had begun officially encouraging the procedure even before the smallpox epidemic of 1767–68 that precipitated such action in several other states. Addressing the problem of smallpox was part of a broader public health agenda adopted by the Francophile margrave, who was admired for his enlightened approach to government throughout his sixty-five year rule (1746–1811) that brought great benefits to Baden.[31] Carl Friedrich's medical reforms included two decrees

---

27 Seitz, "Impfen," 420–1.

28 Friedrich Eser, *Aus Meinem Leben (1798–1873)*, ed. P. Beck (Ravensburg: Alber, 1907), 8–9.

29 Dietrich Tutzke, *Christian August Struve (1767–1807): Leben und Werke eines Görlitzer Arztes im Dienste des Humanismus der Aufklärungszeit* (Görlitz: Town Council, 1957), 51; Apx 2: Heinsius (1780), 140.

30 Apx 2: Baylies (1776), 8–9.

31 Karl W.L.F. von Drais, *Geschichte der Regierung und Bildung von Baden unter Carl Friedrich*, vol. 1 (Karlsruhe: Müller, 1818), 1–3, 190–99.

aimed at encouraging inoculation, which were among the first laws of that kind in Europe. In August 1766 he decreed that all medical students from Baden were to place special emphasis on inoculation procedures, and in October he decreed that students from Baden studying surgery in France and Berlin were to be notified of the statutory requirement to have special training in smallpox inoculation. Once the trained doctors and surgeons were in place and inoculation was available to families at all social levels, the margrave actively encouraged the practice.[32] His novel approach of drawing attention to the unscarred complexions and robust health of the inoculated women in his extended family reportedly had the desired effect of increasing inoculation rates in the territory.[33]

Carl Friedrich's efforts to curb the impact of smallpox included an advice circular compiled by *Landphysikus* Gustav Friedrich Jägerschmid that recommended up-to-date smallpox treatments and warned parents to avoid customary home-remedies. A decree issued in December 1768 required pastors and other officials in rural areas to distribute the circulars along with warnings to parents to adhere to the advice and avoid smallpox treatments that led to children's deaths.[34] Meanwhile, the margrave perpetuated his grandfather's initiative of gathering data on environmental and living conditions that could help in formulating future policies to deal with smallpox and other infectious diseases. The uninterrupted long duration of the readings, initiated in 1724, placed Baden ahead of most other territories in having locally-compiled data to guide policy-making in public health matters.[35] Carl Friedrich also took the lead among German rulers in initiating systematic cowpox vaccination, which commenced in Baden in 1801.[36]

Duke Carl I of Brunswick-Wolfenbüttel adopted quite a different approach to the encouragement of inoculation, though he began in the usual way by alerting the public (1767) to a successful inoculation in his own family. The official announcement that "Prince Carl Georg August … just two years old … was inoculated with smallpox in London" assured the public of the ruling

32 Carl F. Gerstlacher, ed., *Sammlung aller Baden-Durlachischen Anstalten und Verordnungen*, vol. 1 (Karlsruhe: Schmieder, 1773), 527–8.

33 Christian L. Schweickhard, *Ueber den Zustand des Wundarzneiwesens im Badischen* (Karlsruhe: Müller, 1787), 36.

34 Gerstlacher, ed., *Sammlung*, 1:528–9.

35 Jan Brügelmann, "Observations on the Process of Medicalization in Germany, 1770–1830, based on Medical Topographies," in *La Medicalization de la Société Francaise 1770–1830*, ed. Jean-Pierre Goubert (Waterloo, Ontario: Historical Reflections Press, 1982), 133–4.

36 "Margrafschaft Baden, Kuhpocken," *Schwäbische Chronik*, July 31, 1801, 287; "Regierungsblatt, no. 22 (November 19, 1803)," in *Kur-Badisches Regierungsblatt*, vol. 1, nos. 1–26 (1803).

family's confidence in the practice.[37] A local commentator called attention to the successful inoculation of the little prince, in an appeal (1768) to parents to follow the example set by the crown prince and his British wife Augusta, a sister of King George III. For added encouragement, he praised the skill of the local practitioners while also highlighting the inoculation of royal children in France and the great strides inoculation was making in Britain and Sweden.[38] Another commentator made mention of the remarkable progress of inoculation in Vienna where many doctors had opposed the practice until the imperial family gave their official approval.[39] Those articles were two of nine about inoculation that appeared in 1768 in the twice-weekly government-issued *Gelehrte Beyträge zu den Braunschweigischen Anzeigen* (GB), underscoring the strong focus on the topic among local commentators.[40] In the previous year in the same journal, the surgeon J.G. Bütesisch made a public-spirited offer of free inoculation for the poor.[41] A similar initiative by the government commenced in 1768 at the public inoculation facility, which consisted of one room for inoculation and another for patient after-care, at the new hospital for the poor. The service was overseen by the surgeon Eckermann who was soon receiving effusive praise for his inoculation skills "in the English manner."[42] Though the practice came to a halt following three fatalities in 1769, its eventual recommencement and expansion led to the tally of inoculations in Brunswick reaching six hundred by 1787.[43]

Duke Carl I of Brunswick-Wolfenbüttel, a grandfather, was an inoculation enthusiast from a generation known for its general scepticism of the innovation.[44] The ruler of the neighbouring territory of Stolberg-Wernigerode, Count Heinrich Ernst, was one of the sceptics. The Count and his wife believed that inoculation was "morally and physically wrong," according to their son Christian Friedrich who wanted to have his own children inoculated yet failed to do

37 Cited in Albrecht, "Mühen," 129.
38 Apx 2: "Weitere Nachricht" (1768): 57–64.
39 Apx 2: "Nachricht von der hieselbst wieder" (1768): 723–4.
40 See Apx 2 for seven other articles in *GB* 8 (1768): "Des berühmten Herrn d'Alembert," 25–32; Pott, 289–92; "Nachricht von den fernern," 345–60; Brückmann, 425–36; Rahwes, 449–54; "Nochmalige," 679–88; Topp, 725–28.
41 Apx 2: Bütesisch (1767), 311–12.
42 Apx 2: "Nachricht von dem fernern" (1768), 356 (quote). August Hinze, *Lexicon aller Herzogl. Braunschweigischen Verordnungen welche die medicinische Policey betreffen* (Stendal: Franzen und Grosse, 1793), 113.
43 Hinze, 113–4.
44 Apx 2: Sintenis (1790), 109. Review of *Abhandlung über die Einimpfung der Blattern, als sittliche Pflicht betrachtet und empfohlen* (Dortmund: Mallinckrodt, 1800), by Benjamin C. Sowden, *RA* 2 (1800): 2554.

so out of respect for the views of his father. Christian Friedrich and his wife could at least take pleasure in the news in 1774 of the successful inoculation of the children of his sister Luise Ferdinande and her husband Count Friedrich Erdmann of Anhalt-Pless.[45] Friedrich Erdmann was much more aware than his father-in-law of the need to protect his heirs from smallpox, having inherited his own title through the smallpox deaths of his uncle Leopold of Anhalt-Köthen and of Leopold's only son (and a daughter), which caused the title to pass to his father.[46] Such family histories were a great incentive for the extensive German ruling class to embrace inoculation as a way of preventing smallpox from sweeping away their heirs, as had occurred so often in the past.

At the time Duke Carl I was encouraging inoculation in Brunswick-Wolfenbüttel, the practice was initiated in Saxe-Weimar where he was the co-regent with his widowed daughter, Duchess Anna Amalia. The first inoculation at the Weimar court was carried out in 1768 by Anna Amalia's *Leibarzt* Carl Friedrich Kaltschmid, on the nephew of Count Johann Eustach von Görtz, tutor to eleven-year-old Duke Carl August and his brother Friedrich Ferdinand. Wider reverberations from the inoculation of Louis von Görtz emanated from the close links between the court and the territory's university at Jena, where not only *Leibarzt* Kaltschmid was a professor but also the court pastor Ernst Jacob Danovius who reportedly embarked on a personal campaign to advertise the benefits of inoculation to anyone who would listen. The mathematics professor, Schmidt, highlighted the value of inoculation too, by designing a statistics exercise requiring his students to calculate the population increase that would result from reducing smallpox mortality through the adoption of the practice.[47]

Subsequent *Leibärzte* expanded inoculation in Saxe-Weimar in the following years, beginning with Johann Friedrich Hufeland who was appointed by Anna Amalia after Kaltschmid's death in 1769. Before being elevated to his new role, Hufeland had been offering inoculation for quite some time to clients attending his Weimar practice, equipping him well for the task of inoculating the two princes.[48] The increased public acceptance of the new smallpox prophylactic following the successful inoculation of Anna Amalia's children in 1771 highlights once again the importance of high-profile examples in encouraging

---

45 *Briefe und Journale der Fürstin Luise Ferdinande zu Anhalt-Cothen, der Gräfin Auguste Friederike zu Isenberg-Büdingen und der Gräfin Auguste Eleonore zu Stolberg-Wernigerode, aus den Jahren 1764–1784*, part 3: 1774 (Dresden: Henkler, 1785), 38.

46 *Die Europäische Fama, welche den gegenwärtigen Zustand der vornehmsten Höfe entdecket*, part 318 (Leipzig, 1729), 536.

47 Apx 2: Weinland (1770), 140–1.

48 Johann J. Sachs, *Christoph Wilhelm Hufeland: Ein Rückblick auf sein siebenzigjähriges Leben und Wirken* (Berlin: Hirschwald, 1832), 5–6.

emulation. Yet the fragility of public confidence was soon on display when publicity about a number of previously inoculated children catching smallpox largely halted the practice in Weimar. Another opportunity to underscore the benefits of inoculation came with the reappearance of smallpox during the rule of Anna Amalia's son Grand-Duke Carl August, prompting his *Leibarzt* Johann Christian Stark to inoculate a new generation of princely children.[49] That occasion in 1788 was "a great example that gained many followers," according to the Jena professor Christoph Wilhelm Hufeland. *Leibarzt* Stark, also a professor at Jena, attributed the renewed public interest to the ruling family's confidence in the benefits of inoculation, which he himself had highlighted with his own publicity campaign drawing attention to the recovery of young Prince Carl Friedrich and Princess Caroline Luise, rather than to his inoculation of the children *per se.* The reversal of the public negativity toward inoculation was clearly evident in Hufeland's description of a Weimar streetscape, where "the roads and paths were filled with smallpox-afflicted children" after "almost one hundred were inoculated" in the wake of the grand-duke's example. Yet the mingling of the infected children in public had the adverse impact of causing a smallpox epidemic – a timely reminder of the contagiousness of inoculation and the need for a more cautious approach.[50] By then, inoculation had been banned in a number of European cities including Paris, Dijon, Lyon, and Bern, except during smallpox outbreaks.[51]

2 High-Ranking Mothers

Protestant Germany with its plethora of princely families ruling various patches of territory was a popular source of wives for British aristocrats. Letters from relatives or friends reporting family inoculations, or offering advice on the procedure brought the reality of inoculation to high-ranking women in Germany, as did some journals for women.[52] Whichever opinion of the

49 Christoph W. Hufeland, "Erklärung," *Intelligenzblatt der* ALZ, no. 71 (1795): 567–8; Johann C. Stark, "Widererklärung," *Intelligenzblatt der* ALZ, no. 89 (1795): 712.

50 Stark, 712; Apx 2: Hufeland, *Bemerkungen* (1789), 2 (quotes).

51 *Real-Zeitung*, no. 52 (Erlangen), July 2, 1763, 402–3; Schweickhard, *Medicinish-Gerichtliche Behandlungen*, 594; "Verordnung der Kammer, des Conseils und der Stadt-Obrigkeit und Gemeinde zu Dijon, vom 25 September 1779," AFS 2 (1781): 250–2.

52 *Correspondance*, eds. Preuss and Menzel, 47; Jürgen Konert, "SA Tissot und sein Einfluß auf den 'Dessau-Wörlitzer Kulturkreis,'" *Gesnerus* 49 (1992): 41; King George I to his daughter Sophia Dorothea, Queen of Prussia, May 26, 1724, MS 9212/1, Box 229, Shelfmark PP/CRI/M/2/3, Archives and Manuscripts, Wellcome Library, London; "Von der Inoculation

procedure they chose to accept, elite women could hardly ignore the increasing adoption of inoculation by their peer group, and the survival of the vast majority of inoculated children without the scarring that was a common consequence of naturally-acquired smallpox.[53]

The action of the Princess of Wales, Caroline of Ansbach (Figure 4), in having her daughters inoculated in London in 1722 had a wider influence by inspiring her Hanover-based eldest son Frederick Lewis to have himself inoculated. Unwilling to take unnecessary risks with the life of the future Prince of Wales, King George I sent one of the most experienced inoculators in Britain at the time, Charles Maitland, to inoculate his eldest grandson in Hanover.[54] In a letter (1724) to his daughter Queen Sophia Dorothea of Prussia, the king expresses his delight at the successful outcome of the prince's inoculation, also raising the issue of the smallpox susceptibility of his Prussian grandchildren.

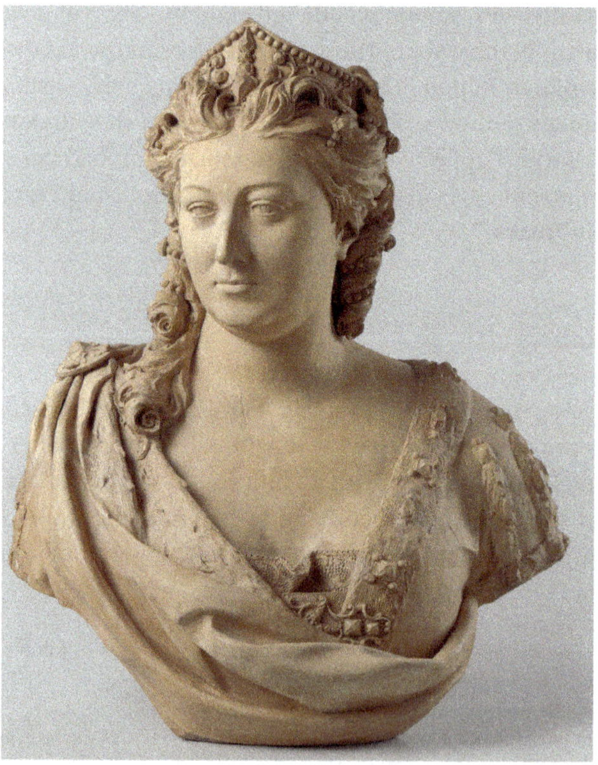

FIGURE 4
Caroline of Brandenburg-Ansbach, 1738. Terracotta sculpture by J.M. Rysbrack
RIJKSMUSEUM, AMSTERDAM: BK-NM-5760

der Kinderblattern," *Für die Frau* 1 (1756): 97–112; "Nachricht von einer Art der Einpfropfung," *Für die Frau*, no. 46 (1757): 363–6; Apx 2: Hufeland et al., "Empfehlung" (1789), 79–86.

53 Apx 2: Büchner (1762), *RNS*, 175–6; Hufeland et al., "Empfehlung" (1789), 82–5.

54 Miller, *Adoption*, 96–7, 176.

He makes particular mention of Crown Prince Friedrich's (later Frederick the Great) recent recovery from smallpox as a prelude to recommending inoculation to his daughter for her seven other children.[55] Though it was theoretically quite easy for the Prussian queen to accept her father's advice, since Dr. Johann Theodor Eller, who had successfully inoculated five children in Bernburg in 1721, was a physician at the Prussian Royal Court, it was not so easy in practice. Eller had been forced to abandon inoculation when he accepted the appointment, owing to a regulation prohibiting court officials from having any deliberate contact with smallpox. King Friedrich Wilhelm I was perhaps even unaware of his court physician's inoculation credentials.[56]

Another relative of Caroline the Princess of Wales, her widowed sister-in-law Margravine Christiane Charlotte of Brandenburg-Ansbach, was so impressed by the inoculation of her nieces in London and nephew in Hanover that she decided to carry out a test when smallpox arrived in Ansbach in 1725. Using her authority as the regent during her son's minority, she gave her court physician Christian Ludwig Rosa instructions to inoculate twelve children and report the outcome. Yet the mixed result, in that six of the candidates developed smallpox and recovered while the other six showed no symptoms, discouraged any further experiments in the territory at the time.[57] Inoculation was revived forty years later under Christiane Charlotte's grandson Margrave Carl Alexander whose *Leibarzt* Carl Ludwig von Breyer became a well-known inoculator among the Ansbach elite in the late-1760s.[58]

The inoculation in Hanover in 1724 of the soon-to-be Prince of Wales, Frederick Lewis, initiated a generational cascade of inoculated royal children after the prince married Princess Augusta of Saxe-Gotha in 1736. The inoculation of the second generation began seven years later with the eldest of the couple's seven children, Augusta, after her five-year-old brother the future King George III contracted smallpox.[59] Augusta later helped to consolidate inoculation among a third generation of the princely familes of Europe, after she married Crown-Prince Carl Wilhelm of Brunswick-Wolfenbüttel and the couple had their baby son inoculated in London in 1767.[60] Four years later, when

55 King George I to his daughter Sophia Dorothea.

56 Johann T. Eller, *Observationes de cognoscendis et curandis morbis, praesertim acutis* (Königsberg and Leipzig: Woltersdorff, 1762), 151–3.

57 Apx 2: "Methode" (1726), 130.

58 Johann B. Fischer, *Geschichte und ausführliche Beschreibung der markgräflich-Brandenburgischen Haupt-und Residenz-Stadt Anspach* (Ansbach: Fischer, 1786), 7–8; Apx 2: Weinland (1770), 139.

59 *Daily Advertiser* (London), November 15, 1743.

60 *Hamburger Relations-Courier*, no. 98 (Hamburg), June, 1767.

a number of skilled British inoculators were practising in northern Europe, Carl Wilhelm and Augusta invited the Sutton-trained Andrew Hewit to travel from The Hague to their Brunswick court to inoculate their younger children.[61] Augusta's youngest sister, too, helped to perpetuate inoculation, having herself undergone the procedure in 1754 along with three of her siblings.[62] Caroline Matilda and the future King Christian VII of Denmark and Norway were indeed the only royal couple both inoculated as children, when they married in 1766.[63] Their son Crown Prince Frederick joined his cousins in 1770 as another of the third generation of inoculated royals, under the skilful hand of King Christian's ill-fated German *Leibarzt* Johann Friedrich von Struensee.[64]

King George III of Great Britain added to the tally of the third generation of inoculated royal children after he married Charlotte Sophia of Mecklenburg-Strelitz and the couple produced a brood of fifteen.[65] Yet the unfortunate death of four-year-old Octavius following his inoculation in 1783 issued a sobering reminder to other parents, of the risks involved. Though some European aristocrats planning to have their children inoculated paused to reflect on the little prince's sad demise, they knew they had little choice other than to go ahead with their plans, since merely awaiting smallpox posed a far greater danger.[66]

When aristocratic mothers in Europe began to take an interest in inoculation in the mid-eighteenth century, the practice was sufficiently familiar to the elite medical fraternity that advice could be obtained from well-known inoculation advocates. One of the first German mothers to follow that course was Luise Dorothea, the wife of Duke Friedrich III of Saxe-Gotha-Altenburg. The duchess was well-aware of the benefits of inoculation from reading Voltaire's works, and from the inoculation in 1754 of her British royal nieces and nephews, the children of her husband's sister Augusta the Princess of Wales.[67]

61 "Inoculation," *Journal Oeconomique*, 321–2.

62 *London Evening Post*, no. 4209, October 31 – November 2, 1754.

63 The future Christian VII was inoculated in 1760: La Condamine, *Histoire*, 259.

64 Franklin Kopitzsch, "Die Durchsetzung der Pockenimpfung. Zu Strategien und Mitteln aufgeklärter Reform in Hamburg und Schleswig-Holstein," in *Das Volk im Visier der Aufklärung*, eds. Anne Conrad, Arno Herzig, and Franklin Kopitzsch (Hamburg: LIT, 1998), 231; *Schriften, die in die Sachen des ehemalige Grafen Johann Friedrich von Struensee, bey der königliche Inquisitions-Commission zu Copehagen übergeben sind* (1772), 98.

65 Samuel G. Vogel, *Handbuch der practischen Arzneywissenschaft zum Gebrauche angehende Aerzte*, 2nd ed. (Stendal: Franzen and Grosse, 1794), 126.

66 George A.-E. Dover, 1st Baron, ed., *Letters of Horace Walpole, Earl of Orford, to Sir Horace Mann* (Philadelphia: Lea and Blanchard, 1844), 109–10.

67 Cotoni, *Correspondance*, 11; *Whitehall Evening Post, or London Intelligencer*, no. 1318 (London), October 26–29, 1754. Augusta of Saxe-Gotha-Altenburg was the wife of Prince Fred-

In 1757 when inoculation was still in its infancy in Germany, Luise Dorothea acted promptly to have her youngest son August inoculated after her elder children Ernst and Friederike contracted smallpox. Following August's recovery, the duchess proudly proclaimed in a letter to Voltaire that having her son inoculated "shows us to be modern and unprejudiced." Her eldest son Crown-Prince Ernst, having noted the mildness of his brother's inoculated smallpox and the successful inoculation of his British royal cousins, took the precaution of arranging the inoculation of his own bride Charlotte soon after their marriage in 1769.[68]

Electress Maria Antonia of Saxony (Figure 5) was another German aristocratic mother who embraced inoculation soon after she learned of it. Having received a high-level education that honed her talents as a musician, during her upbringing as a Bavarian princess, she was an enlightened addition to the Saxon Royal Court when she married Prince-Elector Friedrich Christian in 1747.[69] Yet, as an open-minded mother in a conservative Catholic royal house, her path to the inoculation of her children was by no means straightforward. As she admits in a letter (1763) to her cousin Friedrich II of Prussia thanking him for his advice about inoculation: "it was your words that encouraged me, and persuaded the Prince-Elector to permit it ... my doctors, and above all the priests here, did not want to allow it."[70] Other comments in Maria Antonia's letter suggest that the inoculation of her children had a quite profound wider influence in Saxony at that time:

> I owe you the preservation of my children, and Saxony owes you the lives of about a thousand children whose parents followed my example ... since it was a kind of authorisation ... all the nobility here soon followed my lead.[71]

Soon after his children, Anton and Amalia, recovered from their inoculation, Prince-Elector Friedrich Christian issued a clarion call in the *Leipziger Intelligenzblatt* – "An Alert to Saxons from the Prince-Elector, Regarding Smallpox

---

erick Lewis (†1751), who predeceased his father King George II (†1760), placing his eldest son (George III) next in line for the throne.

68 Cotoni, 10 (quote); Moritz G. Thilenius, *Medicinische und chirurgische Bemerkungen* (Frankfurt am Main: Brönner, 1789), 337.

69 Cordula Bischoff, "Aufklärung in Sachsen? Das höfische Familienporträt zwischen Staatsrepräsentation und Empfindsamkeit," *Das Achtzehnte Jahrhundert: Aufklärung und Hofkultur in Dresden* 37, part 2 (2013): 204–5.

70 *Correspondance,* eds. Preuss and Menzel, 9:47. The letter was dated August 5, 1763.

71 *Correspondance*, 9:47.

Inoculation."[72] That entreaty to emulate the princely couple's action may have been prompted by the realisation that saving lives from smallpox could help to restore the population of Saxony, which had suffered heavy losses during the Seven Years War.[73] Some impact among the broader public is indeed suggested by the Sorau (Saxony) *Physikus* Johann August Heinsius's reflection in 1780 that "the inoculations through the example of ... the Saxon Electoral house

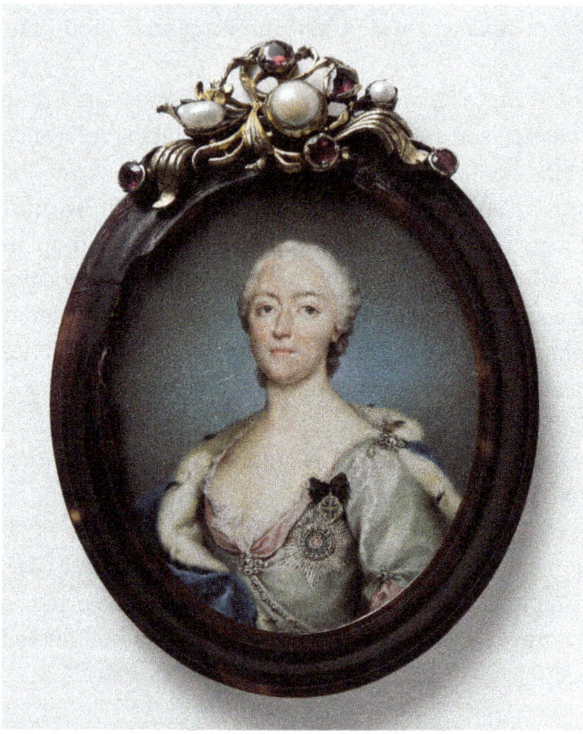

FIGURE 5
Maria Antonia Walpurgis, Electress of Saxony. Watercolour on parchment miniature, attributed to Anton Raphael Mengs
PHOTO BY BODIL BECKMANN. NATIONAL MUSEUM OF STOCKHOLM: NMB 2661. WIKIDATA.ORG

achieved a great deal." Maria Antonia was the primary influence.[74]

Paradoxically, Maria Antonia's husband Friedrich Christian died from smallpox in December 1763, just six months after permitting the inoculation of two of his children, and seventy-four days after his elevation to Elector of Saxony.[75]

---

72 "Landesfürstliche Aufmunterung an Sachsen, zur Einpfropfung der Pocken," *LI*, no. 21, June, 1963. Two further articles in the newspaper in the subsequent year reminded parents about inoculation: *LI*, no. 48, December, 1763; *LI*, no. 12, March, 1764, 116–7.

73 Franz A.J. Szabo, *The Seven Years War in Europe 1756–1763* (Harlow: Pearson Longman, 2008), 430.

74 Apx 2: Heinsius (1780), 140.

75 Carl Gretschel, *Geschichte des sächsischen Volkes und Staaten*, vol. 3 (Leipzig: Hinrichs, 1853), 178.

That calamity when his eldest son was still five years short of his majority highlighted the value of inoculation for dynastic stability. Yet the deceased elector's brother Franz Xaver, who gained the authority over Maria Antonia's children as the closest male relative and co-regent, showed little interest in inoculation even though the inoculator of two of his brother's children was conveniently at the court as his *Leibarzt*. Perhaps the child's death in Bohemia that tainted Dr. Christian Gottlob Demiani's reputation as an inoculator had caused a loss of faith in the practice at the Saxon court.[76] Whatever the reason for the oversight, three of Maria Antonia's sons and her youngest daughter were still un-inoculated when deadly smallpox swept through Saxony in 1766. After the two youngest princes Karl and Maximilian contracted the disease, little Anna was inoculated with some urgency.[77] However, Crown-Prince Friedrich August remained un-inoculated until he eventually underwent the procedure in 1768 after reaching his majority and being elevated to Elector of Saxony.[78] His brother Anton was seemingly less attentive to the dangers of smallpox – his young wife Maria Karoline sadly died from the disease in 1782 after just one year of marriage.[79] The eighteen-year-old princess's father King Victor Amadeus III of Sardinia had clearly failed to follow the example set by his fellow-Catholic sovereigns, the Duke of Parma and Empress Maria Theresa, who both had their children inoculated in the 1760s amid great publicity, after losing others to smallpox.[80]

The Austrian empress Maria Theresa had every reason to embrace inoculation, after seeing smallpox claim several of her children and their marriage partners. The first of those victims was her eldest son Carl Joseph; next came her daughter Maria Gabriela, and then her pregnant daughter-in-law Empress Isabella. More anguish was in store after those deaths during 1761–63, when her daughter-in-law Maria Josepha, Emperor Joseph II's second wife, contracted smallpox and passed the disease to Maria Theresa herself.[81] The simultaneous life-and-death struggle of the two empresses in mid-1767 cast a pall of gloom over not only Austria but also Bavaria, the home of Maria Josepha before her marriage to the Holy Roman Emperor. While the Bavarians were soon in mourning for 'their' empress, the sombre mood of the Viennese turned

76 Gretschel, 3:297; La Condamine, *Histoire*, 267–68.
77 Apx 2: Heinsius (1780), 140.
78 Tutzke, *Struve*, 51.
79 Gretschel, *Geschichte*, 3:199.
80 La Condamine, *Histoire*, 272–3; Anton J. Rechberger, *Vollständige Geschichte der Einimpfung der Blattern in Wien* (Vienna: Grässer, 1788), 7–8.
81 Frank T. Brechka, *Gerard van Swieten and his World, 1700–1772* (The Hague: Martinus Nijhoff, 1970), 115, 118.

to disbelief when Maria Theresa too received the last rites, then widespread joy erupted at the news that their beloved empress had recovered.[82]

Maria Theresa's survival was rare good news in her family's dreadful 1767; they were plunged into mourning again when another of the empress's daughters, Maria Josepha, died from smallpox in October. Two more daughters, Maria Elisabeth and Maria Anna, were soon to emerge from the disease so badly scarred that they retreated from public life.[83] Until then, the empress had taken advice on the matter of smallpox from her physicians, who had steered clear of inoculation, which was not being practised in Austria.[84] Though her *Leibarzt* Gerard van Swieten was not so much opposed to the procedure as too cautious to recommend it, his influential associate Professor Anton de Haen was a staunch opponent who argued that inoculation was not warranted because so few people died from smallpox, and that the practice spread the contagion.[85] Though the latter argument was well justified, the empress was so shocked by the latest death and damage to her children that she came to view inoculation as the best way to protect not only the rest of her family from smallpox but also the broader population.[86]

Austrian officials focused on Britain in their search for an inoculator with proven skills and experience, initially seeking affirmation from the royal physicians that the Suttons's high reputation was warranted.[87] Yet when the ambassador approached the Suttons on the matter of inoculating the empress's family members, the fee they quoted was deemed so excessive that he resumed the search.[88] On the recommendation of the king's *Leibarzt* Sir John Pringle, the assignment was offered to the British-trained inoculator from the Netherlands, Dr. Jan Ingen-Housz, who hastened to Vienna at the beginning of April 1768. Following his arrival on May 14 after encountering some delays and spending

82 "Aus Oesterreich," *Der poetische Zeitungsfabrikant, oder des Münchnerischen Wochenblatt in Versen*, ninth year, no. 1 (1767): item 24 (unnumbered pages).

83 Hopkins, *Smallpox*, 62–3.

84 Johannes Wimmer, *Gesundheit, Krankheit, und Tod im Zeitalter der Aufklärung. Fallstudien aus den Habsburgischen Erbländern* (Vienna, Cologne: Böhlau, 1991), 116–7.

85 Gerhard van Swieten, *Erläuterungen der Boerhaavischen Lehrsätze von Erkentniß und Heilung der Krankheiten* (Frankfurt and Leipzig: Krauß, 1775), 216–9; Anton de Haen, *Réfutation de l'Inoculation servant de réponse a deux pièces qui ont perçu cette année 1759* (Vienna: Trattner, 1759), 58–60, 127–8.

86 Rechberger, *Geschichte*, 7–8.

87 "The Opinion of his Majesty's Physicians and Surgeons, given Jan. 23, 1768, in regard to Messrs. Sutton's Practice of Inoculation, in Consequence of a Letter from Sir John Pringle," *Gentleman's Magazine* 38 (1768): 74–5.

88 "Auszug eines Schreibens von Wien, vom Juli, 1780," *Medizinisches Wochenblatt für Aerzte, Wundärzte, und Apotheker* 2 (1781): 111.

a few days visiting his family in Breda, he was graciously received by Maria Theresa and was soon carrying out hundreds of inoculations to demonstrate his technique to the empress and to the local physicians who were initially mistrustful and antagonistic.[89] He received such widespread approval for his many inoculations with very few casualties that other high-ranking medical men gained the empress's permission to inoculate, and were soon doing so successfully in Vienna and Karlsbad.[90] Ingen-Housz's inoculation of Maria Theresa's youngest sons Ferdinand and Maximilian and granddaughter Theresa, Emperor Joseph II's only child, eventually went ahead on 29 September and the success was celebrated with a *Te Deum* and the issuing of a commemorative medallion.[91] Inoculation then began to expand more broadly, with the establishment of a facility at the St. Veit summer palace to cater to the upper-class, while various medical men offered competent inoculations to the general population. The public could also participate in the annual springtime inoculations supported by the empress at her small Hetzendorf palace.[92] Yet despite Maria Theresa's encouragement and offer of ten Thaler to every soldier who had a child inoculated, the people showed little interest. Nor did the inoculation institute for the poor established by Joseph II in 1786 prove very popular.[93]

Catherine II, the Empress of Russia, officially adopted inoculation in 1768 too, though the practice was by then well-established in the Russian Baltic province of Livonia where it was initiated in 1756.[94] Her decision to not only have her son Paul, the Tsarevitch, inoculated but also to undergo the procedure herself seems to have been inspired by her long-term correspondence with Voltaire, and by her admiration for the *philosophes'* support for inoculation in France.[95] Yet she was warned by Friedrich II of Prussia not to proceed, which seems surprising considering that he was well-known as an inoculation

89 Jan Maarten Ingen Housz, Norman Beale, and Elaine Beale, "The Life of Dr Jan Ingen Housz (1730–99), Private Counsellor and Personal Physician to Emperor Joseph II of Austria," *Journal of Medical Biography* 13 (2005): 17–18.

90 Rechberger, *Geschichte*, 8–10.

91 "Die Merkwürdigsten am Kaiserlich-Königlichen Hof 1768," *FGN*, part 96 (Leipzig: Heinsius, 1769), 798–9.

92 Anton von Störck, *Abhandlung von der Einpfropfung der Kindsblattern* (Vienna: Trattner, 1771), 5–6; "Auszug eines Schreibens," 112.

93 Arnold C. Klebs, *Die Variolation im achtzehnten Jahrhundert: ein historischer Beitrag zur Immunitätsforschung* (Gießen: Töpelmann, 1914), 51; Apx 2: Weinland (1770), 137.

94 Dr. Schulinus from Dorpat who initiated inoculation in Livonia in 1756 had carried out 1,032 inoculations by 1768: Apx 2: "Die Geschichte" (1787), 172–3.

95 Philip H. Clendinning, "Dr. Thomas Dimsdale and Smallpox Inoculation in Russia," *JHM* 28 (1973): 116–7.

enthusiast. His warning seems to have been based on a conviction that the procedure was too risky for adults, which had previously led him to dissuade his niece, Friederike Sophia of Orange, from having herself inoculated.[96] Catherine was not so easily deterred from her course of action.

Just as Maria Theresa's officials had done, Catherine turned to Britain to secure a suitably skilled inoculation specialist. Yet in her case, the chosen candidate needed to be willing to travel all the way to St. Petersburg to carry out the imperial inoculations. The Russian ambassador in London eventually approached Thomas Dimsdale, the well-respected Quaker doctor from Hertfordshire, who accepted the lucrative assignment.[97] Dimsdale's first move after settling in and recovering from his journey to the Russian capital, where he arrived in late-August 1768, was to inoculate several children and teenagers to test the local conditions. The next of his candidates was the empress, who was inoculated at her palace in Tsarskoe Selo, near the capital, where she remained for the duration of her illness.[98] On her return to St. Petersburg three weeks later, Catherine's restored health was celebrated with thanksgiving services, though further festivities were put on hold until her son recovered from his inoculation in the first week of November. The welcome announcement of Grand-Duke Paul Petrowitz's recovery was a time of great celebration, with dedicated church services and an elaborate feast held at the court, along with the illumination of most houses in the city to mark the occasion. The recovery of the imperial pair was such an important event for the empress that she nominated the date for future annual celebrations.[99] Such regular festivities that kept inoculation before the public gaze was a way of encouraging Russians to follow the example set by their imperial leaders, which was facilitated by Catherine's establishment of inoculation centres across Russia. The first was founded near St. Petersburg in 1769, and the second in Irkutsk (Siberia) four years later, while local officials organised public inoculations in Kiev (Ukraine) and Kasan (Tatarstan).[100] As an enticement for parents to take their children to her centres for inoculation, Catherine offered a payment for each child who participated, resulting in 1,358 procedures being carried out at the St. Petersburg centre by 1780, and the far greater tally of 15,380 at Irkutsk.[101]

---

96 Gotthold L. Mamlock, "Friedrich der Grosse und die Einführung der Impfung in Berlin," *ASZ* 10 (1904): 40–1.

97 "Die Regierungs-Geschichte der Russischen Kaiserin im Jahre 1768," *FGN*, part 97 (Leipzig: Heinsius, 1769), 11.

98 Apx 2: "Die Geschichte" (1787), 173–4.

99 "Regierungs-Geschichte," 11–12.

100 Apx 2: "Die Geschichte" (1787), 174–7, 186–7.

101 "Die Geschichte," 175, 191.

The successful inoculation of the Russian empress and her son was celebrated not only in Russia but also in Northern Germany where Catherine had been raised, and where her son Paul Petrowitz held the title and ancestral lands of the Duke of Holstein-Gottorp. While Paul's links to that aristocratic lineage came primarily from Catherine's deceased husband Tsar Peter III, Catherine's mother too was a Holstein-Gottorp.[102] Paul's and Catherine's close connection with the family's ancestral homeland was cause for Paul's local retainers to celebrate the imperial inoculation success. They did so with an elaborate thanksgiving at the great lecture theatre at the University of Kiel, which was situated on Duke Paul's patrimonial lands, and Paul's local Master of the Hunt even composed the cantata performed as part of the festivities.[103] The second aria and the chorus from Peter von Bredal's obsequious cantata provide a sense of the sentiments expressed:

Aria	
Preist den Segen des Geschickes,	Praise the blessings fate has brought,
Preist die Fülle eures Glückes	Praise the fullness of your luck,
Und weiht der Freude eure Brust.	And devote the happiness in your heart.
In glücklicher Verbindung	United in good fortune,
Erfüll euch die Empfindung	Fill yourselves with feelings
Der Dankbarkeit und holder Lust.	Of thankfulness and sweet delight.
Chorus	
Lebe o Fürst! Den wir ehren!	Live, oh prince, whom we honour!
Lebe, die Wohlfahrt Russlands und	Live, to increase Russia's prosperity
Cimbriens stets zu mehren.[104]	And the good fortune of Cimbria, too.

Those celebrations highlighting the successful Russian imperial inoculations, at a time of high smallpox mortality in the Baltic lands, may have served as inspiration for several inoculations among Catherine's relatives and other elite

102 Paul's great-great-grandfather, Christian Albrecht of Holstein-Gottorp, founded the university in 1665 on his patrimonial lands: Johann Hübner, *Reales Staats-Zeitungs und Conversations-Lexicon* (Regensburg and Vienna: Baders, 1765), 568. Paul's lineage is shown in Michail Lukitschev and Reimer Witt, eds., *Die Gottorfer auf dem Weg zum Zarenthron. Russisch-Gottorfische Verbindungen im 18. Jahrhundert* (Schleswig, 1997), 194–5.

103 Peter von Bredal, *Cantate welche bey der, wegen glücklicher Wiederherstellung Sr. Kaiserl. Hoheit aus den Allerhöchstdenenselben eingeimpften Blattern, von dem Herrn Jagd-Junker von Bredal, am 14ten Jenner 1769, in dem grössern Academischen Hörsaal gehaltenen Rede, aufgeführet wurde* (Kiel: Bartsch, 1769), 1–3.

104 Bredal, 2–3.

families in the Holstein region. Ulrike Friederike, the wife of Catherine's uncle, Duke Friedrich August I of Holstein-Oldenburg, adopted a course of action that was remarkably similar to Catherine's approach: the duchess invited a highly-skilled British inoculation specialist to travel to her court to inoculate her children. The Sutton-trained Dr. Andrew Hewit, resident in The Hague, undertook the journey in 1771 and inoculated not only the duchess's children Peter Friedrich and Hedwig Elizabeth but an additional forty-or-so individuals from other elite families, who took the opportunity to capitalise on the British doctor's expertise. Duchess Ulrike assured Hewit in her letter of thanks that "all of those you inoculated in our lands are very well."[105]

Some of Hewit's other clients on that trip were at the Danish Royal court in Copenhagen, a city where confidence in inoculation had been languishing despite an optimistic start in 1754, and where smallpox had wreaked havoc in the severe epidemic of 1769.[106] The initial positive publicity in the 1750s was generated by the German-born Countess Charitas Emilie von Buchwald's action in having herself inoculated by a British specialist, Dr. Argent, with the assistance of the royal physician Johahnn Justus von Berger and the court surgeon Christian Friedrich Wohlert. That courageous act by the wife of the high-profile Foreign Minister Johann Hartwig von Bernstorff, a countryman and longstanding friend of the German-born Dr. Berger, became a focal point for attracting royal support for an expansion of inoculation.[107] Bernstorff and Berger were the prime movers in the establishment of the Royal Inoculation House in Copenhagen that opened its doors to the public in 1755. Yet a number of highly-publicised fatalities four years later among elite citizens inoculated privately, which were incorrectly blamed on the procedure, caused such a loss of public confidence that only 170 individuals had taken advantage of the service by 1766. Not even the celebrated success in 1760 of the inoculation of the crown prince, the future Christian VII, could convince the people to re-engage with inoculation.[108]

Inoculation began to attract official attention in Sweden at much the same time as in Denmark, and a woman was again at the centre of the action. She was Baroness Katarina Charlotte de Geer (Ribbing) who was officially honoured in 1756 with the issuing of a commemorative medallion for having her

---

105 Fréron, "Arrivée," 195, 199, 200 (quote).

106 Apx 2: Heinsius (1780), 134–5. In Copenhagen in 1769, 27.5 per cent of all deaths were recorded as smallpox: see the table in Peter Kübler, *Geschichte der Pocken und der Impfung* (Berlin: Hirschwald, 1901), 80.

107 Anne Eriksen, "A Case of Exemplarity: C.F. Rotböll's History of Smallpox Inoculation in Denmark-Norway, 1766," *Scandinavian Journal of History* 35 (2010): 352–3.

108 Condamine, *Histoire*, 259; Apx 2: Heinsius (1780), 134.

children inoculated. Although two other states also produced medallions to honour particular mothers for their adoption of inoculation, Katarina Charlotte stands out prominently for not only her modest profile compared to the mothers similarly celebrated – Empresses Maria Theresa of Austria and Catherine of Russia – but also for being acknowledged more than a decade earlier than her illustrious counterparts.[109] Yet inoculation never gained acceptance in Sweden beyone elite circles, despite Queen Luise Ulrike's encouragement of the introduction of the practice into schools.[110] The inoculation of the royal children by the British-trained professor David Schultz in 1769 was very likely instigated by Crown Prince Gustav, who underwent the procedure along with his wife Sophia Magdalena, his brothers Charles and Frederick, and his sixteen-year-old sister Sophia. The action was very likely inspired by the highly-publicised inoculation of the royal children's cousin, the Russian empress, and her son. Gustav continued to support inoculation after succeeding his father in 1771, by establishing a public inoculation facility in Stockholm (1774) and issuing a regulation requiring the *Collegia medica* to promote inoculation while ensuring that the contagion would be contained.[111]

The orphaned teenage Holstein-Gottorp princes Peter Friedrich and Wilhelm August were among the other cousins of Empress Catherine II inoculated in the late-1760s. At that time, the princes were under Catherine's guardianship being escorted by their tutor Carl Friedrich von Staal on an eight-year (1765–73) educational tour that took them from Eutin in northern Germany through to Switzerland and Italy, eventually ending up in St. Petersburg.[112] A smallpox outbreak while they were being hosted by Count Heinrich XI of Obergreiz, who had five teenage children to entertain them, led to the visiting princes being inoculated by the count's *Leibarzt* Johann Gottlob Sturm, an experienced practitioner described by Thomas Dimsdale as one of the "busy" inoculators in the region.[113]

---

109 Heinsius, 131–2. Queen Ulrike was a sister of King Friedrich II (the Great) of Prussia: *Brandenburgs Kurfürsten, Preussens Könige, Deutsche Kaiser* (Karwe: Edition Rieger, 2005), 35.

110 Peter Skold, "From Inoculation to Vaccination: Smallpox in Sweden in the Eighteenth and Nineteenth Centuries," *Population Studies* 50 (1996): 249–51.

111 Ludwig von Hess, *Freymüthige Gedanken über Staatssachen* (Hamburg: Bode, 1775), 50; Apx 2: Heinsius (1780), 133. The children's father, King Adolf Frederick, was an uncle of Empress Catherine II of Russia: Lukitschev and Witt, *Gottorfer*, 194–5. The new king was Gustav III.

112 *The Annual Register, or a View of History, Politicks, and Literature, for the Year 1768* (London: Dodsley, 1768), 138; Joachim Rees et al., "Reisen im Erfahrungsraum Europa. Forschungsperspektiven zur Reisetätigkeit politisch-sozialer Eliten des Alten Reichs (1750–1800)," *Das achtzehnte Jahrhundert* 26, part 1 (2002): 59, n. 69.

113 Apx 2: Weinland (1770), 139; Dimsdale (1768), ix.

The well-known inoculation promoter from Halle, Professor Johann Christian Wilhelm Juncker, and the Mayor of Königsberg, Theodor Gottlieb von Hippel, both acknowledged the Austrian and Russian Empresses as the highest-ranking European mothers to not only have to their own children inoculated but also to extend the benefits to the people. As well as giving credit to the empresses for their contribution to fostering a positive attitude to inoculation, those eminent men praised the many other high-profile women who took leadership roles in not only inoculation but also in the betterment of society more generally.[114]

3 Successive Prussian Kings' Strategies

The Prussian kings who held the reins of power successively during the second half of the eighteenth century all acknowledged that prophylaxis was the only way to reduce the smallpox suffering and deaths. The first of those kings, Friedrich II (the Great), was inclined to follow the French *philosophes'* embrace of inoculation as a humanitarian ideal, though he was also mindful of the economic benefits of reducing the deleterious impacts of smallpox.[115] The king responded to the Magdeburg *Stadtphysikus* Johann Daniel Kessler's report in December 1755, alerting him to the successful inoculation of six children, with a recommendation that Kessler be congratulated and encouraged. He also asked his officials why doctors with responsibilities at Berlin orphanages and poor-houses were not inoculating the children, considering the newspaper reports of inoculations being carried out in such institutions elsewhere.[116]

The Berlin churchman and pioneer of public health policymaking, Johann Peter Süßmilch, shared the king's enthusiasm for inoculation. After calculating from the published London mortality rolls for the 1728–57 period that smallpox caused one-twelfth of all deaths in the city, and comparing that figure to his approximation of one in three hundred deaths from inoculation, he wrote: "should one not make use of this great benefit … out of love for humankind, for oneself, and for the fatherland?" He went on to recommend that rulers try to bring inoculation into common use, highlighting the moral rectitude of a

114 Johann C.W. Juncker, *Gemeinnützige Vorschläge und Nachrichten über das beste verhalten der Menschen in Rücksicht der Pockenkrankheit. Erster Versuch, für die mittlern Stände, nebst einem Anhange für Aerzte* (Halle, 1792), 138; Theodor G. von Hippel, *Über die bürgerliche Verbesserung der Weiber* (Berlin: Voß, 1792), 62.

115 Apx 2: de Redern (1765), 81–2.

116 Gustav Behrend, "Ueber Variolation," *DMW* 20 (1896): 309. Friedrich II was born in 1712 and reigned from 1740–86.

parent avoiding the greater danger to their children by choosing a lesser one.[117] Yet Süßmilch's faith in inoculation was not widely shared in Berlin. His attempt in 1756 to have twenty-four orphans inoculated was thwarted somewhere in the orphanage's chain of responsibility involving a board of governors, a medical director, and doctors. He was inclined to blame anti-inoculation prejudices among medical men and the public for the blocking of such initiatives.[118] Nor were the king's efforts to introduce inoculation to Berlin orphanages in that year any more successful, though he managed to overcome the resistance at the Charité Hospital by bringing in the well-respected army doctor Ludolff to do his bidding. Count Sigismund de Redern, a royal official in Berlin, even suggested (1758) that if the king were not engaged in a war involving all of Europe, he "would have already proposed a law obliging Prussians to have their children inoculated at a suitable age."[119]

After the Seven Years War Friedrich made moves to encourage inoculation in Silesia, where three wars during 1740–63 had caused a considerable loss of population.[120] His order in 1765 for the Breslau Medical Board to ensure that inoculation commenced in local hospitals apparently provided sufficient encouragement for it to be reiterated three years later for the town of Thorn. More directives in 1770 required all doctors in Breslau to promote inoculation and to report their inoculations immediately, or incur a fine, and all children of soldiers and the poor to be inoculated at public expense with their parents' or guardians' permission. Another new regulation required officials to take the inoculated children from house to house when they were no longer infectious but still bore signs of recent smallpox, as a way of demonstrating the success of their 'cure,' in order to boost the collection of funds for further free inoculations. Magistrates, for their part, were to ensure that church services were held to give thanks for the successful inoculations, so that pastors and priests would have an opportunity to discuss the matter with their parishioners, and could work toward overcoming the common religiously-based prejudices against the practice.[121] To facilitate such discussions, the Breslau Medical Board recommended that the clergymen be given the sermon preached in 1768

117 Süßmilch, *Ordnung*, 2:417, 440 (quote) –43.
118 Süßmilch, 1:533–4.
119 Apx 2: de Redern (1765), 81–2, 87.
120 "Circulare wegen Einführung der Blatter-Inoculation," *Sammlung aller Ordnungen, Edicte, Mandate, Rescripte, etc. der Regierung Friedrichs II*, vol. 12 (Breslau: Korn, 1770), 47–54.
121 Karl F.W.A. Vater, *Preussisch-Schlesische Civil Medicinal- and Sanitäts-Verfassung*, part 2 (Breslau: Korn, 1800), 540–3.

by the Saxon prelate Gotthilf Friedemann Löber, which was an overt inoculation promotion.[122]

In Berlin, inoculation rates were increasing steadily among the elite until a number of fatalities in 1765 brought the practice to an abrupt halt. The deaths of six of nine children inoculated in a brief period by the royal court physician, Friedrich Hermann Muzell, and by Professor Johann Friedrich Meckel from the University of Frankfurt (Oder) not only shattered public confidence in inoculation but also alerted the king to the urgent need for improvements in the procedures used by Prussian medical men.[123] The severe 1766–67 smallpox epidemic that caused one in six of all deaths in Berlin, including the king's favourite nephew, Heinrich, was the apparent catalyst for Friedrich to initiate his plan to bring state-of-the-art inoculation practice to Prussia. His awareness of the Suttons's pre-eminence led him to ask his ambassador in England, Count Joachim Karl von Maltzan, to arrange for two doctors trained by the Suttons to come to Berlin to teach their exemplary technique to Prussian medical men.[124] Yet, when the unnamed doctors arrived in late-1767 and the matter of remuneration was discussed, he sent them away.[125] As he explained to Maltzan: "they requested 32 thaler of our money for each infant inoculated, which would mean that for 300 children … they would take 9,000 thaler to England."[126] Such an outflow of currency at that time would effectively contradict his order to his General Directorate to try to attract money from abroad to help the struggling Prussian economy recover from the costly war.[127] By then, the urgency for inoculation had diminished anyway, with the waning of smallpox.[128]

A new opportunity to improve inoculation standards in Prussia presented itself when William Baylies (Figure 6) visited Berlin in 1774. The Dresden-based former 'travelling inoculator' was invited to the city by Julius August von der Horst, a government minister whose enthusiasm for inoculation had withstood the loss of two children to Meckel's ill-fated inoculations in 1765.[129]

---

122 "Circulare," 52–3.

123 La Condamine, *Histoire*, 265–6; Apx 2: Baylies (1776), 4–6.

124 Mamlock, "Einführung," 39–40. See Kübler, *Geschichte*, 88, for the mortality rates.

125 The unnamed Sutton-trained doctors were undoubtedly Andrew Hewit and Alexander Sutherland, who were granted permission to inoculate in The Hague after leaving the Prussian Royal Court in Berlin: "Inoculation," 322.

126 Cited in Mamlock, "Einführung," 40. The exemplary Scottish doctor inoculating in the Königsberg region in the early-1770s, George Motherby, charged 6 ducats (17 thaler) per person for a group inoculation and undoubtedly much more for private clients: Ebstein, "Motherby," 37.

127 Theodor Schieder, *Frederick the Great*, trans. and eds. Hamish M. Scott and Sabina Berkeley (London and New York: Longman, 2000), 192.

128 See the mortality table in Kübler, *Geschichte*, 88.

129 La Condamine, *Histoire*, 266.

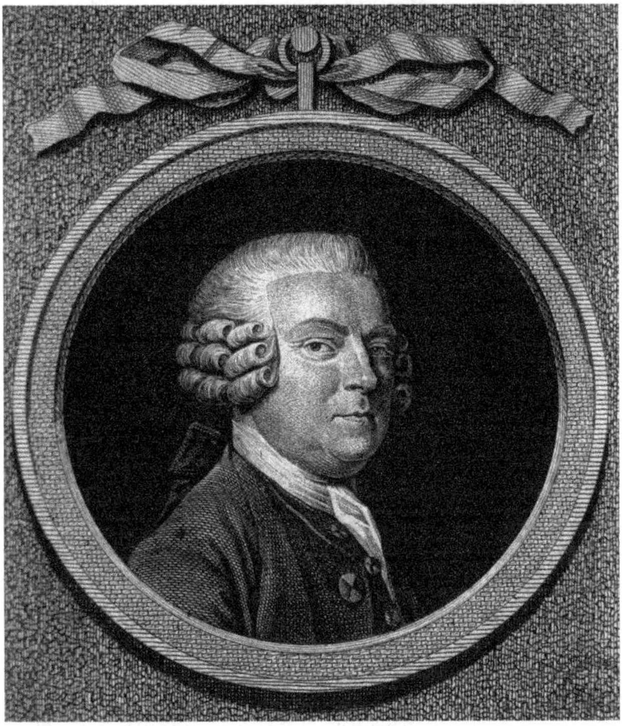

FIGURE 6
William Baylies.
Engraving by D. Berger
after J.H. Schmid
U.S. NATIONAL LIBRARY
OF MEDICINE: B02526

Impressed by friends' reports of Baylies's expertise, the minister hoped that the English doctor's visit would enable not only his own daughter and niece to be inoculated safely but also the children of several elite acquaintances who were keen to take advantage of the opportunity.[130] Yet high-ranking opponents of inoculation in the Berlin medical establishment had other ideas. Determined to thwart any expansion of inoculation in the city, they arranged for Count von Reuß, the secretary of the Prussian *Ober-collegium medicum,* to send Baylies a letter informing him of the need for 'foreigners' to obtain the king's permission to inoculate. They were probably also responsible for an article in a Leipzig newspaper arguing that inoculation was clearly unnecessary because smallpox was not a fatal illness, as 'proven' by the survival of a group of cadets who came through the disease in a Berlin garrison. Those influential doctors also spread rumours of Baylies having a poor inoculation record, and criticised his practice of allowing inoculated children out in the fresh winter air, which they claimed would force the smallpox back into the blood and leave the children susceptible to future smallpox.[131] Since Baylies used the same recuperation approach

130 Apx 2: Baylies (1776), 10–11.
131 Baylies, 12–14.

as the Suttons, his opponents were pointedly taking sides in the widespread medical debate about the Suttons's innovative procedures.[132]

The tactics aimed at discrediting Baylies failed to deter the king from granting him permission to inoculate. Indeed, Friedrich was so impressed with Baylies that he offered him an eventual pension were he to move his medical practice to Berlin, which Baylies gratefully accepted.[133] Having finally secured an English doctor with extensive inoculation experience, Friedrich reinvigorated his plan to have Prussian medical men taught a state-of-the-art British inoculation technique. He invited fourteen provincial doctors as well as local medical men and regimental surgeons to an inoculation demonstration by Baylies scheduled for March 1775.[134] Yet the value of that exercise was compromised by the unpopularity of inoculation in Berlin, and by Friedrich's apparent failure to communicate what he actually wanted Baylies to demonstrate. The first problem encountered was Baylies's inability to convince parents to permit their children to be inoculated, even by an expert offering payment. During the nine-day delay while other children were found, Dr. Friedrich Christian Opitz from Minden requested the king's permission to return home to attend to his affairs, as did some other provincial invitees unable to afford the extra time. Opitz had little to learn from Baylies's demonstration anyway, having already published a book describing his own inoculations using Angelo Gatti's simplified method.[135]

The king's intervention to secure permission for the inoculation of children at the Friedrichs Orphanage eventually enabled the demonstration to proceed. Having selected a group of children showing no signs of previous smallpox, Baylies prepared to inoculate them using "threads impregnated with fresh smallpox material from the London Smallpox Hospital," which he had received by post. He describes laying "small portions of the previously mentioned threads …, moistened, in two different shallow incisions in each arm of each child."[136] Yet that method bore little resemblance to the state-of-the-art procedure so admired by the king. The incision-and-thread approach was not only much more dangerous than the Suttons's mere prick of the skin with a lancet dipped in fresh smallpox pus, but was also more prone to failure. Incisions were regarded as one of the greatest hazards of inoculation because they

132 Apx 2: Körber (1769), 74.

133 Apx 2: Baylies (1776), 14. Johann D.E. Preuss, *Friedrich der Grosse, eine Lebensgeschichte* (Berlin: Nauck, 1833), 292.

134 Apx 2: Baylies (1776), 122–4; de Villiers (1776), 57–8.

135 Baylies, 124; Gotthold L. Mamlock, *Friedrichs des Grossen Korrespondenz mit Aerzten* (Wiesbaden: Sändig, 1966), 109–11; Apx 2: Opitz (1774), 43.

136 Baylies, 127–8; Apx 2: de Villiers (1776), 58–64.

tended to heal slowly and to become infected, sometimes causing fatal ulcers.[137] Inactive threads were a common problem with that method too, as Professor Triller pointed out:

Die Fäden sind vielleicht, zu trocken, dürr, und alt,	Maybe the threads are too degraded, old, and dry,
Daher verlieren sie die kräftige Gewalt,	That is why they lose the power that's required,
Wenn man sie eingelegt, die Pocken zu erregen;	To bring about the smallpox symptoms when they are inserted:
Ein längst verrauchtes Gift hat weiter kein Vermögen:	A long-degraded poison has no likelihood to work:
Wie man es denn schon oft, drey biß viermahl, versucht,	Even when such threads are placed three times and sometimes four,
Und Fäden eingelegt: jedennoch ohne Frucht.[138]	As has happened oft,' no smallpox was endured

Triller could well have been presaging the outcome of Baylies's demonstration. All twelve orphans failed to develop smallpox after either one inoculation or a repeat with smallpox-impregnated threads from second batch. Suspecting that his threads were at fault, Baylies appealed successfully to the Berlin president to find a donor of fresh smallpox material.[139] Yet his demonstration of an inoculation procedure using the fresh material failed to produce smallpox in nineteen children, seven of whom he had not previously inoculated. Baylies finally concluded that the "various children must have all had smallpox before, in the natural way."[140] His chances of success would undoubtedly have been better if the orphanage had not limited the children available for inoculation to those over the age of four.[141] Even though Baylies chose children showing no signs of previous smallpox, all but one was old enough to have lived through all three of the smallpox epidemics that swept through Berlin in 1765–67, 1770, and 1773.[142] Baylies's failure to consider much earlier in the proceedings that

---

137 Angelo Gatti, *Nouvelles réflexions sur la practique de l'inoculation* (Brussels: Musier, 1767), 73–8; Apx 2: Schröter (1773), 21–3.

138 Apx 2: Triller (1766), 23.

139 Apx 2: Baylies (1776), 129–31.

140 Baylies, 132, 133–4 (quote).

141 Baylies, 125. The children's ages ranged between 8 and 16: de Villiers, *Handschrift*, 59.

142 See Kübler, *Geschichte*, 88, for a table of annual smallpox mortality in Berlin during the 1760s–70s.

the children were likely to be immune is indicative of the general confusion at the time about causes of failed inoculations.[143]

Dr. Johann Christian Meier, a witness to Baylies's second demonstration, posed the question: "whose fault is it that inoculation is not more prevalent in the Prussian lands?" In his view, the failure of the initiative of "the great Friedrich, the father of his folk" to "save many lives through inoculation" was due to the prominent publicity given to an unnamed, highly-respected Berlin doctor's assertions "that smallpox was not so deadly; that it is a matter of the treatment; that no smallpox patient entrusted to his care had died during his rather long practice, … and that inoculation should not be permitted."[144] To a public with a longstanding dislike of the practice, the mere suggestion that inoculation was unnecessary was not only readily accepted but also heartily welcomed. Friedrich nonetheless continued his efforts to improve the inoculation skills of Prussian medical men; the new regulations he issued in 1776 required all *Physiki* practising inoculation to pass an examination on the procedure or incur a fine of two *Reichsthaler*, and all private practitioners to follow a set of rules governing inoculation, which were yet to be formulated.[145] That those rules failed to appear before the end of Friedrich's reign but were issued by his successor in 1789 underscores the enduring influence of the high-ranking opponents of inoculation in Friedrich II's *Ober-collegium medicum* and in the Berlin medical establishment more generally.[146]

The Prussian Medical Board appointed by the incoming King Friedrich Wilhelm II (r. 1786–97) attempted to encourage inoculation while preventing the spread of smallpox, which was quite a change from the obstructionist approach adopted by the previous Board. The new king, like his uncle Friedrich II, was a strong supporter of inoculation, and was well-aware of the importance of high-level examples and positive publicity in encouraging emulation.[147] He ensured that the Prussian people were made aware of his utmost confidence in the practice by having four of his children inoculated (1789) and requiring all churches across the vast extent of Prussia to hold thanksgiving services

143 Apx 2: Gardane (1775), xi–xii; Klärich (1778), 219–220.

144 Johann C.W. Juncker, *Archiv der Aerzte und Seelsorger wider die Pockkenoth*, vol. 5 (Leipzig: Weygand, 1798), 93–4.

145 Vater, *Verfassung*, 2:544–5. *Physiki* were government-appointed doctors.

146 Vater, 2:545; Ernst L. Heim, "Ueber die Diagnostik der falschen Pokken mit Hinsicht auf die neuerlich behaupteten Fälle von echten Pokken nach vorhergegangener gelungener Vaccination," *Archiv für medizinische Erfahrung* 2 (1809): 186.

147 Apx 2: Schwager, "Diesmalige" (1790), 26–9.

celebrating the successful 'event.' The Berlin Synagogue joined the celebrations too.[148]

While churchgoers in the larger centres were likely to have known about inoculation beforehand, the many country-folk who had never encountered the procedure must have been wondering what the service was all about.[149] They were left in no doubt that the royal children's survival from inoculated smallpox was the focus of attention, after being regaled with the new hymn "The Joy of the Patriots" composed especially for the occasion by a royal official, Joseph Aloysius Mercy. The nine verses highlight the deadly toll from smallpox, the importance to Prussia of protecting the young princes by having them inoculated, and the king's far-sightedness in encouraging inoculation among the broader population. The following two verses illustrate the general tone of the work:

Du bist nun unser, Friedrich, Bewunderer	You are now ours, oh Friedrich, fond admirer
Des großen Oheims! unser aufs neue seyd	Of your great-uncle! Also ours are you,
Ihr, Ludwig, Heinrich, Wilhelm, alle	Oh Ludwig, Heinrich, Wilhelm, all
Künftige Helden und Menschenfreunde.	Future heroes and friends of mankind.
Triumph, Triumph, sie leben! und Tausenden	Rejoice, rejoice, they live! And Friedrich Wilhelm
Wird Friedrich Wilhelm's Weisheit Errettung seyn,	Will save thousands more through his wise action,
Die, furchtsam ohne kühnes Beyspiel,	Without bold examples, the fearful ones
Früher dem Schicksal erliegen würden.[150]	Would succumb to their fate so much sooner.

Ludwig von Baczko, the Königsberg historian whose sight was destroyed by smallpox as a teenager when he was about to embark on a naval career, joined

148 Review of "Deutsche Monatsschrift," *ALZ*, no. 182 (1790): 734; Napthali H. Wessely, *Dankfeyer auf die Genesung der Königlichen Kinder, nach glücklich erfolgter Blattern-Einimpfung: gehalten in der Synagoge der Judenschaft zu Berlin, am Sabat-Abend 18 Dezember, 1789* (Berlin, 1790).

149 Juncker, *Archiv*, 3:136; 5:120.

150 Joseph A. Mercy, "Freude des Patrioten. Ein Hymnus gesungen im Neujahr, 1790," *DMS* 1 (1790): 105–6.

the rejoicing with his poem acknowledging God as the arbiter of his own and the royal children's very different smallpox experiences:

Er, der mit Freuden seine Schöpfung füllt:	God, who fills his creatures with joy:
er hies dem Uebel mich zu Boden drücken,	he meant the evil to cast me down,
hies ihm die theuren Prinzen fliehn,	he meant it to flee from the valuable princes,
und ließ für Sie, um Völker zu beglücken,	and, in order to make the folk happy,
die Fülle der Genesung blühn …	he let them bloom, completely recovered …
Jauchzt, Völker, jauchzt zu Gott, dem Freudengeber,	Cheer, you people, cheer God who brings joy,
der die Genesung unsern Prinzen gab.[151]	who ensured that our princes recovered.

Baczko's suggestion that his blindness was a sign of God's disapproval, and that the royal children's recovery signalled God's approval of inoculation was an approach with the potential to break down the enduring religiously-based doubts about inoculation.[152] Increased demand for inoculation in Prussia in the wake of the royal example was indeed noted by Dr. Elias Henschel from Breslau and by Pastor Johann Moritz Schwager from Joellenbeck.[153] By 1796 inoculation was even gaining increasing acceptance in Berlin, according to the king's *Leibarzt* Ludwig Formey, which marked quite a shift in sentiment since the 1780s when opposition was still widespread in the city.[154] Renewed confidence in inoculation among medical men and the public may reflect a willingness of a younger generation of doctors and parents in Berlin to accept the simpler, safer inoculation procedures during periods of high smallpox mortality such as 1789–90, 1792, and 1795.[155] On the other hand, concerns were

151 Apx 2: Baczko (1791), 436–7.

152 Apx 2: Bail (1796), 219–28.

153 Apx 2: Henschel (1795), 24; Schwager, "Inoculationsgeschichte" (1790), 27–8.

154 Ludwig Formey, *Versuch einer medicinischen Topographie von Berlin* (Berlin: Felisch, 1796), 165; Fritze, "Eine Blatterimpfung," *Neues Magazin für Aerzte* 9 (1787): 213; Heim, "Diagnostik," 186.

155 See Kübler, *Geschichte*, 91, for smallpox mortality tables for 1782–1800.

growing about the contagiousness of inoculation, and *Leibarzt* Formey was among the critics blaming inoculation for spreading smallpox.[156]

4 The Rural Nobility

By the 1790s inoculation had become commonplace among the German aristocracy and nobility, and was increasingly being adopted by the rural landowning class to protect their future work-force from smallpox.[157] While encouragement at the highest level came through publicity such as the statewide thanksgiving services for the Prussian royal children's recovery in 1789, such occasions when evidence of the benefits filtered from the prince to the public were quite rare.[158] As inoculation spread into rural Prussia in the late 1780s-90s, some regional noblewomen showed an ability to deliver positive messages using a personal touch and degree of subtlety that no prince could achieve ensconced in his capital.

One such instance was the Dowager Countess von Dohna's celebration in 1799 of the inoculation of her son's new bride Amalie von Kospoth. The festivities began with all ninety-seven children from the Malmitz village school, dressed in their best and adorned with flowers, parading from the school to the dowager countess's palace led by their teachers, and accompanied by musicians from the palace orchestra. Once assembled in the gardens before an audience of hundreds, the children performed a song, followed by eighteen of their number delivering formal expressions of delight at the successful inoculation of Count Fabian's new bride, and offering the couple their best wishes. While the adults stayed at the manor to participate in an annual festival, after cake was served, the children returned to the school where the dowager countess marked the festive occasion with a donation of a library of books.[159] The children were reminded that the honourable lady was "a concerned mother who very much took care of the welfare of the schools under her authority." The dowager countess was also known for providing money for the schooling of every child from a poor family, as well as free books to those who needed them.[160] At the end of that day, neither the children participating in the celebration nor

156 Formey, "Versuch," 168–71.

157 Juncker, *Archiv*, 4:13–14; Apx 2: "Nachricht" (1791), 515–6.

158 Review of "Deutsche Monatsschrift," 731–4.

159 Weinhold, "Schul Feierlichkeit," *SP* 30 (1799): 456–7.

160 Weinhold, 457–8 (quote), 459.

the attendees at the annual festival at the von Dohna palace, held afterwards, could have failed to hear about the inoculation of the incoming countess.

The novelist Augusta von Goldstein (von Wallenrodt) was another inoculation promoter belonging to the minor nobility from the Breslau region of Prussia. She delivered her 'messages' about smallpox and inoculation in her writing, particularly in her romantic novel *Das Mädchen Wunderhold* (The Wonderfully Charming Girl), which she published anonymously, presumably to counter the societal disapproval of women participating in the literary milieu.[161] The goings-on among the landed nobility, at the heart of her novel, were familiar territory for Goldstein who had spent years working as a tutor-governess to a noble family in Neumark (Brandenburg).[162] Her depiction of the inoculation activities of the household physicians at a fictional count's country-palace suggests that the German nobility was very familiar with the procedure. Indeed, the physicians in her story hold inoculation in such high regard that they set up an isolated house in the palace grounds where they prepare to inoculate and care for the young house-guests arriving for the spring festivities. As a reminder of the simplicity of inoculation, and to reinforce her 'message' about the contagiousness of inoculated smallpox and the need for its containment, Goldstein creates a drama surrounding the inoculation of a fictional foreign prince and his sister. While the inoculated pair were recovering, another guest almost dies from smallpox after visiting them in their isolated abode, confident that he was immune to smallpox after having a mild bout during childhood.[163] This episode was an implicit warning of not only the danger of smallpox transmitted from inoculated individuals but also of presuming that a mild pustular disease in childhood was actually smallpox. Perhaps the most high-profile case of mistaken assumption of immunity to the disease was the agonising demise of the French king Louis XV from smallpox in 1774, after believing throughout his life that he had the disease in his youth.[164]

Other noblewomen in regional Prussia involved themselves in inoculation 'hands-on,' in various ways. The local government official from Madlitz (Brandenburg), Countess Ernestina Carolina Finck von Finckenstein, was so familiar with inoculation after seeing Professors Kölpin and Berends from the

161 W. Daniel Wilson, "Eighteenth-century Germany in its Historical Context," in *German Literature of the Eighteenth Century: The Enlightenment and Sensibility*, ed. Barbara Becker-Cantarino (Rochester: Camden House, 2005), 278.

162 Karl G. Nowak, *Schlesisches Schriftsteller-Lexicon*, part 5 (Breslau: Korn, 1841), 50–1.

163 Augusta F. von Goldstein, *Das Mädchen Wunderhold. Eine abendländische Romanesk in neuern Styl* (Leipzig, 1810), 99–100, 108–9.

164 Voltaire, *Collection Complette des Oeuvres de M. Voltaire*, vol. 27, *Histoire du Parlement de Louis XV, Fragmens* (Geneva, 1776), 285.

University of Frankfurt (Oder) inoculate seven of her children, that she inoculated her youngest daughter in 1788 without any assistance. More notable was her offer of her expertise to the locals, resulting in her successful inoculation during 1789–96 of seven children of the parents who accepted her offer: a tailor, a coachman, and a rural landlord. Another remarkable aspect of the countess's activities was the detailed ten-page report she sent to Professor Juncker in Halle describing not only her own inoculations but also those carried out on her children by various doctors.[165]

Groups of noblewomen in other parts of Prussia contributed to the spread of inoculation by volunteering to assist local peasant mothers in caring for their inoculated children. Three von Rochow and von Luck ladies and their friend, Fräuelin von Stechow, volunteered to assist in the inoculation of thirty-four peasant children in 1797 at Nennhausen, near Rathenow. While three of the ladies met daily with the peasant mothers to ascertain the progress of the children's recovery, which they reported to the inoculator *Stadtphysikus* Johann Christian Meier, another of the ladies joined Pastor Lympius and the doctor in making regular visits to ensure that the recovering children received appropriate care.[166] Another group of noblewomen offered a similar kind of support for a much larger initiative involving 114 peasant children scattered across the towns and villages of an estate near Züllichau. Following the inoculation of the children in 1799 by Dr. Christian Samuel Ungnad, four von Riedesel ladies and four von Reuß sisters provided the mothers and their inoculated children with three daily meals from their own manor kitchens, as well as taking care of the laundry and helping Pastor Poeler and his wife make notes on the children's progress for a report to the doctor.[167]

The collective contribution of the Prussian rural noblewomen to the promotion of inoculation in their localities, particularly the ladies who provided their personal assistance to the peasants, highlights the sense of community goodwill engendered by the compassionate actions of those generous ladies. Such co-operation between the landowning nobility and the peasants involved

165 Juncker, *Archiv*, 5:110–17.

166 "Nachricht von der Pockeninokulation zu Nennhausen bei Rathenow," *Jahrbücher der preußischen Monarchie unter der Regierung Friedrich Wilhelms des Dritten*, vol. 2 (Berlin: Unger, 1798), 97–9. Caroline von Rochow (born von Briest), Friedrike and Karoline von Luck, and Fräulein von Stechow were the ladies named.

167 Christian S. Ungnad, "Nachricht von einer zahlreichen Blatter-Impfung auf dem Lande," *Jahrbücher der preußischen Monarchie unter der Regierung Friedrich Wilhelms des Dritten* (1800), 3:306–8. Lieutenant General von Riedesel's widow Friederike (born von Massow), her three then unmarried daughters: Friederike, Caroline, and Amerika von Riedesel, and Friederike's married daughter Countess Gustava von Reuß were the ladies named.

in those inoculation 'events' shows that not all rural estates at the time conformed to the stereotype of dissonant social-class relationships. The efforts of the pastors and their wives deserve acknowledgement too, as just one example of the contribution of the vast cohort of rural pastoral couples to the well-being of the peasant population.

Not many years after those group inoculations in rural Prussia, inoculation gave way to cowpox vaccination. Friedrich Wilhelm II's successor, his son Friedrich Wilhelm III (r. 1797–1840), was among the first of the European leaders to have his children vaccinated, and he established the Royal Prussian Vaccination Institute at much the same time (1802).[168] The king encouraged the public to adopt vaccination, by means of publicity campaigns and offers of free vaccination for the poor rather than by implementing compulsory vaccination for all individuals who had not experienced smallpox, as some other territorial governments chose to do. In the long run, his softer approach of enforcing vaccination only for the people in the vicinity of a smallpox outbreak seems to have been just as effective as the general compulsory vaccination implemented in other territories.[169]

168 Michael J. Bennett, *War Against Smallpox. Edward Jenner and the Early Global Spread of Vaccination* (Cambridge: Cambridge University Press, 2020), 187.

169 Claudia Huerkamp, "The History of Smallpox Vaccination in Germany: a First Step in the Medicalization of the General Public," *JCH* 20 (1985): 622–5.

CHAPTER 3

Academics and Medical Men

Professors at German university medical schools were among the first Europeans to take a serious look at inoculation as a means of ameliorating smallpox.[1] Quite unconnected to that 1720s scholarship was the flurry of actual inoculation practice in Germany, which was prompted largely by curiosity about inoculation among princes and their physicians.[2] Those streams of theoretical and practical interest merged during the second half of the eighteenth century when the professors themselves became inoculation practitioners, and were in some cases appointed as *Leibärzte* while continuing their academic pursuits.[3] Most medical school professors were enthusiastic about the new age of disease prevention promised by inoculation, and all were keen to see the end of smallpox. By teaching inoculation procedures to their students, certain professors helped to expand the number of practitioners with the skills and confidence to offer inoculation to their clients with a reasonable chance of success. Yet the public needed to be convinced of the safety and efficacy of inoculation, which had gained a bad reputation in some circles through the harmful effects of poor technique.[4] By the 1790s, when it was widely acknowledged that inoculation was too contagious to prevent smallpox on a wide scale, medical men were nonetheless grateful for having the tool, imperfect though it was, which could at least ameliorate the worst impacts of the disease in individuals while the contagion could be contained through the use of suitable isolation measures.[5]

Doctors shared the business of inoculation with surgeons, the only other 'healers' authorised to inoculate in Germany.[6] Yet competition between the two

---

1 Almost one-fifth of the 41 inoculation-related dissertations published by German universities in the eighteenth century were produced during 1720–29 (Apx 1).

2 Johann T. Eller, *Observationes de cognoscendis et curandis morbis, praesertim acutis* (Königsberg and Leipzig: Woltersdorff, 1762), 151–3; Apx 2: Wreden (1723, 1724); "Methode" (1726); Seip (1727).

3 Johann C. Stark, "Widererklärung," *Intelligenzblatt der* ALZ, no. 89 (1795): 712; Apx 2: Weinland (1770), 138, 140.

4 Johann C.W. Juncker, *Archiv der Aerzte und Seelsorger wider die Pockennoth,* vol. 5 (Leipzig: Weygand, 1798), 213; Apx 2: Migula, "Noch etwas" (1787), 422–3; Thebesius (1788), 126–7.

5 Ernst B.J. Hebenstreit, *Lehrsätze der medicinischen Policeywissenschaft* (Leipzig: Dyk, 1791), 178–9; Johann C. Scherf, *Archiv der medizinischen Polizey und die gemeinnützigen Arzneikunde*, vol. 2 (Leipzig: Weygand, 1783), 239–42.

6 Midwives, bath-masters, and apothecaries were classified as 'healers' too, but were not permitted to inoculate: Moritz Pistor, "Geschichte der preussischen Medizinalverwaltung," DVG 40 (1908): 780–1.

 | DOI:10.1163/9789004465374_005

groups was minimal, since the elite tended to gravitate toward doctors while the less affluent preferred surgeons. The social discrepancy was rooted in the doctors' social ranking as part of the university-educated class, whereas barber-surgeons were classified as craftsmen by virtue of their training through an apprenticeship under the auspices of the craft guilds. The longstanding public perception of surgeons' social inferiority extended to those emerging from the highly-regarded medical-surgical academies that were increasing in number at the end of the eighteenth century. Even though the graduate surgeons were equipped with a high-standard medical education as well as superior surgical skills, the notion of surgeons' social inferiority was perpetuated with the help of the doctors who feared the growing competition.[7]

The social ranking of doctors, in their turn, was regarded as lower than that of the wealthy townsfolk and minor nobility who were their usual clients, placing the doctors under considerable pressure to display correct manners.[8] The prospect of inoculating healthy upper-class children with potentially deadly smallpox added to the stress, though the usually generous remuneration and the boost that successful outcomes would bring to a doctor's career prospects tended to make the anxiety worthwhile. In the last decades of the eighteenth century when aristocratic and elite parents were increasingly having their children inoculated, a doctor known for his skill in carrying out the procedure could even aspire to an appointment as a physician at one of the many princely courts, or to a much higher rung of the career-ladder as *Leibarzt* to a prince.[9]

1 University Medical Schools

Professors at university medical schools, particularly those at the larger schools, were well-placed to influence the spread of inoculation through their teaching and encouragement, if the prince sponsoring the university was of

7 Sabine Sander, *Handwerkschirurgen: Sozialgeschichte einer verdrängten Berufsgruppe* (Göttingen: Vandenhoek & Ruprecht, 1989), 57–9, 134; Thomas Broman, "Rethinking Professionalization: Theory, Practice, and Professional Ideology in Eighteenth-Century German Medicine," *Journal of Modern History* 67 (1995): 849, 863–4.

8 Ute Frevert, *Krankheit als politisches Problem 1770–1880. Soziale Unterschichten in Preußen zwischen medizinischer Polizei und staatlicher Sozialversicherung* (Göttingen: Vandenhoek & Ruprecht, 1984), 41–2; Claudia Huerkamp, "The History of Smallpox Vaccination in Germany: a First Step in the Medicalization of the General Public," *JCH* 20 (1985): 621.

9 Moritz G. Thilenius, *Medicinische und chirurgische Bemerkungen*, 3rd ed. (Frankfurt am Main: Brönner, 1814), xx-ii; Samuel-Auguste D. Tissot, *Leben des Ritters von Zimmermann, Hofrath und Leibarztes zu Hannover* (Hannover: Hahn, 1797), 143.

the same mind. Inoculation was well supported at the University of Halle, which housed the largest of the three university medical schools in Prussia.[10] The first inoculation-related doctoral dissertation from Halle (1760) was by Friedrich Ludwig Kessler who later became a well-known practitioner like his father Johann Daniel Kessler, the Magdeburg *Stadtphysikus* congratulated in 1756 by the Prussian king for his pioneering inoculation activities.[11] A student two years ahead of Kessler was an enthusiast too:

> I was embarking on my practical training in 1758 when some of the best publications about inoculation appeared, describing with inspirational fire the overwhelming advantages of it … As a young doctor I was burning with enthusiasm to use this advantageous method, and keenly awaited the first smallpox epidemic in order to collect the material for storage.[12]

The former student who wrote those reminiscences in 1788, Adam Samuel Thebesius, was supervised in his doctoral studies by Professor Andreas Elias Büchner, an inoculation promoter likely to have directed his students toward the publications that Thebesius found so compelling. By then, inoculation had been described and discussed in a plethora of books and articles.[13] Professor Büchner made his own significant contribution with four articles (1762 and 1766) aimed toward educating the public about inoculation, as well as a dissertation (1766). Professors Johann Peter Eberhard and Philipp Adolph Böhmer were two colleagues who followed his lead by submitting promotional articles to the local newspaper during 1768, after which interest in inoculation faded with the waning of severe smallpox.[14] When the disease returned with a vengeance in the 1780s, a new generation of Halle professors was promoting inoculation. Philipp Friedrich Meckel became a well-known inoculation practitioner, while his colleague Johann Christian Wilhelm Juncker wrote extensively about ways of dealing with smallpox, and led a smallpox eradication campaign during 1796–1800 with a core strategy of safe inoculation practices.[15]

---

10 The other Prussian medical schools in the 1760s were at the Universities of Königsberg and of Frankfurt (Oder).

11 Gustav Behrend, "Ueber Variolation," *DMW* 20 (1896): 309; Apx 1: Kessler (1760).

12 Apx 2: Thebesius (1788), 125.

13 See references listed in Apx 2.

14 Apx 1: Büchner (1766); Apx 2: Büchner (1762, 1766); Böhmer (1768). Wolfram Kaiser and Kurt Werner, "Die Anfänge der Pockenschutzimpfung in Halle und Umgebung," *ZGH* 19 (1973): 809–10.

15 Kaiser and Werner, 811.

At least three professors from the University of Leipzig (Saxony) Medical School supported inoculation too. Christian Gottlieb Ludwig and Georg Christian Reichel were well-known inoculators among the local elite during the 1760s, while Carl Christian Krause supported the practice as well.[16] Yet Leipzig professors and students published no inoculation-related dissertations at all during 1763–1800, a period when twenty-five were published collectively by eleven other German universities.[17] Perhaps positive messages about inoculation such as those delivered at Halle were drowned out at Leipzig by sceptics in the professorial ranks, of whom Ernst Platner was arguably the most influential. During his rise through the ranks from doctoral graduate in 1767, to professor in 1770, to rector of the university in the 1780s, and to dean of the medical faculty in 1796 Platner made no secret of his opposition to inoculation.[18] Such a long career offered ample opportunity to stifle inoculation progress at Leipzig for decades, as was the case at the smaller Saxon medical school at the University of Wittenberg where the staunch inoculation opponent Daniel Wilhelm Triller (see Figure 3 on p. 26) was in the professorial ranks from 1747–82. During that period the Wittenberg Medical School failed to build on its proud reputation for inoculation scholarship acquired in the 1720s through Abraham Vater, the highly-regarded anatomy professor who produced not only the first publication about inoculation from a German university (1720) but also two of the earliest books on the topic (1721 and 1723). Triller's lengthy poem about inoculation (1766), by comparison, adopted an entirely negative standpoint.[19]

Ernst Gottfried Baldinger was an inoculation advocate from the outset of his professorial career that commenced in 1768 at the University of Jena Medical School. His name became indelibly linked to inoculation through his translation (1768) of the Swiss physician Samuel-Auguste Tissot's well-known book highlighting the value of inoculation and describing the method.[20] A number of Baldinger's former-students too showed a profound interest in inoculation methods, reflecting their mentor's renowned ability to impart his enthusiasm for a topic. One of those graduates, Johann Christian Ackermann, translated Thomas Bond's description of a new inoculation method used in Philadelphia,

---

16 Apx 2: Hensler, vol. 1 (1765), 126. Apx 1: Krause (1762).

17 Dissertations listed in Apx 1.

18 Anton von Haen and Ernst Platner, *Anton von Haen's kaiserlichen Leibarztes Heilungsmethode, in dem kaiserlichen Krankenhaus zu Wien*, vol. 5 (Leipzig: Weygand, 1782), 397–434; Samuel G. Vogel, *Handbuch der practischen Arzneywissenschaft zum Gebrauche angehende Aerzte* (Vienna: Trattner, 1789), 117.

19 Apx 1: Vater (1720); Apx 2: Vater (1721 and 1723); Triller (1766). Kurt Sprengel, *Versuch einer pragmatischen Geschichte der Arzneikunde*, part 5 (Halle: Gebauer, 1803), 606.

20 Apx 2: Tissot, trans. Baldinger (1768).

which helped him to a professorial appointment at Altdorf (Bavaria). Another of Baldinger's former students, Johann Christian Scherf, included a lengthy section on inoculation in the extensive public health policy proposal he formulated during his service as a court physician of the Count of Lippe-Detmold.[21] Dr. Joseph Lenhardt had already shown an interest in inoculation during his student years at Jena, when he produced his own dissertation on the topic for his doctorate (1770) rather than taking the usual course of defending a dissertation written by a professor.[22] He subsequently gained sufficient experience as an inoculator while working as a medical practitioner in Quedlinburg (Prussia), to be confident in making pointed recommendations of certain inoculation procedures in his medical advice book (1787), while warning against others.[23]

A decade after Baldinger's departure from Jena in 1773, Professor Johann Christian Stark was teaching a new generation of students about inoculation. One of Stark's more talented students, Johann Friedrich Panzerbieter, took a particular interest in the issue of the prohibition of inoculation in smallpox-free areas, arguing in his doctoral dissertation (1782) that inoculation should be permitted as long as it were offered free to all people in the area who had not previously experienced the disease.[24] Stark not only agreed with that recommendation but took action along those lines, offering inoculation free of charge at the university's teaching clinic. Those public inoculations served the additional purpose of providing practical demonstrations of the procedure to Jena medical students.[25]

The larger medical schools were not the only ones in which professors helped to spread inoculation by imparting their knowledge and enthusiasm to their students. Several of the much smaller schools were influential in that regard too.[26] Professor Ludwig Philipp Schröter from Rinteln (Schaumburg-Lippe) and Carl Gottlieb Wagler from the Brunswick Medical College deserve particular mention as the first German professors to urge the change from

21 Apx 2: Bond (1787). 215–41. Scherf, *Archiv*, 2:215–41.

22 Apx 1: Lenhardt (1770). Arvo Tering, "The Dissertations of Doctors of Medicine Active in Estland, Livland, and Courland defended at European Universities in the Eighteenth Century," *Ajalooline Ajakiri*, 133–4 (2010): 376–7.

23 Joseph Lenhardt, *Arzneyen ohne Maske* (Leipzig, 1787), 215–41.

24 Apx 1: Panzerbieter (1782), 14.

25 Johann C. Stark, *Auszüge aus dem Tagebuch des herzoglischen Jenaischen klinischen Instituts* (Jena: Cuno, 1789), 144–145, n.

26 Professors Johann Gottfried Morgenbesser from Breslau, and Johann Friedrich Ackermann from Kiel published notable works about inoculation during the 1750s–70s: Apx2: Morgenbesser (1768); Ackermann (1771, 1773).

inoculation with incisions to the needle-prick methods (early-1770s).[27] At the University of Tübingen medical school, which had an enrolment of just seven to ten students per semester, Professors Ferdinand Christoph Oettinger, Carl Philipp Diez, and Christian Friedrich Reuß were all involved in inoculation in one way or another.[28] Just as remarkable as the high concentration of professors interested in inoculation at such a small medical school was the achievement of three students from a single Tübingen graduation class, in not only reaching the top rungs of the career-ladder but also in making their mark as inoculation promoters and practitioners. One of those noteworthy doctoral graduates, Carl Ludwig von Breyer, became known as inoculator among the Ansbach elite while serving as *Leibarzt* to Margrave Carl Alexander of Brandenburg-Ansbach during the late-1760s, after which he moved on to other posts before acting for many years as a trusted medical adviser to the Prince of Thurn and Taxis.[29]

Another of the Tübingen 'class of 64,' Friedrich Samuel Kretschmar, made his mark as *Leibarzt* to Duke Leopold III Friedrich Franz of Anhalt-Dessau, particularly through his medical reforms during the late-1760s-80s.[30] Better known as a promoter than a practitioner of inoculation, Kretschmar tried to remind the public about the importance of protecting their children, by including a "report and procedure for the inoculation of smallpox" in the 1769 and 1770 editions of the widely-consulted Dessau *Kalender* that reached country-folk as well as townsfolk. Another of his initiatives was a mass-inoculation in 1780 aimed at preventing smallpox from spreading through the progressive educational institution, the Dessau Philanthropium, which led to inoculation becoming a requirement for student enrolment.[31] A third notable doctoral graduate from Tübingen in 1764, Johann Friedrich Cloß, was a medical adviser to Prince William V, the Regent of the Netherlands, when he published a book describing his own smallpox 'cure' (1769). Yet Cloß admitted that his 'cure' was no substitute for inoculation, explaining that he worked toward finding a cure for smallpox only because the benefits of inoculation were not being

---

27 Apx 2: Gatti and Wagler (1772, 1782); Schröter (1773).

28 Klaus D. Mörike, *Geschichte der Tübinger Anatomie* (Tübingen: Mohr, 1988), 33; Apx 2: Weinland (1770), 138–9. Apx 1: Oettinger (1762); Diez (1768).

29 Weinland, 139; Friedrich Schlichtegroll, ed., *Nekrolog auf das Jahr 1799* (Gotha: Perthes, 1805), 72, 75.

30 Arina Völker, "Johann Christian Wilhelm Juncker (1761–1800) und die Dessauer Impfpropagisten," in *Johann Juncker (1679–1759) und seine Zeit*, eds. Wolfram Kaiser and Hans Hübner (Halle-Wittenberg: Martin Luther University, 1979), 91–4.

31 Georg C. Hamberger and Johann G. Meusel, *Das gelehrte Teutschland* (Lemgo: Meyer, 1776), 597; Erhard Hirsch, "Naturwissenschaftlicher Unterricht am Dessauer Philanthropium," in *Johann Juncker (1679–1759) und seine Zeit*, eds. Wolfram Kaiser and Hans Hübner (Halle-Wittenberg: Martin Luther University, 1979), 62.

fully realised owing to deeply-entrenched prejudices among the public, and because princes were reluctant to implement compulsory inoculation.[32]

Professors at the George Augustus University medical school at Göttingen (Hanover) showed the strongest focus on inoculation of any group of German academics, particularly during the mid-1750s-60s. Indeed, the sheer number of inoculation-related dissertations from Göttingen during that period was almost as great as the total from all of the other German universities combined, and a steady flow of publications on the topic from Göttingen academics and medical graduates continued until the mid-1790s.[33] Since the university established by its namesake King George II in his ancestral territory of Hanover proved to be a magnet for foreign students, the Göttingen medical school was well-placed to influence the spread of inoculation in the broader region, given the right kind of academic leadership.[34] Albrecht Haller, the foundation professor of anatomy, provided that leadership. The Esslingen (Württemburg) lawyer, Erhard Friedrich Weinland, made this appraisal of Haller's influence on the reinvigoration and spread of inoculation:

> It was like a mere glimmer of fire still lying beneath the ashes, ... our German Aesculapius splendidly took it upon himself to move forth with the tinder, and set it all alight. Haller's great students went out from Göttingen, and in that way it soon spread in all lands.[35]

The activities of Johann Justus von Berger and Georg Christian Oeder exemplify the anatomy professor's influence in expanding inoculation. Both of those former students of Haller became inoculation practitioners in Copenhagen in the 1750s while holding appointments at the Danish Royal Court. When virulent smallpox swept across Europe, Berger used his influence as a royal physician to bring about the establishment in 1755 of the Royal Inoculation House to offer the benefits of inoculation to the public.[36] Oeder made his

---

32 Johann F. Cloß, *Neue Heilart der Kinderpocken* (Ulm: Bartholomai, 1769), 3, 7–9; *Württemburgisches gelehrten Lexicon, so viel die jetztlebende Württemburgische Schriftensteller betrift* (1772), 87–8.

33 Apx 1: Röderer (1757); Murray (1763); Wrisberg (1765); Schröder (1766 – two dissertations); Vogelsang (1788); Hager (1795). Apx 2: Haller and Röderer (1757); Matthiä (1761); Hensler (1765); Linekogel (1766); Wichmann (1766, 1767, 1773; trans. of Monro 1766; trans. of Chais 1770); Murray (trans. of Rosenstein 1768, 1778; trans. of Schultz 1768, 1769; 1773, 1779); Klärich, 1778); Hufeland (1789, 1793); Gramberg (1787); Girtanner (1796).

34 Peter Watson, *The German Genius* (London: Simon & Schuster, 2010), 50–3.

35 Apx 2: Weinland (1770), 135–6. Haller was from Bern, in the Swiss Confederation.

36 Arnold C. Klebs, *Die Variolation im achtzehnten Jahrhundert: ein historischer Beitrag zur Immunitätsforschung* (Gießen: Töpelmann, 1914), 48, 52

mark in Denmark in quite a different way by pioneering the inoculation of cattle against the debilitating infectious disease referred to in his native German as *Hornviehseuche,* a prophylactic that proved beneficial for the maintenance of dairy herds.[37] Another former-student of Haller, Johann Friedrich Meckel, began inoculating in 1756 among the elite of Berlin while his counterpart Johann Georg Runge was doing likewise in Bremen.[38] Haller's countryman and protégé Johann Georg Zimmermann became involved in inoculation too, as an adviser.[39] Zimmerman's high reputation made such an impression on another Swiss doctor rising to prominence, Samuel-Auguste Tissot, that in 1755 Tissot sent him a copy of his now classic defence of inoculation, *L'inoculation justifiée,* which refuted pointed assertions by the high-profile opponent of the practice, Anton de Haen. Tissot's biography of Zimmermann published in the 1790s shows how well the two men became acquainted in the intervening years.[40]

Professor Johann Georg Röderer was the leading influence in encouraging inoculation among the Göttingen students after Haller's departure in 1753. Under his guidance, the doctoral graduate Leberecht Friedrich Lentin gained the inspiration to commence inoculating in Danneberg (Hanover) during the 1756 smallpox epidemic, while another of his former-students, Johann Samuel Berger, was similarly engaged not far away in Zelle.[41] Röderer was well supported in his teaching by two new appointees (1755) with an interest in inoculation, Rudolf Augustin Vogel and Georg Matthiä. Professor Vogel chose to follow the clinical path taken by Röderer, which involved setting up a medical practice where he offered instruction to the students, including inoculation procedures, and he also treated poor townsfolk for an hour twice per week.[42] Professor Matthiä contributed to the public inoculation discourse as an authoritative voice in support of the practice, with his persuasive arguments countering common concerns raised by doctors and other contributors.[43]

Several of Röderer's former students from the 1760s became known as inoculators, having gained a solid grounding from their teachers. Among

37 Georg C. Oeder, "Ueber die Inokulation der Hornviehseuche," *DM* 1 (1776): 409–10; Gottfried C. Reich, "Etwas über die Hornviehseuche," *MCZ* 4 (1796): 381–2.

38 "Geschichte der Staaten. Aus Teutschland," *Berlinische privilegirte wöchentliche Relation der merkwürdigsten Sachen,* no. 10 (1756): 74–5; Apx 2: de Redern (1765), 83.

39 Albrecht Rengger, *Johann Georg Zimmerman's Briefe an einige seiner Freunde in der Schweiz* (Aarau: Sauerländer, 1830), 186.

40 Tissot, *Zimmermann,* 56–7.

41 Apx 2: Hensler (1765), 1:126.

42 Johann S. Pütter, *Versuch einer academischen gelehrten-Geschichte von der Georg-Augustus Universität Göttingen* (Göttingen: Vandenhoek, 1765), 292, 293, n.

43 Apx 2: Matthiä (1756, 1761).

them was Philipp Gabriel Hensler who gained his initial clinical experience in 1762 by assisting in the inoculation and treatment of patients at Röderer's practice while preparing his doctoral dissertation on the topic of smallpox disease characteristics. Hensler remarks on the 'secret medicine' they used for 'preparing' candidates for inoculation, of which the composition was known only to Röderer and to Professor Büttner who concocted the mixture.[44] He also mentions having discussions about inoculation with his Swedish friend Johann Andreas Murray, who was busily translating the published inoculation methods of two prominent Swedish practitioners.[45] Another fellow-student, Heinrich August Wrisberg, was involved in Röderer's inoculation business too, checking annually on the smallpox status of five sisters the professor tried to inoculate unsuccessfully on four occasions in 1758, using a different set of smallpox-impregnated threads each time.[46] Röderer's concern over the sisters' failure to develop smallpox was indeed warranted. Not only did they all come down with severe smallpox in 1763 but their plight became a *cause célèbre* for inoculation opponents arguing that inoculation was futile because 'artificial' smallpox failed to protect against 'real' smallpox.[47]

After Röderer's untimely death in 1763 at age thirty-seven, Hensler praised his mentor as "a true genius who had many new ideas and turned old ideas in a new direction in his writing and speaking," pointing out too that Röderer's teaching had fostered his own interest in inoculation.[48] While working as the *Stadtphysikus* in Segeberg (Holstein) and later in Altona (near Hamburg) Hensler gained a strong reputation as a skilled inoculator, enhancing his standing with his informative two-volume work about smallpox and inoculation (1765–66) that helped him to an eventual professorship at the University of Kiel.[49] Five other students among the twenty-five attending Röderer's lectures in physiology during 1760–62: Wagler, Schlözer, Wichmann, Wrisberg, and Murray similarly furthered their careers by publishing books or articles about one or other aspect of smallpox or inoculation.[50]

44 Apx 2: Hensler (1765), 2:259–60.

45 Apx 2: Hensler, 2:261; Schultz, trans. Murray (1759, 1762).

46 Hensler, 2:261–2.

47 *Mémoires pour l'histoire des sciences et beaux-arts*, vol. 1 (Paris, 1766), 1116–7; Apx 2: Heinsius (1780), 77–8; Henschel (1795), 50–51.

48 Apx 2: Hensler (1765), 2:259.

49 Scherf, *Archiv*, 2:218–20, 224.

50 August L. Schlözer, *Von Russland's Bevölkerung überhaupt. Erster Theil. Von der Unschädlichkeit der Kindsblattern oder Pocken daselbst* (St. Petersburg: Royal Academy, 1768); Heinrich A. Wrisberg, *Beytrag zur Pocken-Geschichte* (Göttingen: Vandenhoek, 1770); Apx 2: Gatti and Wagler (1772, 1782); Wichmann (1766, 1767, 1773; trans. of Monro 1766; trans. of

Carl Gottlieb Wagler had his name more indelibly linked to the practice of inoculation than any of his former-classmates, after rapidly racing up the career-ladder to an appointment in 1763 as Professor of Obstetrics at the Brunswick Medical College, followed three years later by his elevation to the esteemed role of *Leibarzt* to the Duke of Brunswick-Wolfenbüttel.[51] As an inoculator himself, Wagler recognised that Angelo Gatti's simple 'needle-prick' procedure should be made readily available to German doctors still using the more invasive methods. His translation (1772) of Gatti's straightforward French description of a simple method, alongside his own insightful comments, was soon being praised by not only doctors but also by laymen with limited medical experience who found the 'Gatti-Wagler' method well within their capabilities.[52]

Wagler's close friend August Ludwig Schlözer, Professor Röderer's son-in-law, published his own book about smallpox after moving to Russia to pursue a career in philosophy. Even though he had abandoned his medical studies shortly before completion, his interest was reawakened by a smallpox epidemic that struck St. Petersburg not long after his arrival. Schlözer's study of the disease and the treatments used by Russian medical men culminated in a book in which he made the controversial claim that smallpox was not a deadly disease in Russia.[53] After returning to Göttingen, Schlözer adopted a protective stance toward his father-in-law's legacy, levelling unjustified criticism at local practitioners for abandoning the late Professor Röderer's incision-and-thread procedure in favour of the "so-called newer methods." His claim that just as many local children had died from inoculation in 1777 as from the naturally-acquired disease was contested by one of the doctors he criticised, who pointed out Schlözer's hypocrisy in having his own children inoculated, in the light of such unsubstantiated assertions.[54]

Johann Ernst Wichmann headed to London after gaining his doctorate at Göttingen in 1762 alongside Hensler and Wagler. Helped by the contacts forged

---

Chais 1770); Murray (1773, 1779; trans. of Schultz 1759, 1762, 1769; trans of Rosenstein 1768, 1778).

51 Christian von Schlözer, *August Ludwig von Schlözer's öffentliches und Privatleben* (Leipzig: Hinrichs, 1828), 137–8.

52 Apx 2: Gatti and Wagler (1772, 1782). For doctors' praise for Wagler's book, see in Apx 2: Hannes (1773), 309; Schröter (1773), 18; Opitz (1774), 3; Ziegler (1776), 22; Fritze (1787), 213; for laymen's praise, see in Apx 2: Klose (1786), 396; Schwager, "Patriotische" (1786), 236; Migula, "Noch etwas" (1787), 410.

53 Schlözer, *Unschädlichkeit*, 88–90, 100–101.

54 C. von Schlözer, *August*, 64; Apx 2: Klärich (1778), 210 (quote), 209–11, 222.

by his father, a surgeon at the Royal Hanover Court, Wichmann mingled in elite medical circles where he befriended Sir John Pringle whose special interest in infectious fevers and inoculation he shared.[55] After returning to Hanover, Wichmann set about translating the Scottish doctor Alexander Monro's book about inoculation (1766) and a journal article from London comparing Thomas Dimsdale's method with that of the Suttons. The latter publication was prompted by intense public curiosity about the composition of the Suttons's 'secret medicine' and other potential reasons behind the phenomenal success enjoyed by the Sutton father-and-sons inoculators.[56] Wichmann's involvement in treating orphans and the poor in Hanover when smallpox arrived in 1767 offered him the opportunity to put theory into practice, and he carried out many successful inoculations.[57] His translations, together with the assistance he received from the esteemed old *Leibarzt* Paul Gottlieb Werlhof at the Royal Hanover Court, helped Wichmann secure a position as court physician that paved the way for his eventual promotion in 1796 to *Leibarzt* to King George III.[58]

Heinrich August Wrisberg was another Göttingen student who took a close interest in inoculation. The topic he chose for his doctoral dissertation, supervised by Röderer, was a comparison of instruments for creating inoculation incisions of a defined depth (Figure 7), one designed by Dr. Ambrose Hosty and the other by Dr. Angelo Gatti.[59] Since his supervisor should have arranged the inoculations using those devices, Röderer's sudden death in April 1763 derailed Wrisberg's project. Forced to take decisive action to keep his doctorate on track, Wrisberg established a medical practice in Göttingen that enabled him not only to continue his study but also to compete for the clinical teaching position vacated by his late mentor. A period teaching anatomy and physiology under a special concession led to his appointment as Professor of Obstetrics and of Anatomy soon after being awarded his doctorate in late-1764.[60]

Alongside his teaching, Wrisberg pursued his interest in a hot topic engaging many investigators in many places at that time: the influence of local weather on disease. To gather data for Göttingen, Wrisberg recorded the daily atmospheric pressure, temperature, wind direction, and cloud conditions, which

55 Friedrich Schlichtegroll, ed., *Nekrolog der Teutschen für das neunzehnte Jahrhundert* (Gotha: Perthes, 1805), 3:165–72.
56 Apx 2: Monro (1766); Wichmann (1766), 433–6, 817–40.
57 Schlichtegroll, *neunzehnte Jahrhundert*, 173–4; Apx 2: Hufeland (1793), 224.
58 Schlichtegroll, 187–8.
59 Apx 1: Wrisberg (1765), 22, 27.
60 Pütter, *Versuch*, 190–1.

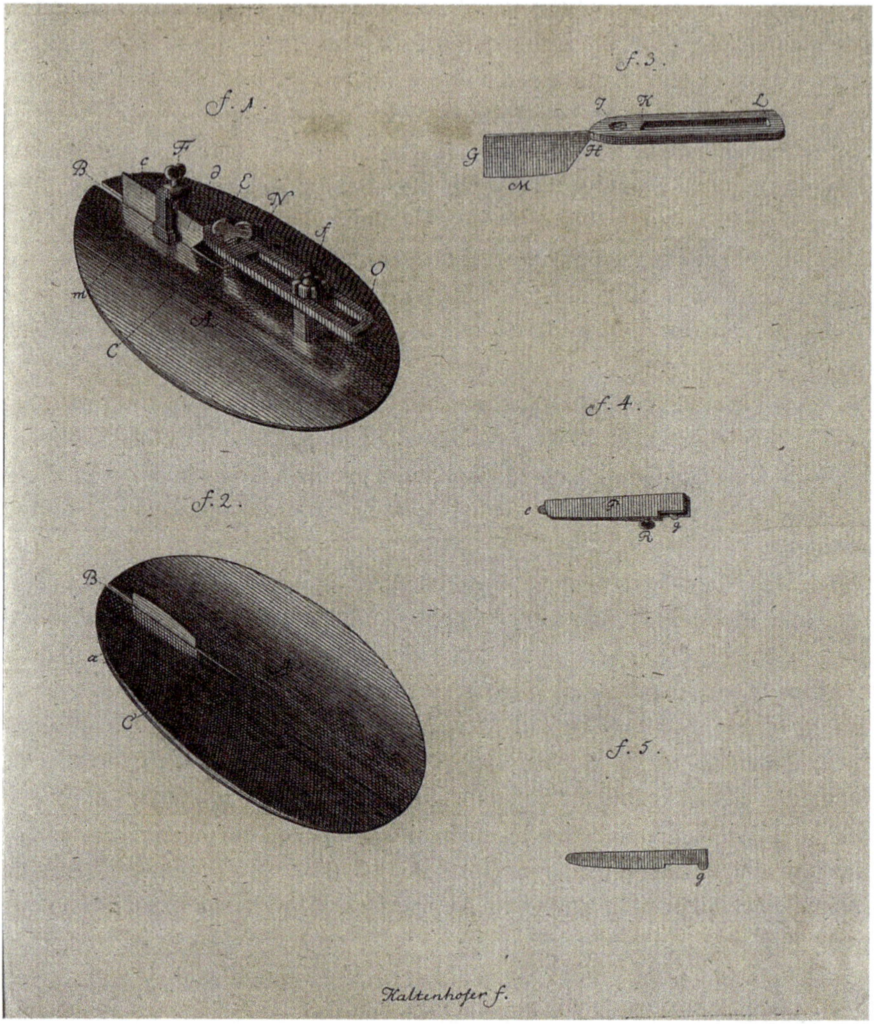

FIGURE 7 Diagram of Ambrose Hosty's (f. 1–3) and Angelo Gatti's (f. 4–5) instruments for making inoculation incisions of a defined depth. Page 29 from Heinrich A. Wrisberg, *Dissertatio de insitione variolarum* (Göttingen, 1765)
NIEDERSÄCHSISCHE STAATS- UND UNIVERSITÄTSBIBLIOTHEK GÖTTINGEN: HTTP://RESOLVER.SUB.UNI-GOETTINGEN.DE/PURL?PPN716997231 (ACCESSED 18 JUNE 2021)

he correlated with prevailing diseases. A twelve-month period of his readings happened to coincide with the smallpox epidemic in Göttingen during 1766–67, enabling him to associate the disease with mainly overcast weather tending to rain, with an unusually low number of sunny days. Although his findings were in agreement with much of the other published data, contrary results from other investigators confused the issue.[61] No consistent answers emerged from comparisons of many studies of that kind.[62]

The talented Swedish student Johann Andreas Murray was another of those taught by Röderer, who produced a doctoral dissertation on an inoculation-related topic. Murray was also offered an immediate professorial appointment at Göttingen (1763), by which time he already had three publications to his credit: two translations of Swedish inoculation methods, and his dissertation examining the introduction of inoculation to Sweden. Murray's prolific vein of inoculation-related publications continued for another sixteen years, while he gave lectures about inoculation in the medical history subject and in the special medical therapies.[63] Professor Philipp Georg Schröder, who came to Göttingen from Marburg, complemented Murray's theoretical teaching with 'hands on' tuition. A former Göttingen student at the time, Gerhard Anton Gramberg, reminisced (1787) that "I inoculated myself in 1765 at Göttingen under the supervision of ... Professor Schröder." Schröder published case-studies of three other self-inoculated students in the form of a dissertation (1766) examining the disease course of inoculated smallpox in adults, which was defended by the three subjects of the study: Johann Philipp Rüling, Moritz Friedrich Houth, and Friedrich Ludwig May.[64] The focus shifted away from inoculation with the waning of smallpox soon afterwards, and the topic never regained its former prominence among Göttingen professors after the deaths during 1772–74 of three of its strongest supporters: Schröder, Matthiä, and Vogel. Göttingen graduates nonetheless continued to make their mark as inoculation promoters and practitioners.[65]

The most prominent eighteenth-century medical graduate from Göttingen was arguably Christoph Wilhelm Hufeland (Figure 8). Among his many accomplishments, Hufeland was a leading authority on inoculation and containment measures for smallpox, and one of the first German doctors to recognise the

---

61 Wrisberg, *Beytrag*, 47–55, 87–8; Apx 2: Opitz (1774), 3; Möhsen (1775), 107–9, 145–7; Hufeland (1793), 41.

62 Volker Hess, "Vom Miasma zum Virus," in *Pocken zwischen Alltag, Medizin und Politik*, ed. Ragnhild Münch (Berlin: Engel, 1994), 16–19; Andrea A. Rusnock, *Vital Accounts. Quantifying Health and Population in Eighteenth-Century England and France* (Cambridge: Cambridge University Press, 2002), 129–33.

63 Apx 1: Murray (1763); Apx 2: Murray (1773, 1779; trans. of Schultz 1759, 1762, 1769; trans. of Rosenstein 1768, 1769, 1778). Pütter, *Versuch*, vol. 2 (Göttingen: Vandenhoek and Ruprecht, 1788), 142.

64 Apx 2: Gramberg (1787), 75; Apx 1: Schröder (1765, 1766 - two dissertations).

65 See note 33 above.

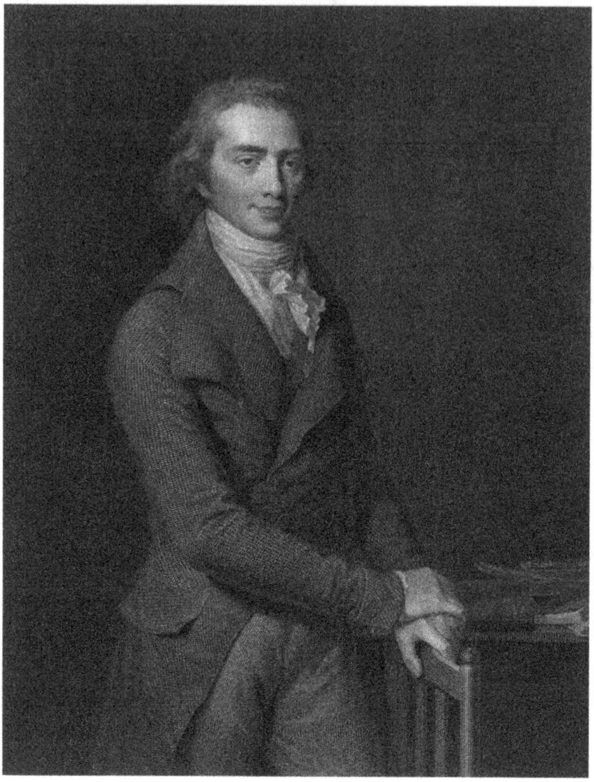

FIGURE 8
Portrait of Christoph Wilhelm von Hufeland. Engraving by J.F. Müller after J.F.A. Tischbein, 1802
RIJKSMUSEUM, AMSTERDAM: RP-P-1906-93

promise of Edward Jenner's cowpox vaccination, as well as a foremost influence in bringing the new prophylactic to the Prussian people.[66] While his career seemed to be going nowhere after he graduated with a doctorate in 1783, when he was obliged to assist in his father's medical practice in Weimar, he gained a professorial appointment at Jena ten years later with an impressive list of publications to his name. Hufeland's subsequent meteoric rise to prominence is reflected in not only his dual appointments in 1800 as Director of the Prussian *Collegium Medico-Chirurgicum* and Chief Physician at the Charité hospital in Berlin but also by his elevation in the following year to *Leibarzt* to King Friedrich Wilhelm III.[67]

66 Apx 2: Hufeland (1789 – one article and one book; 1793). Christoph W. Hufeland, "Neuer Vorschlag zur Verhüting der Blattern durch Inoculation der Kuhpocken," *JAW* 6 (1798): 907–9; Christoph W. Hufeland, "Neue Aussicht zur Vertilgung der Blattern," *TM* 4 (1786): 167–81, 253–63; Johann J. Sachs, *Christoph Wilhelm Hufeland: Ein Rückblick auf sein siebenzigjähriges Leben und Wirken* (Berlin: Hirschwald, 1832), 24.

67 Sachs, 8–9, 12–13, 21–3.

2 *Physiki* Lead the Way

Doctoral graduates aiming to climb the career ladder outside academia usually sought a position as a *Physikus,* a government appointment that provided a platform for further advancement. *Physiki* generally held two offices simultaneously, one as a town-based *Stadtphysikus* and the other as either a *Kreisphysikus* covering a district, a *Landphysikus* covering a large rural area, a *Bergphysikus* attending to miners, a *Garnisonsphysikus* looking after the health of a garrison, or a *Physikus* responsible for some other section of the population. *Physiki* were required to treat the poor without charge, oversee public health, supervise surgeons and bath-masters, examine midwives and barber-surgeon apprentices, and oversee hospital care and apothecaries, as well as carrying out other duties relevant to their locality, including "the eradication of the *Quacksalber*."[68] A conscientious *Physikus* also kept up with new developments in the scholarly literature and published his observations, which was essential if he were seeking higher office without the backing of an influential patron.[69]

As local public health officials responsible for containing and curbing infectious diseases, the *Physiki* were at the forefront of the long battle against smallpox, and were quick to recognise the promise of inoculation as a means of ameliorating the severity of the illness. *Stadtphysikus* Kessler from Magdeburg and *Kreisphysikus* Rehfeld from Prenzlau (Brandenburg) were among the first doctors to respond to the mid-1750s smallpox epidemic by carrying out inoculations.[70] Many other *Physiki* adopted the practice later, particularly in the northern half of Germany where inoculation was generally more readily accepted than in the southern regions.[71] Inoculation could be quite a daunting prospect for a doctor uncertain about not only which method to follow but also about the identification, collection, and storage of infectious material at the correct state of 'ripeness.' During the 1760s-70s when the smallpox-impregnated thread method was widely favoured, many *Physiki* and other medical

---

68 Ernst Schwabe, *Anweisung zu den Pflichten und Geschäften eines Stadt-oder Land-Physikus,* vol. 1 (Erfurt: Keyser, 1786), 121–41, 256 (quote), 257. *Quacksalber* were unauthorised 'healers.'

69 Mary Lindemann, *Health and Healing in Eighteenth-Century Germany* (Baltimore and London: Johns Hopkins University Press, 1996), 72–80; Broman, "Professionalisation," 842.

70 Pistor, "Geschichte," 779–80.

71 *Physiki* who carried out inoculations in the 1750s–60s include Johann F. Bolten (Hamburg), Johann G. Hopfengärtner (Stuttgart: Württemburg), Gustav F. Jägerschmid (Karlsruhe: Baden), J.F.K. Jäschke (Spandau: Brandenburg-Prussia), Leberecht F.B. Lentin (Danneberg: Hanover), Carl G. Magnus (Torgau: Saxony), and P.H.G. Möhring (Jevern: Anhalt-Zerbst): Apx 2: Hensler (1765), 1:126.

men sought advice from the more experienced practitioners, and were usually gratified with useful tips. Some were also given a supply of dried, smallpox-impregnated threads for their initial inoculations. Dr. Rudolf Christian Opitz in Minden was assisted in that way in 1762 by the Magdeburg *Stadtphysikus* Kessler, and the Nördlingen *Stadtphysikus* Stang was provided with threads by the Erlangen professor Heinrich Friedrich Delius in 1768. A decade later, the Weimar *Stadt-* and *Landphysikus* Paul Johann Helmershausen received prepared threads from Dowager Duchess Anna Amalia's *Leibarzt* Johann Friedrich Hufeland, and the Göttingen doctor Friedrich Wilhelm Klärich was likewise assisted by the Duke of Saxe-Gotha's *Leibarzt* Johann Caspar Sulzer and by Polykarp Friedrich von Leyser from Zelle (Hanover), *Leibarzt* to the disgraced former Queen of Denmark Caroline Matilda.[72] The recipients of material assistance from such well-recognised practitioners clearly expected their inoculations using the experts' threads to succeed. However, the well-publicised case of Professor Röderer's failed inoculation of five sisters on four occasions, and the girls' subsequent affliction with severe smallpox confirmed that even the experts' smallpox-impregnated threads could be unreliable.[73]

Several *Physiki* were among the leaders of the change to the simpler, less-invasive inoculation procedures, a move expedited by Professor Wagler's publication in 1772 of the so-called Gatti-Wagler method.[74] During the following two years in Prussia, the Wesel *Stadt-* and *Landphysikus* Christian Rudolf Hannes used that method to introduce inoculation to Kleve, and *Stadtphysikus* Christian Friedrich Opitz did likewise in Minden, as did *Stadtphysikus* Johann Gottlieb Fritze in Halberstadt. Fritze made a further contribution to the dissemination of simplified inoculation procedures by translating the French doctor Jacques-François de Villiers's eyewitness account of the procedure that the Suttons made famous but failed to publish until 1796.[75] Yet even when the simple 'needle-prick' procedures were being increasingly accepted, parental fears and anti-inoculation prejudices continued to thwart attempts to introduce inoculation to local communities.[76]

Physiki were often unable to convince parents to adopt inoculation, even if they offered the procedure at no cost. *Kreisphysikus* Müller in Wohlau (Silesia)

---

72 Juncker, *Archiv*, 1: 183; Apx 2: Opitz (1774), 35; "Zu der Geschichte" (1770), 186; Klärich (1778), 220.

73 Apx 2: Hensler (1765), 2:257–63; Heinsius (1780), 77–8.

74 Apx 2: Gatti and Wagler (1772, 1782).

75 Johann G. Fritze, "Eine Blatterimpfung," *Baldinger's neues Magazin für Aerzte* 9 (1787): 213; Apx 2: Hannes (1773), 309; de Villiers (1776); Opitz (1774), 3rd page of introduction.

76 Apx 2: Schröter (1773), 8; Baylies (1776), 124. Juncker, *Archiv*, 2:261; 3:22; 5:120, 234, 237. Daniel Sutton, *The Inoculator, or Suttonian System of Inoculation* (London, 1796).

blamed entrenched prejudices for the poor response in 1790 to his "promise to people of the lower-classes to provide their children with the benefits of inoculation free of charge."[77] *Kreisphysikus* Märcker in Marienwerder (Prussia) noted that the people in his region largely rejected inoculation because they regarded it as "somewhat of a new fashion," or as "a sin and interference in Providence," or were concerned that "smallpox must have a certain 'ripeness' that is impossible to determine," or that inoculation "does not protect from a natural infection," or that "inoculated people are not as healthy and will not grow to old age." Other locals were concerned that "another disease can be inoculated with the smallpox," which was indeed quite likely if donors of smallpox material were not carefully selected.[78] *Stadtphysikus* Georg Christoph Conradi from Northeim (Hanover) addressed the issue of parental resistance to inoculation (1782) by recommending that correct information about the procedure and about appropriate smallpox treatments be included in the annual *Kalender* of advice for day-to-day living.[79]

The Quedlinburg *Stadtphysikus* Christian Jacob Ziegler lamented (1776) that even his better-educated acquaintances ignored his protestations that common prejudices about inoculation were misconceived. He also noted that his successful inoculation of his own child and of Pastor Steinhausen's children helped to overcome such prejudices.[80] The Lauterbach (Hesse-Kassel) *Stadtphysikus* Moritz Gerhard Thilenius similarly saw an initial increase in demand for inoculation after parents saw the mildness of the inoculated disease in his children. He also noted that in later smallpox epidemics, when inoculation was more widely adopted, the survival of the inoculated children while many of their un-inoculated counterparts succumbed to smallpox provided a tragic 'lesson' that helped to break down local anti-inoculation prejudices.[81]

Since the office of *Physikus* was more of step toward further advancement than a well-paid position, *Physiki* generally needed to attract private clients to make ends meet. Yet the social taint of caring for the poor as a primary part of their duties was a distinct disadvantage for *Physiki* competing for a limited number of well-off clients, particularly in towns with an over-supply of doctors.[82]

77 Apx 2: Scheliha (1790), 367.

78 Juncker, *Archiv*, 5:237.

79 Juncker, 2:279; Georg C. Conradi, "Unterricht über die Behandlung der Blattern und Empfehlung der Inoculation, dem Landmanne bestimmt," *Neuer Volkskalender* (Hanover: Hahn, 1795), 242.

80 Apx 2: Ziegler (1776), 5–7.

81 Moritz G. Thilenius, *Medicinische und chirurgische Bemerkungen*, 2nd ed. (Frankfurt am Main: Brönner, 1809), xxxviii-ix.

82 Broman, "Professionalization," 842–3, 855; Lindemann, *Health*, 13, 79–80; Frevert, *Krankheit*, 42, 58.

Inoculation could be a very useful skill in such situations. Even princes were more inclined to call in a *Physikus* or other local practitioner known for his inoculation expertise than to entrust the task to a less experienced household physician or *Leibarzt*, judging by the experiences of the Lauterbach *Stadtphysikus* Moritz Gerhard Thilenius (1745–1808; Figure 9).[83] Thilenius's account of his own career reveals not only the social challenges confronting a humble *Physikus* called upon to inoculate high-born children, but also the reality that a conscientious *Physikus* could attain the higher rungs of the career ladder even without an upper-class background.

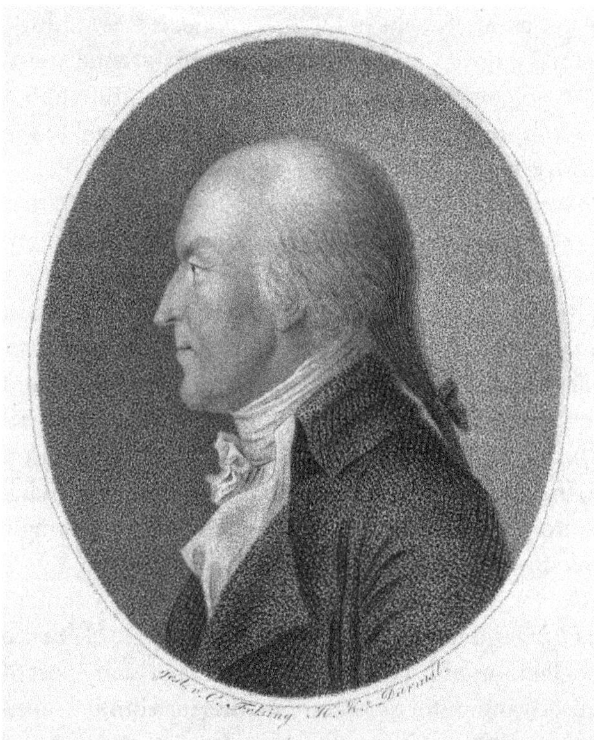

FIGURE 9
Moritz Gerhard Thilenius. Stipple engraving by C. Felsing
RIJKSMUSEUM, AMSTERDAM: RP-P-1914-2866

As the son of a provincial apothecary from Hesse-Kassel who gained a medical licence by passing the requisite examination, Moritz lacked the elite family-background, patronage, influential connections, and post-graduation travel to assist his career. Yet the young Moritz made the most of a good basic education, and with added diligence he emerged from the Göttingen medical school in 1765 with a doctorate, having made a good impression on his teachers. At

83 Vogel, *Handbuch*, 116; Thilenius, *Bemerkungen* (1789), 433–40.

that point, compulsory army service followed by an obligation to assist in the family medical practice forced him to put his career on hold until his father's death in 1769 set him free to pursue more ambitious goals. His former teachers at Göttingen helped to further his career by recommending him to an official inquiring about a suitable candidate for appointment as the *Stadt-* and *Landphysikus* at Lauterbach, in his home-territory of Hesse-Kassel. By then, Thilenius had a recent publication to boost his credentials for the position, which he accepted when it was offered.[84]

After moving to Lauterbach in 1770, Thilenius soon found that many of his patients' illnesses were caused by the after-effects of the smallpox epidemic that struck the region two years earlier. That realisation prompted him to discuss inoculation with his new acquaintances, most of whom agreed to have their children inoculated when smallpox returned. Yet the mothers' fears resurfaced when the disease arrived in 1777, and no children were inoculated. He was left with few other options to prepare for the epidemic than to compile a circular advising the best treatment for smallpox, which was printed and distributed by Johann Wilhelm von Riedesel zu Eisenbach, the owner of the lands in his *Physikat*. Determined to promote inoculation as effectively as possible when smallpox returned, Thilenius examined relevant publications by Wagler, Dimsdale, and Petrus Camper to acertain procedural details and guidelines for judging the suitability of candidates. His successful inoculation of his own six children in 1783 prompted sufficient demand to bring his tally of inoculations to 121 during the next four months as smallpox swept through the region.[85]

Thilenius's reputation as a skilled inoculator soon reached a relative of the Lauterbach estate owner, *Oberjägermeister* Volprecht von Riedesel in Darmstadt who was concerned about his children contracting the smallpox approaching the town. When he received the *Oberjägermeister's* letter asking him to travel to Darmstadt to inoculate his children, Thilenius responded with extreme caution. He was acutely aware that inoculating during a smallpox outbreak was very risky, particularly since the recent deaths of two local children who had inadvertently contracted smallpox in the few days before being inoculated by the surgeon Lorenz.[86] In his reply to the *Oberjägermeister*, Thilenius pointed out that his busy schedule would not allow an idle week waiting for smallpox symptoms to appear, were he to travel to Darmstadt to inoculate the children. As an alternative, he offered to send fresh smallpox material

84 Thilenius, *Bemerkungen* (1814), x, xv–xvi.

85 Thilenius, *Bemerkungen* (1789), 341, 343–59; Apx 2: Dimsdale (1768, 1769, 1782); Gatti and Wagler (1772, 1782).

86 Thilenius, 408–10.

and the inoculation method so that the household physician could carry out the procedure, and to arrive a week later to oversee the children's recovery.[87] That plan ensured that the risks and responsibility were borne not by himself, a comparatively lowly *Physikus,* but by the physician employed on a much higher salary specifically to care for the *Oberjägermeister's* family. As it turned out, the household physician, L.L. Bader, was also reluctant to inoculate the three children, since he handed the task further down the pecking order to a regimental surgeon named Ruben who successfully carried out the procedure under Bader's supervision.[88]

While Thilenius was in Darmstadt and the *Oberjägermeister's* children were recovering well, he received a request from Crown Prince Ludwig of Hesse-Darmstadt, who lived nearby, to determine the fitness of his three children for inoculation. Thilenius agreed to examine them, and judged only the eldest child to be sufficiently robust, yet he would not agree to inoculate the boy until his responsibilities were clearly defined. At a meeting with the crown prince and his wife, he agreed to supervise the inoculation and after-care of young Prince Ludwig, with the assistance of the *Oberjägermeister's* physician, Bader, but only after returning home to attend to his affairs. It was also agreed that Dr. Bader would inoculate the prince if the proximity of smallpox warranted urgent action while Thilenius was away. Meanwhile, the crown prince's physician Theodor Friedrich Balser carried out the usual preparations for high-profile procedures: he inoculated his own children and others to gain valuable experience and a supply of fresh smallpox material from a known source. The inoculation of the prince went ahead successfully after Thilenius's return, and he recovered well amid concerns about a measles outbreak in the area.[89]

The situation in which Thilenius found himself in 1783 when negotiating the responsibility and risks associated with the inoculation of high-born children was parodied in a work of fiction published in the same year by August Gottlieb Meißner, the Privy Council Archivist at the Saxon elector's court in Dresden. Part of the story, *Gustav Lindau,* was set in a fictional ducal court where the physicians hatch a plot to avoid any responsibility for inoculating the duke's only legitimate heir, a sickly young boy. They initiate their strategy by spreading around the court the name of a local doctor with a supposed reputation as an experienced inoculator, ensuring that their hints gain the duke's attention. Naturally, the duke proceeds to ask the unnamed doctor to inoculate his son, and the remnant feudal social traditions demand that the doctor regard the

87 Thilenius, 410.
88 Thilenius, 410–11.
89 Thilenius, 412–17.

request as a command he is unable to refuse. Fortunately for the doctor and for the frail prince, the inoculation is successful, and the doctor receives the duke's undying gratitude along with the promised generous payment. Yet his achievement arouses intense jealousy among the court physicians concerned that the duke may offer the post of *Leibarzt* to the outsider ahead of one of them. In order to dissuade the interloper from considering any such offer, the physicians and their cronies bombard him with disdainful invective and reminders of his social inferiority, during his weeks overseeing the prince's recovery. Of course, the supercilious physicians are quite unaware that the doctor's experience of life at the court, even before their spiteful attacks, had inspired only his longing to return to blissful mediocrity.[90]

Back in real life, *Stadtphysikus* Thilenius announced with great pride and relief his "recent inoculation of the heir to Hesse-Darmstadt ... with the greatest success," referring also to another 148 of the procedures he undertook in 1783, which all went well. Just as successful was his inoculation in 1785 of the Crown Prince of Hesse-Darmstadt's younger children Louise and Georg, which he carried out with no hesistation in the knowledge that smallpox was absent from the area and that the children were in good health.[91] His reputation gained such a boost from his successful inoculations among the aristocracy, reflecting the crown prince's faith in his skills, that he received several offers of higher positions. The first two came in 1786 from officials in Darmstadt and Frankfurt, with more arriving from Wetzlar, Kiel, Fulda, and Wiesbaden during the following decade, including some repeat enticements after the publication (1789) of his lengthy medical and surgical observations. Eventually, when the rigours of travelling around his large *Physikat* became too demanding, he accepted Duke Friedrich August of Nassau's offer of an appointment as physician at the mineral springs and court in Wiesbaden. By then (1795), he had 1,800 inoculations to his credit as well as eight publications.[92]

Thilenius's life took another turn in 1799 when war with France made life in Wiesbaden untenable. Following his retreat to Lauterbach, the lawyer Carl Georg von Riedesel found him a sedentary position at the Imperial Law Courts in Wetzlar where he remained until the Duke of Nassau enticed him back to Wiesbaden in 1803, after peace was restored. In his new role as *Leibarzt,*

---

90 August G. Meißner, "Gustav Lindau, oder der Mann, der keinen Neid ertragen will. Fragment aus Branko's Reisejournal," in *Meißner's Erzählungen und Dialogen*, vol. 1 (Karlsruhe: Schmieder, 1783), 118–21.

91 Moritz G. Thilenius, "Lauterbach, am Vogelsberg, December 5, 1783," *Politisches Journal* 2 (1783): 1227 (quote); Thilenius, *Bemerkungen*, 433–40.

92 Thilenius, *Bemerkungen*, 3rd ed. (1814), xxi–ii.

Thilenius was required not only to look after the duke's health but also to serve as medical adviser to the visitors being hosted at the court during their trips to the nearby mineral springs for the health benefits. With such high-ranking figures as the Regent of the Netherlands, Empress Josephine, and the Duke of Coburg among his patients, Thilenius had reached a very high rung of the career ladder indeed, even without an elite family background, through his diligence, competence, professional publications, and formidable reputation as a skilled inoculator.[93]

3 Social-Class Considerations – Doctors versus Surgeons

Social commentators advertising the benefits of inoculation in some cases highlighted the boost to a state's prosperity that could be gained by reducing population losses from smallpox.[94] Yet few had the courage to point out that the inoculation of the productive class would be more beneficial than preserving upper-class lives. Dr. Johann Clemens Tode was a notable exception. The eminent Tode laments that the daughters of the common man, who sewed, spun, and worked for a living, had much lower inoculation rates than comparatively unproductive upper-class women. Citing cost as one of the main obstacles to the expansion of inoculation among the working class, he accuses his peers of being so enticed by money and obsessed by income that they inoculated only those with the ability to pay.[95]

By the 1790s when inoculation was becoming more widespread and authorities in some areas wanted to offer the procedure for free to the poor, local benefactors or the practitioners themselves covered the costs.[96] Yet finding a doctor to carry out inoculations was becoming increasingly difficult, according to Dr. Christian Samuel Ungnad from Züllichau (Prussia) who lamented (1798) that younger doctors lacked interest in inoculation, perhaps owing to laziness or fear of failure.[97] An alternative reason for doctors' increasing reluctance to inoculate (1797) was the contagiousness of the practice. In the experience of Dr. Waghas from Dramburg (Prussia), parents with children who had never been infected with smallpox barred him from entering their houses, forcing him to face the reality that his *clientèle* was dwindling because of his inoculation

---

93 Thilenius, xxii–iv.

94 Apx 2: Weinland (1770), 155–6; Möhsen, part 2 (1775), 8–9.

95 Apx 2: Tode (1785), 24–7, 32, 37–41.

96 Juncker, *Archiv*, 2:261; 5:97; 6:218; Apx 2: "Pokkeneinimpfung" (1796), 164; "Ein Wort" (1797), 142.

97 Juncker, 5:20, 234.

activities, and that unless he changed course his livelihood would depend largely on clients seeking inoculation.[98]

Parents who wanted their children inoculated by a qualified practitioner but were unable to afford a doctor's fees or secure a free inoculation had the choice of a range of surgeons trained in various ways.[99] Surgeons tended to offer cheaper inoculations because of their inferior social status compared with the doctors, who collectively belonged to the *Gelehrtenstand* by virtue of their university education.[100] Doubts about the competence of surgeons was another issue that came into play, though Pastor Christian Gottfried Klose from Domanze (Silesia) regarded the surgeons' poor reputation as undeserved, and expressed disappointment that some of his parishioners would not permit a surgeon to inoculate their children.[101] Other parents were quite confident in taking their children to a surgeon, some of whom were well-regarded for their general skills.[102] Such differing opinions reflect the variable standards of surgical training, which relied largely on an apprenticeship scheme whereby ownership of a barber-shop was the qualification required to teach apprentice barber-surgeons. The lack of a medical education, and the expectation that the apprentices would acquire the necessary anatomical knowledge from reading recommended texts suggests a scheme designed to produce barber-surgeons capable of carrying out quite straightforward procedures such as routine bloodletting, but nothing with any complexity.[103]

The highly-skilled surgeons in Germany in the first three decades of the eighteenth century were usually doctors who added surgery to their repertoire of talents, or surgeons trained at one of the foreign academies. One of the best was Gabriel Senff, an exceptional barber-surgeon in the Prussian army who was sent to Paris by King Friedrich Wilhelm I to undertake additional specialised surgical training. While Senff's subsequent teaching of surgery to doctors at the Charité Hospital in Berlin provided the great benefit of expanding the supply of skilled surgeons in Prussia, the 'soldier king,' so-named because of his love and support for his army, wanted a reliable supply of expert military surgeons too.[104] In order to achieve this aim, he set up his own training scheme

98 Juncker, 2:262.

99 Juncker, 5:83, 197; Apx 2: "Bericht" (1788), 293–5.

100 Broman, "Professionalization," 841, 863; Apx 2: Schwager, "Patriotische" (1786), 216.

101 Apx 2: Klose (1786), 404.

102 Vogel, *Handbuch*, 116; Apx 2: Weinland (1770), 141; "Blattern-Inoculation" (1788), 165; "Nachricht von den fernern" (1768), 353–6.

103 Sander, *Handwerkschirurgen*, 84–6; Broman, "Professionalization," 841, 863.

104 Gerhard Jaeckel, *Die Charité. Die Geschichte eines Weltzentrums der Medizin von 1710 bis zur Gegenwart* (Berlin: Lehmanns Media, 2018), 44; Jörg Heinrich, *Johann Theodor Eller.*

along the lines of the French and British surgical academies that provided students with not only high quality practical surgical training but also a medical education.[105] The Berlin medical-surgical school, which turned out its first graduates in 1730, became widely recognised in Germany for producing surgeons with superior skills and competence. Yet the number of graduates was so small compared to the number of barber-surgeons that the overall surgical landscape remained largely unchanged for most of the eighteenth century until other German princes emulated the Prussian model.[106]

Surgeons became involved in inoculation from the outset when the use of incisions was the norm and the medical regulations deemed such 'external procedures' as a surgeon's responsibility.[107] The Hamburg surgeon Wallis attracted a number of doctors to his services by equipping himself in the 1760s with a *Rotterdammer Instrument* for making inoculation incisions of a defined depth, while the surgeon Döring in Zittau (Saxony) made small incisions for inoculation in a more conventional fashion (1771) for the local doctor Karl August Richter.[108] As inoculation became more widely practised, surgeons increasingly inoculated independently, sometimes at the behest of the local *Physikus* when his hands were full with patients.[109] Among the surgeon-inoculators remembered with reverence were "the famous Rephalides" in Augsburg in the 1760s, and surgeon Flügel from Wallendorf (Schwarzburg-Rudolstadt) who inoculated many young people in the late-1770s. Flügel's efforts were so successful that when smallpox swept through the area in 1796, those he inoculated who had by then become parents were well-aware of the importance of ensuring that their own children were inoculated.[110] The surgeon Richter in Schandau (Saxony) was similarly praised (1800) for inoculating every child whose parents gave permission, free of charge, and for providing a sheet of instructions about the care of smallpox patients.[111] Levin Ludolph Eckermann, the surgeon at the public inoculation facility in Brunswick in the 1760s-70s,

---

Ein bedeutender Arzt, Wissenschaftler und Medizinalbeamter in Brandenburg-Preussen in der ersten Hälfte des 18. Jahrhunderts (Husum: Matthiesen, 2003), 19–20.

105 Pistor, "Geschichte," 237–8; Broman, *Transformation*, 67–9.

106 Broman, "Professionalization," 863.

107 Pistor, "Geschichte," 234.

108 "Vermischte Nachrichten," *LM*, no. 3 (1771): 45; Apx 2: Hensler (1765), 2:431. Some doctors preferred the incision-and-thread method even after the simpler skin-prick inoculations became popular: Lenhardt, *Arzneyen*, xxxv–vi; Leberecht F.B. Lentin, *Beyträge zur ausübenden Arzneywissenschaft* (Leipzig: Crusius, 1789), 36.

109 August K. Holsche, *Historisch-topographisch Beschreibung der Grafschaft Tecklenburg* (Berlin and Frankfurt: Kunze, 1788), 255–7; Apx 2: Vogler (1799), 691–2.

110 Apx 2: Weinland (1770), 141 (quote). Juncker, *Archiv*, 5:173.

111 "An alle gut gesinnte vernünftige denkende Eltern wegen Einimpfung der Blattern," *RA* 2 (1800): 3148.

was highly-regarded too, as was *Leibchirurgus* Johann Bodo Lampe at the Royal Hanover Court who had five hundred successful inoculations to his credit by 1788.[112] *Landchirurgus* Burmeister from the tiny Duchy of Lauenburg, bordering Meckenburg to the west, accrued a similar tally, and was even called upon to inoculate a princess of Mecklenburg (1780s) despite not holding a court appointment.[113]

Although some surgeon-inoculators gained a high reputation for their competence, a general sense of social and professional superiority among doctors gave rise to generic criticisms. One notable instance was the Bassum (Bremen) doctor Schröter's comment in 1773, in relation to inoculation, that he deplores the spectre of "the surgeon, who appears so frightful to the children, with his cutting instrument."[114] Yet most German doctors at that time also used a cutting instrument for inoculation, to prepare the incisions for the placement of their smallpox-impregnated threads. Moreover, to children unfamiliar with doctors and their mannerisms, an unfamiliar black-suited stranger trying to cut their arms with a lancet would be a more frightening spectacle than a familiar, less formally-attired local surgeon. Indeed, some surgeon-inoculators used more up-to-date methods than doctors. The surgeon Eckermann in Brunswick was already using Thomas Dimsdale's simple method in 1768, five years before Dr. Schröter reported his own abandonment of the incision-and-thread inoculation method, while criticising the methods used by surgeon-inoculators.[115]

In a medical landscape where barber-surgeons with lower levels of skills and competence vastly outnumbered the well-skilled graduates from the medical-surgical schools, *Physiki* were required to oversee surgeons' activities. Surgeons intending to inoculate were usually taught and initially supervised by a doctor, while even the most experienced surgeons required a doctor to check their procedures if any problems arose.[116] An ability to recognise the early signs of smallpox so that a planned inoculation could be abandoned if such symptoms were evident was a crucial skill for independent surgeon-inoculators, as was the medical knowledge to not only identify any additional infections that could be transmitted through inoculation but also to diagnose the donor's pustular disease correctly.[117] The collection of infectious material from a case of measles, chicken-pox, or another illness mistakenly diagnosed

112 Apx 2: "Nachricht von den fernern" (1768), 353–6; "Blattern-Inoculation" (1788), 165.

113 Vogel, *Handbuch*, 116.

114 Apx 2: Schröter (1773), 21. Broman, "Professionalization," 863–4.

115 Apx 2: Schröter, 17–18; "Nachricht von den fernern" (1768), 353–6.

116 Juncker, *Archiv*, 5:237; Thilenius, *Bemerkungen* (1789), 408–9; Apx 2: Klose (1786), 408; Opitz (1774), 104–5; Künzel (1788), 76–7.

117 Christoph L. Hoffmann, *Pathologie der Pockenkrankheit*, part 2, *Abhandlung von den Pocken* (Mainz, 1789), 107; Juncker, *Archiv*, 2:288; Apx 2: Elsner (1787), 33–5. A case of mea-

as mild smallpox was a particular problem when such pustular diseases were epidemic at the time the material for inoculation was being collected.[118]

The range of medical procedures that surgeons and other officially registered 'healers' were permitted to undertake was expanded in many regions by authorities attempting to improve medical care and curb the harmful activities of the *Quacksalber*. As part of that reform, the surgeons were either classified in groups according to their skill level, or each surgeon's particular knowledge and expertise was linked to a personal authorisation.[119] In Prussia, new regulations issued in 1773 permitted surgeons in rural areas to transgress the doctors' usually exclusive right to treat internal diseases, if no doctor were in easy reach, and required *Physiki* to instruct the surgeons accordingly.[120] Official permission for surgeons to inoculate with greater independence, and for *Physiki* to enlist the surgeons' help in caring for patients at busy times such as smallpox epidemics was not only a bonus for the surgeons, in helping them add to their skill set, but also for the *Physiki*.[121]

Reports of inoculations that resulted in death or failed to protect against smallpox aroused the interest of the Halle professor Johann Christian Wilhelm Juncker. Yet Juncker was frustrated at the usual lack of important details such as the inoculator's name and status, which would enable the cause of the problem to be investigated.[122] As a longstanding critic of unauthorised inoculators and of poorly-skilled surgeons, Juncker was perhaps hoping to find that he could attribute the botched inoculations to such practitioners, which would reinforce his controversial push for inoculation to be the sole preserve of doctors.[123] Although collective accounts of deaths following inoculation largely indicate no fault except smallpox having been contracted in the days before the procedure, infected inoculation wounds caused a number of deaths too,

---

sles was reportedly inoculated together with smallpox, and on another occasion erysipelas broke out in a group of children inoculated together: Juncker, 2:279; 4:14.

118 Juncker, 2:279; 6:69, 73–5; Christoph Girtanner, *Krankheiten der Kinder und über die physische Erziehung derselben* (Berlin: Rottmann, 1794), 201, 204–5.

119 Christoph L. Hoffmann, "Ueber die münsterschen Medizinalgesetze," *DM* 1 (1778): 34–6; Sander, *Handwerkschirurgen*, 233; Johann H.L. Bergius and Johann Beckmann, *Sammlung auserlesener Landesgesetze, welche das Policey und Cameralwesen zum Gegenstände haben* (Frankfurt am Main: Andreä, 1791), 44.

120 Frevert, *Krankheit*, 63–4.

121 Juncker, *Archiv*, 3:88; 5:168, 237; 6:36, 226; 7:262; Apx 2: Steiger (1787), 163.

122 Juncker, 3:211–12.

123 Johann C.W. Juncker, *Gemeinnützige Vorschläge und Nachrichten über das beste verhalten der Menschen in Rücksicht der Pockenkrankheit. Erster Versuch, für die mittlern Stände nebst einem Anhange für Aerzte* (Halle, 1792), 95–8; Juncker, *Dritter Versuch* (1796), 47–56.

at the hands of doctors as well as surgeons and laymen.[124] On the other hand, reports of eighteen unexplained deaths and six failures from inoculations carried out in Darmstadt and in Ansbach-Bayreuth (Prussia) during 1798–99 indicate that most of the inoculators in those instances were doctors.[125] Ten deaths from fifty children inoculated in Darmstadt, and eight deaths from seventy-six children inoculated in Ansbach was an unusually high fatality-rate for the late-1790s when inoculation procedures were quite refined. The ten deaths in Darmstadt caused outrage among the local public, prompting a request in the widely-circulated Gotha-based *Reichs-Anzeiger* for an explanation from someone who could shed light on the matter.[126] Although the truth of the various assertions is unclear, some of the Darmstadt children who died after inoculation were reportedly given an extreme form of stimulant treatment, indeed so extreme in one case that the child was said to have consumed twelve bottles of wine during his illness.[127] Such suggestions support claims that the Darmstadt doctors' general belief in the theories of the Scottish doctor John Brown was to blame for the children's deaths. Brown's recommendation for treating illnesses affecting the nerves, the category in which he placed smallpox, was a stimulant regimen that included a diet with a high meat content, consumption of alcoholic beverages, and avoidance of cool conditions.[128] Yet that was exactly the kind of treatment deemed positively harmful to smallpox patients by the vast majority of competent doctors since the 1750s.[129] The inoculators in Darmstadt defended their practices by variously blaming the deaths on the weather and on the nature of the smallpox disease at the time.[130] Since any inoculation fatalities tended to work against further local inoculations for a considerable period, a high level of competence of the majority of inoculation practitioners, whether doctors or surgeons, was crucial if parents were to be convinced of the benefits of the procedure.

124 Thilenius, *Bemerkungen* (1789), 408; Juncker, *Archiv*, 1:179; 2:254, 291; 3:62; 4:20–1; 5:90, 233; Apx 2: Vogel (1787), 19.

125 Juncker, 7:235–48.

126 "Anfrage, die diesjährige Blattern-Impfung in Darmstadt betreffend," *RA* 2 (1800): 2549.

127 "Schreiben, eines Reisenden über die Blattern in Darmstadt," *RA* 2 (1800): 2860.

128 "Schreiben," 2861; "Etwas zur Berichtigung der Anfrage, die diesjährige Blattern-Impfung in Darmstadt betreffend," *RA* 2 (1800): 2857–8; John Brown, *Anfangsgründe der Medizin*, trans. Andreas Röschlaub (Frankfurt am Main: Andreä, 1806), 12, 239–43.

129 Prussian Medical Board, "Kurze Anleitung wie der Landmann und diejenigen, die keinen Arzt erlangen können, bei der grassirenden Pocken sich zu verhalten haben," *HM* 7 (1769): 569–71.

130 "Schreiben, eines Reisenden," 2860–1.

CHAPTER 4

The Discourse in the Print Media

Initial recognition of the importance of inoculation in ushering in a new approach to disease prevention is reflected in the sheer number of eighteenth-century publications on the topic. Of the more than six hundred dissertations, journal articles, books, and reviews about inoculation produced in Germany, the first sixty, published between 1714 and 1750, were largely erudite works aimed toward an audience of mainly academics and professionals. The wider public was subsequently informed about inoculation through newspapers and the generally-targeted journals that kept increasing in number in concert with the expansion of the public sphere.[1] By the time inoculation captured the public interest during and after the severe smallpox epidemic of the mid-1750s, the sense of curiosity pervading the earlier books and articles had largely given way to religious concerns and debates about the morality, safety, and efficacy of the practice.[2]

Inoculation embodied so many facets of human emotion in the balancing act between life and death that Germans from a wide variety of social and professional groups were inspired to put pen to paper. The flow of German publications about inoculation continued almost uninterrupted from 1750 until circa 1801 with intermittent surges at times of smallpox outbreaks, while in Britain and particularly in France the output tapered off more than a decade earlier.[3] The collective body of German publications reveals temporal changes in the style and nature of the commentary as well as in the themes addressed by the various social groups that expressed an opinion. Of course, the authors, translators, journal owners, reviewers, and editors were all in a position to control much of what the journal-reading public was offered. The reading ability of the public to whom the commentaries about inoculation were directed, and the ease with which potential readers could access the journals were other

1 Johann S. Ersch, *Litteratur der Medicin seit der Mitte des achtzehnten Jahrhunderts* (Amsterdam and Leipzig: Kunst-und Industrie-Comptoir, 1812), 261–3; *Allgemeines Sachregister über die wichstigsten deutschen Zeit- und Wochen-schriften* (Leipzig: Weygand, 1790), 400–403; publications listed in Apx 1 and Apx 2.

2 Andreas-Holger Maehle, "Conflicting Attitudes Towards Inoculation in Enlightenment Germany," *CM* 29 (1995): 201–52; Peter Albrecht, "Wie hältst Du es mit der Blatterninokulation? Eine 'Gretchenfrage' im 18. Jahrhundert," *Praxis Geschichte* 5 (1999), 58–60.

3 Maehle, "Attitudes," 201; publications listed in Apx 2.

 | DOI:10.1163/9789004465374_006

important elements in determining the extent to which the 'messages' being delivered in the print media reached their intended targets.

1 The Published Word Spreads News of the Innovation

German readers were first alerted to the use of inoculation for the prevention of severe smallpox in 1714, in a review of an article by Emanuele Timoni, a Greek doctor working in Constantinople. That seminal work was revisited in another journal article in 1717, while a review of a treatise on the topic by Dr. Jacob Pylarini, the Venetian consul in Smyrna (modern Izmir), was published in the same year.[4] First-hand accounts in the 1720s of inoculations carried out in London, Boston, Eperjes (Hungary), Constantinople, and the German territories of Hanover, Brandenburg-Ansbach, and Waldeck alerted German readers to not only the spreading practice of inoculation but also to the procedural experiments being carried out in Britain and occasionally in their homeland.[5] The first personal account of an inoculation in continental Europe was Dr. Johann Adam Reimann's description in September 1721 of his inoculation of his daughter in his home-town, Eperjes.[6] More inoculations were carried out in 1721 by Johann Theodor Eller, at the behest of Duke Viktor Friedrich of Anhalt-Bernburg who had recently appointed Eller as a physician at his court. Yet Eller waited until 1762 before first reporting that occasion when he successfully inoculated five children at the Bernburg court, and indicating that he had previously inoculated an orphan in his care in Paris during a smallpox outbreak.[7] Eller's tardiness places the Hanover military and royal court surgeon Johann Ernst Wreden as the first German to provide a personal account of his own inoculation activities.[8] In an initial publication in 1723 and in a more comprehensive account in the following year, Wreden describes his inoculation of five

4 Apx 2: Review of Timoni (1714); Klaunig and Timoni (1717); Review of Pylarini (1717). Timoni's and Pylarini's works were also published in an abbreviated form in the *Transactions of the Royal Society*: Emmanuel Timoni, "An Account, or History, of the Procuring the Small Pox by Incision, or Inoculation: as it has for Some Time Been Practiced at Constantinople," PT 29 (1714): 72–84; Jacob Pylarini, "A New and Safe Method of Communicating the Small-pox by Inoculation, lately Invented and Brought into Use," PT 29 (1716): 207–10.

5 Genevieve Miller, *The Adoption of Inoculation for Smallpox in England and France* (Philadelphia: University of Pennsylvania Press, 1957), 67–8, 72, 92, 173; Apx 2: Vater (1721; Reimann (1723); Wreden (1723, 1724); "Methode," (1726); Seip (1727).

6 Apx 2: Reimann (1723), 253–5.

7 Johann T. Eller, *Observationes de cognoscendis et curandis morbis, praesertim acutis* (Königsberg and Leipzig: Woltersdorff, 1762), 150.

8 Eller, 151–2.

children and an adult in Hanover, mostly in conjunction with King George I's local *Leibarzt* August Johann Hugo and sometimes with the court physician Christian Siegmund Wolff.[9]

Another contemporary report, by Dr. Johann Philipp Seip, describes the inoculation in 1725 of an orphan in his care in Pyrmont. The smallpox outbreak that prompted Seip's action happened to coincide with one of King George I's visits to the local mineral springs accompanied by his body surgeon, J.E. Wreden's father, who agreed to carry out the inoculation.[10] The requisite permission was obtained from Prince Friedrich Anton of Waldeck and Pyrmont, who showed considerable interest by travelling the 115 kilometres from Waldeck to Pyrmont with several officials to witness the procedure.[11] Later in 1725 another twelve children were inoculated in Ansbach, by the court physician Christian Ludwig Rosa, at the request of the Regent of Brandenburg-Ansbach, Margravine Christiane Charlotte. The details of that group inoculation, which was the largest in Germany at the time, were provided in an anonymous doctor's account published in the following year.[12] The involvement of princely courts was a notable common feature of all of those inoculations reported in Germany during the 1720s.

The Wittenberg anatomy professor Abraham Vater (Figure 10) looms large as a prominent early promoter of inoculation. He was the author of not only the first German book (1721) on the topic but also of the first German dissertation about inoculation, which was defended in 1720 by his students Johann Heinrich Ulrici and Carl Hieronymus Stoll.[13] In his book, Vater recounts the history of inoculation among the Greek community of Constantinople, as told by Dr. Jacob Pylarini. He relates how Pylarini was in the city during the deadly smallpox epidemic of 1701 when he was asked by his friend Caryophyllum, a Greek nobleman, about the traditional procedure used by a culturally distinct group of local women to prevent severe smallpox in their children. Though he had never heard of the procedure, Pylarini saw no reason to advise his friend against trying it. Caryophyllum proceeded to seek out a woman with the requisite experience to inoculate his four daughters, and was gratified and relieved at the successful outcome. As the good news spread around his community, other parents followed his lead and were also pleased with the results,

9 Apx 2: Wreden (1723); Wreden (1724), 60–78; see Wolff (1726), 207–8, for an eyewitness account of Wreden's inoculations.

10 Miller, *Adoption*, 177–8.

11 Apx 2: Seip (1727), 235–41.

12 Apx 2: "Methode," (1726), 130–6.

13 Apx 1: Vater (1720). Apx 2: Vater (1721).

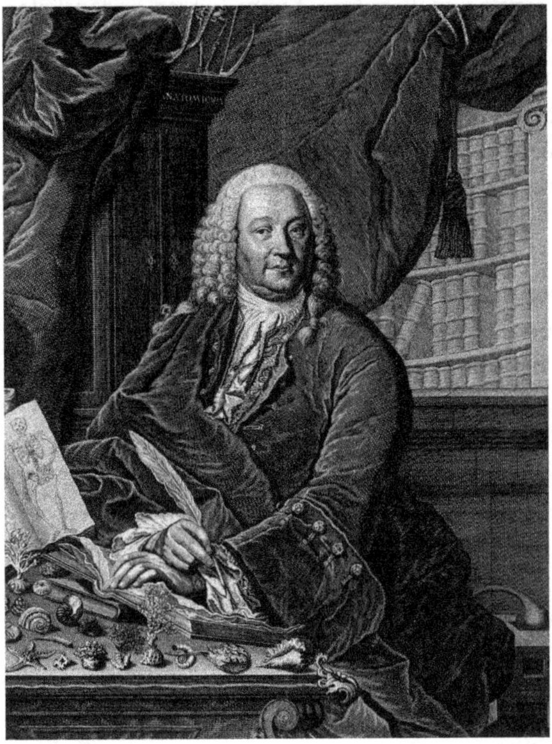

FIGURE 10
Abraham Vater, 1752. Engraving by J.M. Bernigeroth
WELLCOME COLLECTION: 93621. PUBLIC DOMAIN MARK

leading to inoculation practice becoming traditional among Greek mothers in Constantinople.[14]

Vater acknowledges with regret that many of his countrymen believed in not only the plethora of magic 'cures' and superstitious practices related to smallpox but also in the religious preconceptions that contradicted the very idea of prophylaxis. His laments about the nature of some common religious beliefs are supported by a dissertation published in 1713 in which the Urach (Württemburg) *Stadtphysikus* Immanuel Weißman rails at the people's failure to recognise that they themselves controlled the means for preventing smallpox. Weißman pointedly advises them to mend their sinful ways in order to remove any reason for God to inflict smallpox as punishment.[15] Such views being expressed by a *Physikus* with responsibilities for public health underscores the magnitude of the task of persuading the general public that severe smallpox could be prevented by inoculation.

---

14 Apx 2: Vater (1721), 9–11.

15 Immanuel Weißmann, *Fata & imposturae variolosorum. Oder Muthmaßliche Gedanken und Ursachen, Wie? Und Warum? Manche Leute die sogenannte Urschlechten oder Kinds-Blattern als ein Göttliches Straff-Gericht nicht erkennen* (Ulm: Bartholomeo, 1713), 4–11.

At that time, when smallpox was widely believed to be innate, and inflicted by God, Professor Vater asserted that the disease was actually a contagious fever spread by miasma, contact, or sweat, and that inoculation could provide a major benefit by lessening the dreadful suffering from the affliction.[16] He reinforced his pro-inoculation stance by translating (1723) the Reverend Benjamin Colman's detailed account of Dr. Zabdiel Boylston's controversial inoculations in Boston two years earlier, in which Colman highlighted the mildness of inoculated smallpox compared with the severe disease that caused so many deaths among his parishioners.[17] Twenty-four years later, Vater welcomed a new appointee to the professorial ranks at Wittenberg, Daniel Wilhelm Triller, who turned out to be an inoculation opponent and great admirer of the like-minded Professor Anton de Haen from Vienna.[18] Triller scoured not only the medical literature but also religious tracts for evidence to support his own dislike of inoculation, when the procedure was becoming more widely practised. He laid out his objections quite clearly in his lengthy treatise in rhyming couplets, with copious footnotes, in which he asserts repeatedly that inoculation was audacious interference in God's prerogative to inflict smallpox, while also providing valid medical reasons for opposing the practice.[19]

When interest in inoculation began to wane after the intial publication flurry during 1721–26, the focus of the commentary turned to re-visitations of past 'inoculation events.' A particular focus was placed on the 'Newgate experiment' carried out on condemned prisoners in London in 1721, which was first reported in Germany in the following year by two eyewitnesses, the Königsberg doctor Matthias Ernst Boretius and King George I's *Leibarzt* Johann Georg Steigerthal who was involved in the trial.[20] The Duke of Brunswick-Lüneburg's *Leibarzt* Conrad Berthold Behrens revisited the Newgate inoculations, in 1727, and Abraham Vater added the trial to the revised edition (1741) of his book describing inoculation in Turkey that he had published twenty years earlier. The Newgate inoculations were also highlighted by the Prussian court apothecary Caspar Neumann in his brief but glowing assessment of inoculation in early-1720s England, from the viewpoint of mid-1740s Germany where the practice had long been dormant.[21]

16 Apx 2: Vater (1721), 18–19, 34.

17 Benjamin Colman, *A Narrative of the Method and Success of Inoculating the Small-Pox in New England, with a reply to the Objections made against it from Principles of Conscience* (Dublin: Grierson, 1722), 19–21; Apx 2: Colman, trans. Vater (1723).

18 Apx 2: Triller (1766), 155–6, 165, n., 167, n. Kurt Sprengel, *Versuch einer pragmatischen Geschichte der Arzneikunde*, part 5 (Halle: Gebauer, 1803), 606.

19 Triller, 3, 12–15, 42–4, 55–8, 60–1, 111, 135–6, 211–12.

20 Apx 2: Boretius (1722); Steigerthal (1722).

21 Apx 2: Behrens (1727); Vater (1741); Neumann (1745).

Reports reaching Britain in the 1730s showed that inoculation was by no means in abeyance in the American Colonies and the Caribbean, where it was being used quite extensively and was valued for the protection of slaves.[22] The sheer number of candidates involved became clear from Dr. James Kirkpatrick's account, under the name Kilpatrick, of at least 800 inoculations carried out in South Carolina in 1738 by several doctors including himself. A German review of Kirkpatrick's book focusses primarily on the low number of deaths, just eight, among so many inoculated individuals.[23] Kirkpatrick credits Dr. Mowbray with not only introducing the practice in the area at that time but also with the greatest number of inoculations, pointing out too that most were carried out without any prior 'preparation.'[24] Another innovation was the effective use of pustular material from inoculated individuals, the kind of inoculum previously believed too weak to be effective.[25]

Kirkpatrick's arrival in London in 1742 to promote his book helped to encourage renewed demand for inoculation, which was already being reported in parts of southern England and Northern Ireland in response to localised smallpox outbreaks. A deadly epidemic of the disease in Britain during 1751–53 provided further impetus for an expansion of inoculation not only there but also in Europe, where news of the benefits of the practice was also spreading.[26] The resurgence in German publications about inoculation began with a trickle of reviews (1750–51) of new books from Britain, followed by translated publications and more reviews of books from not only Britain but also from America, France, and the Swiss Confederation. The publication flow soon became a flood that reached an initial peak in 1757 as smallpox swept across Europe generating interest in the new method of preventing a severe case of the disease. The subsequent reduction in output as the epidemic faded gave rise to the peak and trough publication pattern that was repeated during and after other severe smallpox epidemics, in the mid-1760s, -1780s, and -1790s.[27]

Translators of the books and articles made a vitally important contribution to the recommencement of inoculation in Germany by making the foreign specialists' methods readily available to interested medical men.[28] Translated

22 Michael J. Bennett, *War Against Smallpox. Edward Jenner and the Early Global Spread of Vaccination* (Cambridge: Cambridge University Press, 2020), 55.

23 James Kilpatrick (Kirkpatrick), *Essay on Inoculation Occasioned by the Smallpox being brought into South-Carolina in the Year 1738* (London: Huggenson, 1743), 34; Review of *Essay*, by Kilpatrick, *Neuer Zeitungen von gelehrten Sachen, Leipzig*, part 1 (1744): 701–2.

24 Kilpatrick, 44.

25 Kilpatrick, 50.

26 Bennett, *War*, 34–7.

27 The peak-and-trough pattern is evident from the publication list in Apx 2.

28 For prominent foreign inoculators' works translated and published in Germany, see in Apx 2, from Britain: James Kirkpatrick (1756), Richard Mead (1756), James Burges (1756),

British accounts of inoculation matters featured prominently in the 1750s-70s, particularly in journals published in towns with close trade, political, and academic links to Britain. Perhaps those British links were instrumental in placing Bremen, Brunswick, Hamburg, Hanover, and Göttingen at the forefront of inoculation practice and discussion when the procedure was still unknown in many other regions. Indeed, journals from those five towns collectively published half of the translated and foreign-language articles about inoculation during the 1750s-70s, and almost two-thirds of the reviews.[29]

Some translators and editors appealed to the public fascination with faraway lands during those interesting times of exploration and discovery, by offering accounts of foreign inoculation customs. The English doctor John Zephaniah Holwell's description of the method used in Bengal, anonymous reports of inoculation practices in China, and an account by Pastor Charles Chais from The Hague of the procedure used on the Barbary Coast and in the East Indies showed German readers that inoculation was far more widely-practised than many would have believed.[30] That perception was reinforced by the British Ambassador John Porter's reports of inoculation in Georgia, accounts of inoculation in Livonia, and a revisitation of Timoni's and Pylarini's respective reports in 1714–15 of inoculation in Constantinople.[31] Aberrant outcomes of inoculations in France described in a journal specialising in exceptional medical cases of general interest attracted attention in the late-1750s, a time when the practice was highly controversial in some regions and still unfamiliar in many others.[32]

Henry Bracken (1758, 1759, 1760), Ebenezer Gilchrist (1758), Alexander Monro (1766), William Watson and Thomas Glass (1769), Thomas Dimsdale (1768, 1769, 1782), William Baylies (1776), John Mudge (1778), Charles Roe (1786), and John Haygarth (1786, 1799); from the Swiss Confederation: Samuel-Auguste Tissot (1756, 1768, 1770, 1778); from Sweden: David Schultz (1762, 1769) and Nils Rosén von Rosenstein (1768, 1778); from Denmark: Christian Friis Rotböll (1767); from The Netherlands: Hieronymus Gaub (1767); from France: Ambrose Hosty (1757, 1758, 1759), and Angelo Gatti (1772, 1782); from Philadelphia: Benjamin Rush (1783), and Thomas Bond (1787).

29 See articles listed in Apx 2, in the following journals: *BM*, from Bremen; *BA* and its successors *GB* and *BRM*, from Brunswick; *HUC, HAM, Neues HAM, Neues MF,* and *HJ*, from Hamburg; *NS* and its successors *HB* and *HM*, from Hanover; *GA*, from Göttingen.

30 Apx 2: "Nachricht" (1756); Holwell (1769); Chais (1770).

31 Apx 2: Porter (1755, 1757, 1758, 1777); Eisen (1771); "Von den Blatterimpfung" (1774); Timoni (1757); "Die Geschichte" (1774).

32 *Sammlung auserlesene Wahrnehmungen aus der Arzneywissenschaft, der Wundarzneykunst und des Apothekerkunst* (*SAW*) was published in Germany in the 1750s and moved in 1761 to Strasburg; see in Apx 2 four articles in *SAW* in 1757, two in 1758, one in 1759, and one in 1760.

German translators tended to show great enthusiasm for inoculation, in the dedication of their works and in their usually lengthy introductions, and seemed very selective about the opinions they chose to translate.[33] The rarity of German translations of works opposed to inoculation is evident in the treatment of the set of questions posed in 1757 by the prominent inoculation opponent Professor Anton de Haen, director of the main hospital in Vienna, in response to the Swiss physician Samuel-Auguste Tissot's tract in favour of inoculation.[34] While de Haen's questions in Latin were translated into French, Dutch, and Swedish, according to the Berlin doctor Johann Georg Krünitz's comprehensive list (1768) of publications about inoculation, Krünitz mentions no German translation. Yet Tissot's pro-inoculation arguments, originally in French, were translated and published in 1756 by Friedrich Simon Morgenstern and by an anonymous author.[35] Similarly, Count Francesco Roncalli-Parolino's Latin tract (1759) arguing that more people died from inoculation than were saved was published in Germany only in a Latin journal, and the reviews were limited to periodicals aimed toward intellectuals. Tissot's defence of inoculation against the Italian doctor's assertions, by comparison, was translated into German in its entirety and published as a book (1771).[36]

The translation of high-profile foreign doctors' pro-inoculation tracts into German but not the anti-inoculation views of their equally high-profile counterparts, at a time when inoculation was a relative novelty in Germany, underscores the powerful position of the translators in shaping attitudes to inoculation among the reading public. Not only the highly-educated translators but also the journal owners and editors would have been well-aware that inoculation-related articles were no longer read exclusively by university-educated men equipped with rhetorical skills. They would have also known that less-educated readers from a public reputed to be easily swayed by prejudice and superstition probably lacked the ability to recognise, evaluate, and

33 Apx 2: Tissot, trans. Baldinger (1768); Dimsdale, trans. Tiemann (1768); Schultz, trans. Murray (1769); Gardane, trans. Opitz (1775); Baylies, trans. Krünitz (1776), de Villiers, trans. Fritze (1776).

34 Anton de Haen, *Quaestiones saepius motae super methodo inoculandi variolas, ad quas directa eruditorum responsa hucusque desiderantur; indirecta minus satisfacere videntur: orbi medico denuo proposita* (Vienna: Trattner, 1757); Samuel-Auguste D. Tissot, *L'Inoculation justifiée, ou dissertation pratique et apologétique sur cette méthode* (Lausanne: Bousquet, 1754).

35 Johann G. Krünitz, *Verzeichniß der vornehmsten Schriften von der Kinderpocken und deren Einpfropfung* (Leipzig: Hilscher, 1768), 121–2, 154–5; Apx 2: Tissot, trans. Morgenstern (1756); "Bestätigende Abhandlung" (1756); reviews of de Haen (1758, 1760, 1764).

36 Krünitz, 147–8; Apx 2: reviews of Roncalli-Parolino (1758, 1761); de Redern's refutation of Roncalli-Parolino (1765); Tissot's refutation of Roncalli-Parolino (1771).

discount unenlightened opinions.[37] A desire to encourage a positive public attitude to inoculation was an obvious motivation for the translators' and publishers' resistance to disseminating views to the contrary. Considering that not only the translators, but also the publishers of the new kinds of generally-targeted journals were usually part of the progressive new intelligentsia known to embrace inoculation like a proud badge of Enlightenment, there was indeed little likelihood that such men would spend their time translating or publishing views with which they disagreed. Possible reputational damage from attaching their name to someone else's negative opinions about inoculation was another consideration.[38] Alternatively, many translators may have grown tired of the seemingly endless debates, believing that readers would prefer to learn of positive personal experiences of inoculation or other aspects of the practice.

The near-disappearance of translated articles about inoculation from German journals by 1784 along with a sharp decline in translated books on the topic left readers largely reliant on reviews to keep abreast of developments in neighbouring and distant states.[39] That trend shifted the power to shape public opinion about inoculation from the translators choosing which works to translate, to the editors deciding which works to publish. Editors of the dedicated review journals that were increasing in number during the 1760s-1800 were in a particularly strong position to influence public opinion, through their ability to not only select which publications their journal would review but also to choose the reviewers. The surge in book production at the time offered those editors even greater influence by limiting the proportion of the new books that their journal was capable of reviewing. [40] Nor was it pure chance that the publishers of the dedicated review journals tended to base their respective enterprises in Protestant university towns, where an abundant supply of potential reviewers held opinions with which the publishers and their editors were likely to agree.[41]

---

37 Laments about prejudice and superstition even extended to doctors' educated acquaintances: Friedrich S. Kretschmar, *Irrthumer, Warnungen, und Lehren* (Würzburg, Bamberg, Fulda: Stahel, 1770), 1–2; G.B. Schäffer, "Ueber medizinisches Aufklärung," *neues HM* 2 (1792): 1393–4; Apx 2: Ziegler (1776), 5–6.

38 For contemporary perceptions of links between Enlightenment ideology and inoculation, see Christoph W. Hufeland, "Neue Aussicht zur Vertilgung der Blattern," *TM* 4 (1786): 167–8; Apx 2: de Reden (1765), 82–3; Tode (1785), 24.

39 Wilhelm G. Ploucquet, *Literatura Medica Digesta*, vol. 4 (Tübingen: Cotta, 1809), 270–8. The trend is also evident in the chronology of references listed in Apx 2.

40 Helga Brandes, "The Literary Marketplace and the Journal," in *German Literature of the Eighteenth Century: The Enlightenment and Sensibility*, ed. Barbara Becker-Cantarino (Rochester: Camden House, 2005), 97.

41 Altenburg, Erlangen, Göttingen, Greifswald, Halle, Helmstedt, Jena, Leipzig, Nuremberg, Rostock, and Tübingen were Protestant university towns hosting publishers of review journals.

A number of the prominent literary review journals shared an underlying agenda to promote secular ideas in line with the humanist philosophy of the Enlightenment. One was *Allgemeine deutsche Bibliothek* (ADB), which was established and controlled along those lines by Friedrich Nicolai from Berlin who was well known as an outspoken defender of free speech and rationalist ideology.[42] The *Göttingische Anzeigen von gelehrten Sachen* (GA) supported similarly progressive ideas from Göttingen academics enjoying the freedom to think and write, which was enshrined in the university's foundation statute denying the theology faculty the traditional right of censorship.[43] The University of Jena's literary review journal *Allgemeine Literatur-Zeitung* (ALZ) had a similarly progressive outlook, having been established with an agenda to promote Kantian philosophy.[44] The strongly secular bias of ADB, GA, and ALZ ensured that the reviewers had little tolerance for religiously-based arguments opposing inoculation. Indeed, they seemed to relish the cloak of anonymity that gave them the freedom to display their well-honed rhetorical skills and linguistic flair in issuing criticisms of opinions they regarded as unenlightened.[45]

The intellectuals who shared the agenda of men such as Nicolai, to implement social change according to such Enlightenment ideals as the subversion of prejudice and superstition by reason, formed a highly influential new stratum in German society.[46] Such men known for holding progressive ideas were commonly employed as officials of benevolent governments, where they wielded a great deal of influence.[47] That well-educated cohort of enlightened intelligentsia included the censors employed by the pro-inoculation government of Brunswick-Wolfenbüttel during the 1760s-70s, who ensured that no articles expressing an anti-inoculation viewpoint were published in the duchy during the mid-1760s-70s when inoculation was being officially promoted.[48]

---

42 Brandes, 96–7; Rainer Baasner, *Einführung in die Literatur der Aufklärung* (Darmstadt: Wissenschaftliche Buchgesellschaft, 2006), 52–4.

43 Emil F. Rössler, *Die Gründung der Universität Göttingen* (Göttingen: Vandenhoek and Ruprecht, 1855), 24–6.

44 Theodore Ziolkowski, *German Romanicism and its Institutions* (Princeton: Princeton University Press, 1990), 235–6.

45 Review of *Sendschreiben, Beantwortung der Frage: Was ist von den Impf-Predigern und von Empfehlung der Blatter-Einimpfung auf der Kanzel zu halten? Von zween Freunden der Wahrheit*, by Christian G. Hauck, ADB 38, part 2 (1779): 445–6; Baasner, *Einführung*, 52–3.

46 Tim C.W. Blanning, *The Culture of Power and the Power of Culture; Old-Regime Europe, 1660–1789* (Oxford: Oxford University Press, 2002), 199–209, 225–6; Peter Watson, *The German Genius* (London: Simon and Schuster, 2010), 53–4, 87–8.

47 Blanning, 206–7.

48 Peter Albrecht, "Von den vergeblichen Mühen, die Bevölkerung der Stadt Braunschweig von der Nützlichkeit des Impfens gegen Blattern zu überzeugen (1754–1787)," in *Gotts*

2 Intellectuals, Doctors, and the Public Have Their Say

Translators with an interest in inoculation presented not only foreign doctors' views and methods to the public but also many commentaries on the ethics and morality of inoculation.[49] The most translated and reviewed tract of that kind was Charles Marie de la Condamine's (Figure 11) address to the Academy of Sciences in Paris in 1754, which gave rise to many other publications emanating from the ideas presented.[50] Indeed, the widespread impact of that address ranks it as arguably the most significant 'inoculation event' in Europe. La Condamine's main points were: whether inoculation produced a 'true' disease that would protect against future smallpox, the possibility of transmitting an additional, unwanted, disease in the inoculum, problems of ulcers and other lasting ill-effects from the inoculation incision, whether the induction of an illness that otherwise arose naturally could be regarded as interference in

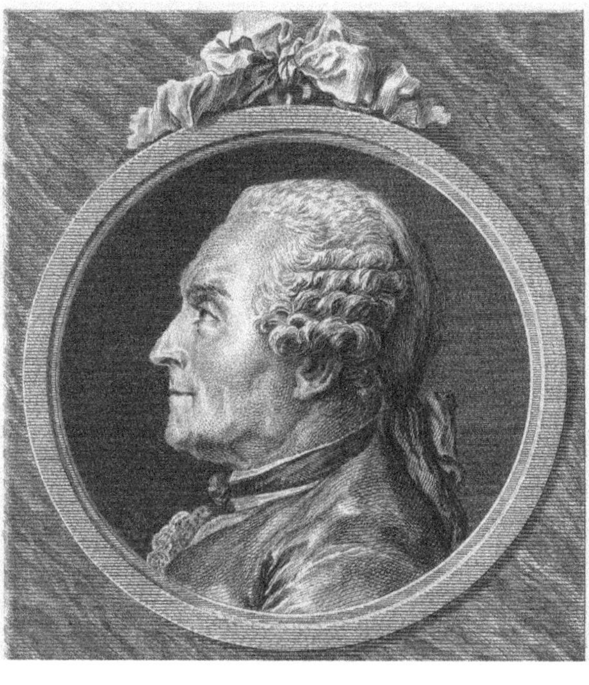

FIGURE 11
Charles Marie de la Condamine. Engraving by C.N. Cochin II, after C.N. Cochin I
RIJKSMUSEUM, AMSTERDAM: RP-P-1908-4598

Verhengnis und seine Straffe – zur Geschichten der Seuche in der frühen Neuzeit, ed. Petra Feuerstein-Herz (Wolfenbüttel: Herzog August Bibliothek, 2005), 128.

49 Apx 2: Bishop of Worcester (1753); La Condamine (1755, 1756, 1762); Chais (1765, 1770, 1774); Cramer (1759, 1760, 1762).

50 Krünitz, *Verzeichniß*, 109–10; Apx 2: La Condamine (1755, 1756, 1762); reviews of La Condamine (1754, 1760); reviews of Cantwell's response (1757); Letter from Mallet (1760).

Providence, and the moral issue of giving a dangerous disease to a child who may otherwise never experience it. In his discussion, he reveals his own view that the advantages of inoculation far outweigh the disadvantages.[51] While his fame as an Amazon explorer and mathematician may have attracted much initial attention to his speech, his intuitive approach to inoculation justified the widespread acclaim. In Germany, where inoculation was hardly known at the time, La Condamine's timely and crucially important exposition of the pros and contras of the practice shaped the inoculation discourse.[52]

La Condamine's presentation of the medical, moral, religious, ethical, and philosophical issues surrounding inoculation prompted responses from a number of high-profile commentators. One German who professed an opinion was Johann Heinrich Gottlob von Justi who later became known as a pioneer of cameralist thought. During the early stage of his career (1755) when he was lecturing at Göttingen, Justi addressed the issue at the heart of La Condamine's speech, giving his own assurances that inoculation would confer total protection from future smallpox.[53] His vote of confidence was undoubtedly an attempt to counter the common assertions that smallpox returned to inoculated individuals, which were used by inoculation opponents to justify their claims that the procedure was futile.[54] Another of La Condamine's points, the moral dilemma of parents endangering their children's lives, was addressed in a translated journal articles by Pastor Johann Andreas Cramer from the Danish Royal Court and by the like-minded Pastor Charles Chais from the French Reformed Church in The Hague.[55] Those pastors' religious arguments in favour of inoculation contributed to the widespread 'inoculation debates' of the 1750s-60s, as did the Swiss mathematician Dr. Daniel Bernoulli's calculations of the increased life expectancy that could be achieved by inoculation.[56]

---

51 Apx 2: La Condamine (1756), 40–62, 74–5.

52 Maehle, "Attitudes," 200; Albrecht, "Blatterninokulation," 59–60. La Condamine's views inspired official 'inoculation action' in Paris, Sweden, and Florence: Miller, *Adoption*, 211; Peter Skold, *The Two Faces of Smallpox, A Disease and its Prevention in Eighteenth and Nineteenth-Century Sweden* (Umea: Umea University Press, 1996), 260; Klebs, *Variolation*, 59.

53 Apx 2: Justi (1755), 169–71. For Justi's later recommendations about curbing infectious diseases as a way of preventing population loss, see Ursula Backhaus, "Johann Heinrich Gottlob von Justi (1717–1771): Health as a part of a State's Capital Endowment," in *The Beginnings of Political Economy*, ed. Jürgen G. Backhaus (New York: Springer, 2009), 181–2.

54 Apx 2: Review of *Noodig Bericht*, by Schwenk (1756), 253–4; Schwager, "Patriotische" (1786), 207; Klose (1786), 414; "Ueber" (1792), 123–4.

55 Apx 2: La Condamine (1755, 1756, 1762); Chais (1765, 1770, 1774); Cramer (1759, 1760, 1762).

56 Sally Blower, "Classic Paper: An Attempt at a New Analysis of the Mortality Caused by Smallpox and of the Advantages of Inoculation to Prevent it, by Daniel Bernoulli," *Reviews in Medical Virology* 14 (2004): 278.

The *philosophe* Jean le Rond d'Alembert's tract, in which he questioned the assumptions on which the probability theory pioneer Bernoulli had based his model, was translated and serialised in four consecutive issues of a broadly-targeted journal from Hanover as well as being summarised in a Brunswick-based journal. D'Alembert's queries gave rise to assumptions that he opposed inoculation, though he had queried only Bernoulli's model and not taken issue with inoculation *per se*.[57]

La Condamine was criticised anonymously (1756) by one German inoculation advocate for failing to discredit the commonly held doubts about the 'cleansing capacity' of mild inoculated smallpox.[58] Such doubts, which were based on the longstanding belief that the biological mechanism of smallpox was to cleanse the body of 'contaminants' thought to predispose to future diseases, were shared by Dr. J.G. Büscher who appealed (1755) for answers from an authority on the matter. The Göttingen professor Georg Matthiä responded to Büscher's concerns with a solid refutation of the popular notion that mild inoculated smallpox lacked the power to achieve complete 'cleansing,' and that the residual 'contaminants' predisposed to acute fevers such as tuberculosis, typhus, ague, and other diseases.[59] Büscher's and Matthiä's informative question-and-answer articles in the Hanover-based *Nützliche Sammlung* (NS) prompted the journal's editors to revisit the matter in 1760–61 with a new set of articles by those authors.[60] Considering that fears of future ill-health were frequently cited as reasons for rejection of inoculation, such discussions and expert explanations in the generally-targeted periodicals were vitally important for allaying public concerns.[61] Of course, not all doctors agreed with Matthiä's opinion. Professor Ernst Platner from Leipzig argued (1786) that inadequate 'cleansing' by inoculated smallpox caused stupidity, lassitude, and infertility in elite adolescents and young adults, an assertion he based purely on the higher inoculation rates among that group in which such characteristics were 'observed' than in other social groups.[62]

---

57 Apx 2: D'Alembert, *HM* (1768); *GB* (1768), 25–32.

58 Apx 2: "Bestätigende Abhandlung" (1756), 1068.

59 Apx 2: Büscher (1755), 747; Matthiä (1756), 1229–31.

60 Apx 2: Büscher (1760); Matthiä (1761).

61 Apx 2: Matthiä (1761), 1225; "Etwas" (1777), 305; Klose (1786), 413–4; Migula, "Noch etwas" (1787), 411–12.

62 Anton von Haen and Ernst Platner, *Anton von Haen's kaiserlichen Leibarztes Heilungsmethode, in dem kaiserlichen Krankenhaus zu Wien,* vol. 5 (Leipzig: Weygand, 1782), 438. For a refutation of Platner's arguments, see in Apx 2: Schwager, "Noch etwas" (1786), 535–40, 544–49.

German churchmen and philosophers considered inoculation too, though their ideas about the ethics and morality of the practice often lay buried for many years. The Göttingen-based Lutheran church historian Johann Lorenz von Mosheim concluded in favour of inoculation as early as 1752, well before La Condamine popularised the topic. Yet his deliberations first emerged eighteen years later in a set of extracts from his seven-volume theological work.[63] Similarly, the Berlin church official Johann Peter Süßmilch's favourable assessment of inoculation (1761–62), culminating in his recommendation of the practice as a means for curbing population loss, was buried in his two-volume tract on the economic benefits of increasing a state's population.[64] The consistorial adviser Johann Jacob Plitt from Frankfurt ensured that his own assessment of the religious and moral issues pertaining to inoculation (1768) was not similarly left to languish, by publishing it under the title "Can Smallpox Inoculation be undertaken in Good Conscience?"[65] Plitt's pronouncements showing that the Christian religion approved of inoculation, along with similar statements from other high-ranking church officials were acknowledged by several doctors who used such authoritative pronouncements to allay religious concerns raised by parents considering inoculation.[66]

A number of other German churchmen promoted inoculation during the 1760s-70s from a humanitarian rather than a religious viewpoint. Pastor Johann Friedrich Danneil from Quedlinburg concluded from his comprehensive comparison of naturally-acquired and inoculated smallpox (1769) that inoculation was an indisputably better choice than passively awaiting the natural disease.[67] His counterpart from Altenburg (Saxony), Pastor Gotthilf Friedemann Löber, recommended inoculation in a context of its importance as an integral part of any approach to addressing the pressing need to care for children's health.[68] The Prussian prelate from Halberstadt, Friedrich Eberhard von Rochow, adopted the novel approach of promoting inoculation in a children's book (1779). He relates a fictional conversation in which a teacher gives a simple explanation of inoculation and its benefits to a father, in response to

---

63 Apx 2: Mosheim (1770), 177–85.

64 Johann P. Süßmilch, *Die göttliche Ordnung in den Veränderungen des menschlichen Geschlechts, aus der Geburt, dem Tode und der Fortpflanzung desselben erwiesen*, 2nd ed., vol. 2 (Berlin: Buchhandlung der Realschule, 1762), 440–3.

65 Apx 2: Plitt (1768).

66 Apx 2: Opitz (1774), 32; Hirschel (1770), 2–3; Baldinger (1768), 16th–17th page of (unnumbered) introduction.

67 Apx 2: Danneil (1769), 53.

68 Apx 2: Löber (1769).

the man's comment about his astonishment at the mildness of his daughter's inoculated smallpox. Rochow intuitively includes multiple references to the pastor's approval of the child's inoculation, as a way of countering the common religiously-based anti-inoculation prejudices.[69]

The economic and humanitarian benefits of saving lives through inoculation was the focus of two very different publications in the 1770s by two prominent lawyers. Erhard Friedrich Weinland from Württemburg proposed an expansion of inoculation as a way of achieving population increase, in his book (1770): "The Benefits to a State from Smallpox Inoculation." He dedicated the work, which explores the links between public health, population, and prosperity, to Duke Carl Eugen of Württemburg in the hope of convincing the duke that inoculation would benefit his state.[70] The high-profile Osnabrück jurist and social commentator Justus Möser underscored the benefits of inoculation in quite a different way, using intuitive satire suggesting that he agreed with the notion of God inflicting smallpox in order to limit population growth. Adopting the device of an open letter to "a young married woman," Möser 'justifies' the argument that "it was not without reason that wise Providence introduced smallpox to the world," with this 'advice' to the fictional young mother:[71]

> Now my dear child! I will say nothing more against it, the earlier the better you let your dozen little children be inoculated with smallpox, all my wholehearted wishes are with you. But afterwards, make sure you find husbands for your eight girls. I shall tell you in advance that not one of them will die; our doctors understand that method so well and are much too competent to give you even one exception. Where will it end, when it keeps going this way; when the children who are now alive reproduce at the same rate and none are killed? Before that, a good mother would thank God when He shared them with her and also took another little lamb.[72]

69 Friedrich E. von Rochow, *Der Kinderfreund, ein Lesebuch zum Gebrauch in Landschulen* (Frankfurt; Eichenberg, 1779), 52–7.

70 Apx 2: Weinland (1770).

71 Apx 2: Möser (1783), 39–43. See p. 37 for other discussion of this publication. Common notions of the divine purpose for smallpox are also noted in Juncker, *Archiv*, 3:113–4, 123–4; Johann C. W. Juncker, *Gemeinnützige Vorschläge wider die Pockenkrankheit. Dritter Versuch, für möglichst alle Aerzte, die der deutschen Sprache kundig sind* (Halle: Hemmerde and Schwetscke, 1796), 353–71.

72 Möser, 39–40.

Möser also lampoons the aristocracy by 'advising' them that inoculating their children would allow the survival of many more male aristocrats than the army could accommodate in the special officers' roles created for them, and would push female heirs even further down the pecking order than usual.[73] His clever irony in 'disapproving' of inoculation with arguments that highlighted and applauded the specialists' skills was indeed an ingenious way of underscoring the lifesaving potential of the practice. Möser's choice of journal for the publication of his article, the *Berlinische Monatsschrift*, which was edited by the secretary of the exclusive Berlin *Mittwochgesellschaft* for 'men of the Enlightenment,' ensured that at least some like-minded readers would correctly interpret and appreciate his irony.[74]

The morality of inoculation was revisited in the 1790s not only in relation to the perennial concern of potential fatal outcomes but also with regard to the spread of the contagion from inoculated individuals.[75] Professor Johann Christian Wilhelm Juncker from Halle sought opinions from Immanuel and Kant and from five of his own counterparts in the philosophy faculty, on the issues of concern. Although he recorded no reply from Kant, he received well-considered responses from the Halle philosophers.[76] Johann Gebhard Maaß expressed his approval of inoculation, though only by doctors, as a way of assuring the best protection of the candidates, and recommended government involvement in ensuring the containment of the smallpox contagion. Johann Christoph Hoffbauer argued that everybody has a duty to protect their own life, thus accepting a lesser danger is preferable to risking a greater danger, and that adults have a duty to apply that principle to children. He also stressed the importance of inoculated individuals not infecting others, as did his colleagues Johann August Eberhard and Ludwig Heinrich Jakob, which was a reflection of the broader late-1790s discourse.[77] Johann Heinrich Tieftrunk was the only one of the five Halle philosophers opposed to inoculation. He too addressed the issue of contagiousness, arguing that inoculation would prevent the achievement of the ultimate goal with regard to smallpox: the eradication of the disease. Another of his objections was that the inoculation of children who had

73 Möser, 40.

74 Richard van Dulmen, *The Society of the Enlightenment, the Rise of the Middle Class and Enlightenment Culture in Germany* (Cambridge: Polity, 1992), 98–9.

75 Apx 2: Michaelis (1792), 313–26. Heinrich Stephani, "Ist die Inoculation der Pocken auch nach reinsittlichen Grundsätzen erlaubt?," *RA* 2 (1798): 2119–21.

76 Johann C.W. Juncker, *Archiv der Aerzte und Seelsorger wider die Pockennoth*, vol. 7 (Leipzig: Weygand, 1799), 62–96.

77 Juncker, 7:57, 61–2, 65, 68–9, 86–9.

no say in the matter was unconscionable.[78] Immanuel Kant (†1804), who was seventy-four years-old when Juncker requested his opinion, had suggested a general disapproval of inoculation in his earlier pronouncements, for reasons other than contagiousness. Fragments of his writings in old age, after the introduction of cowpox vaccination, indicate that he still disapproved of any form of smallpox prophylaxis: "the wise application (of doctors' heroic measures) cannot be expected from individuals but must come from Providence, which seems to have wanted war and smallpox (indeed deliberately) to limit great population increase."[79]

Of course, doctors were among the most prolific commentators on inoculation matters in Germany. Most were supportive of inoculation, and those who opposed the practice usually offered good medical reasons for their stance, including Professor Triller, though Triller was better known for his religious objections.[80] Another inoculation opponent, *Leibarzt* Christian Gottlieb Selle who attended Friedrich II of Prussia in his last years, argued that inoculation may have caused more deaths than were immediately apparent, owing to residual disease-causing contaminants in the body.[81] Dr. Adam Samuel Thebesius from Hirschberg (Silesia) admits to having been an admirer of inoculation until he visited an 'inoculation institute' in Breslau in 1770. Appalled at seeing children at the 'institute' suffering in various ways from adverse effects of inoculation, he developed a sudden dislike of the procedure that was enhanced by reports of inoculated children contracting smallpox.[82] Cases of inoculation failing to offer protection, which were often due to incorrect diagnosis of the donor's pustular disease, continued to be a great concern to inoculation advocates.[83]

Provincial journals in regions where inoculation was undertaken during the 1750s-60s, particularly Hanover, Brunswick, and Hamburg, were a popular forum for doctors and other well-educated citizens to express an opinion,

78 Juncker, 7:75–9.

79 *der weise Gebrauch (von heroischer Mittel der Aerzte) kann nicht von einzelnen Menschen, sondern muß von der Vorsehung erwartet werden, welche Krieg und Kinderpocken (und zwar absichtlich) gewollt zu haben scheint, um groß Vermehrung der Menschen zu beschränken*: Heinrich Bohn, "Ueber Kant's Beziehungen zur Medizin," *Altpreussische Monatsschrift* 9 (1872): 624 (quote) –25.

80 Apx 2: Triller (1766), 12–15, 40–50, 53–8, 111, 135–6, 147, and elsewhere.

81 Christian Gottlieb Selle, *Medicina Clinica oder Handbuch der medicinischen Praxis* (Berlin: Himburg, 1786), 119–20.

82 Apx 2: Thebesius (1788), 125–8. For 1760s reports of inoculated children catching smallpox, see in Apx 2: Linekogel (1766), 447–8; Löber (1767); Andreä and Bolten (1769), 297–8.

83 Apx 2: Wieland (1775): 279–92; Elsner (1787), 5, 27–8; Henschel (1795), 13.

report their inoculation experiences, or ask questions to be answered in a later issue.[84] In some regions where inoculation began expanding later in response to increasingly frequent smallpox epidemics, a range of journals established in the 1780s-90s made a valuable contribution to the local inoculation discourse by encouraging a broader cross-section of society to air an opinion. A temporal geographic shift in general interest in the topic is evident from the regional stamp of the journals that published the greatest number of original German 'inoculation articles' in each decade during 1750–1800.

Table 1 shows that journals from Hanover and Brunswick, which were the most prolific publishers of articles about inoculation during the 1760s-70s, were eclipsed in the 1780s-90s by the new Silesian monthly journal established in 1785, the *Schlesiche Provizialblätter* (SP).

Indeed, the large increase in the total number of articles about inoculation in the 1780s and in the 1790s compared with the previous decades was largely due to the contribution from SP. The impressive initial output of 'inoculation articles' in SP had much to do with the establishment of the journal a year before virulent smallpox caused a great deal of suffering and death in the region. Inoculation was not widely known or practised in Silesia at that time, according to comments from several contributors.[85]

Not only was the regional stamp of the journals changing but also the nature of the 'inoculation articles.' Contributors reporting personal inoculation experiences, airing doubts, offering advice, promoting inoculation, or asking questions became the predominant kind of 'inoculation article' in several provincial journals established during the 1780s-90s, as editors responded to increasing public interest in the topic by encouraging 'average parents' to have their say. Contributors' questions were in many cases answered in a later issue, sometimes prompting debates between supporters and sceptics, which echoed the informative discussions in journals from other regions during the 1750s-60s.[86] Such interactions were valuable for not only informing readers about important aspects of inoculation but also for dispelling myths and rumours, as exemplified by a debate in SP in 1791. That discussion, stretching to

84 Question-and-answer articles from the 1750s–60s, in Apx 2: Büscher, *NS* (1755), and Matthiä, *NS* (1756); Büscher, *HB* (1760), and Matthiä, *HB* (1761); Kleine, *Neues HAM* (1769), and Bolten, *Neues HAM* (1769). Articles responding to matters raised in previous issues of a journal, in Apx 2: Brückmann, *GB* (1768); "Nochmalige," *GB* (1768); Crell, *GB* (1771); "Etwas," *BMN* (1777); Bytanus, *HM* (1776).

85 Apx 2: "Bericht," *SP* (1788), 293–5: "Waldenburg," *SP* (1790), 166; Migula, "Noch etwas," *SP* (1787), 428.

86 Apx 2: "Etwas," *BMN* (1777); Steiger, *SP* (1787); Künzel, *SP* (1788); Fein, *HM* (1788); Sintenis, *Neue BMN* (1790); "Ueber," *LM* (1792); Vasmer, Neues *HM* (1795).

TABLE 1 Journals with the most German articles about inoculation: 1750s–1800

Period	Journal (abbreviation)	Place (years) of publication	No. / total	Av. length
1753–60	*Nützliche Sammlungen* (NS) and *Hannoverische Beyträge* (HB)	Hanover (1756–59) Hanover (1759–62)	6/17	20pp.
	Fränkische Sammlung (FS)	Nuremberg (1755–68)	3/17	3pp.
	Für die Frau (FF)	Leipzig	2/17	8pp.
1761–70	*Gelehrte Beyträge zu den Braunschweigischen Anzeigen* (GB)	Brunswick (1761–88)	8/31	9pp.
	Hannoverisches Magazin (HM)	Hanover (1763–90)	8/31	8pp.
1771–80	*Hannoverisches Magazin* (HM)	Hanover (1763–90)	8/16	11pp.
	Gelehrte Beyträge zu den Braunschweigischen Anzeigen (GB)	Brunswick (1761–88)	3/16	10pp.
1781–90	*Schlesische Provinzialblätter* (SP)	Breslau (1785–1849)	15/41	7pp.
	Hannoverisches Magazin (HM)	Hanover (1763–90)	4/41	15pp.
	Deutsches Museum (DM)	Leipzig (1776–88)	4/41	15pp.
	Annalen der Braunschweig-Lüneburgisches Churlände (ABC)	Hanover (1787–95)	4/41	3pp.
1791–1800	*Schlesische Provinzialblätter* (SP)	Breslau (1785–1849)	18/38	8pp.
	Schleswig-Holsteinische Provinzialberichte (SHP) and *S-H Blätter für Polizei und Kultur* (SHB)	Hamburg-Altona (1791–98) (1799–1800)	5/38	3pp.
	Neues Hannoverisches Magazin (*Neues* HM)	Hanover (1791–1812)	4/38	18pp.

three articles, was pervaded by prejudiced rumours surrounding the death of one of eighteen children inoculated by a doctor in Hirschberg. The dead girl's father ended the blame and negativity with a defence of inoculation, pointing out that his daughter's death was caused by smallpox she contracted in the natural way at around the time of her inoculation.[87] Editors of other Silesian regional journals: *Lausitzisches Magazin* (LM) from Lusatia, the *Bunzlauische*

87 Apx 2: Rimann, *SP* (1791); "Blattern-Einimpfung," *SP* (1791); "Rettung," *SP* (1791); "Pocken-inoculation," *SP* (1791). For an earlier discussion, see in Apx 2: "Auszug," *TM* (1774); "Nöthige," *TM* (1775); Wieland, *TM* (1775).

Monatsschrift zum Nutzen und Vergnügen (BMN) from Bunzlau, and its successor *Neue* BMN attempted to counter common local prejudices about inoculation too, by occasionally publishing logical arguments addressing issues of concern.[88]

In the late-1790s when inoculation was increasingly familiar in Silesia, *SP* published a fictional short-story designed to attract readers' attention to important characteristics of smallpox and inoculation.[89] The anonymous author used the common dilemma of parents' opposing views hampering their decision-making, as a platform to issue several warnings about the destructive capacity and potential lethality of smallpox, and about the vagaries and contagiousness of the inoculated disease. The core theme of this domestic saga is the children's inoculation, which becomes a bargaining chip in a dispute over the wife's vanity and the husband's gambling. The main character is Julie, a mother who regards inoculation as unnecessary for her son and stepdaughter because she believes that a good diet, a healthy upbringing, and attentive nursing would see them safely through smallpox. Since her husband is very much in favour of inoculation, and Julie is seeking a way to convince him to stop gambling, she does him the favour of having the children inoculated while he is away, in the hope of shaming him into giving up his gambling habit.

As it turns out, the teenage Florentine has very mild symptoms while young Gustav has quite a severe disease that he passes to his mother, who barely survives. Julie's severe case of smallpox highlights not only the contagiousness of the inoculated disease but also the potential susceptibility of adults, an important warning considering that the German terms commonly used for smallpox, *Kinderblattern* and *Kinderpocken,* imply an illness of childhood.[90] The advantage of inoculation highlighted in this story is the preservation of women's faces from potentially severe damage; Florentine's beauty is actually enhanced after an inoculation that offers her the added bonus of a love affair and betrothal to the dashing young doctor who inoculates her. Her stepmother's bout of naturally-acquired smallpox, by comparison, has such a disastrous impact on her appearance that she fears becoming yet another victim of abandonment by a husband who cannot tolerate his wife's loss of beauty.[91] Julie's musing about whether her beauty was destroyed as divine punishment for her vanity, and the vehement denial from her husband Reinhold are a reminder

88 Apx 2: "Ueber," *LM* (1792); "Etwas von," *BMN* (1777); "Ueber Blattern," *Neue BMN* (1787).

89 Apx 2: "Die Inokulation" (1799), 499–523. For parental disagreements about inoculation, see in Apx 2: Sintenis (1790), 109–14; "Kurze Geschichte" (1790), 861–3.

90 "Die Inokulation," 501–4, 506, 509.

91 "Die Inokulation," 519.

that the notion of smallpox as divine punishment was no longer acceptable in polite society.[92] For this family, the inoculation episode not only served the purpose of putting an end to Reinhold's gambling, which was Julie's original aim, but it also brought love and happiness to Florentine as well as protecting both children from smallpox. The badly disfigured former beauty, Julie, was the only loser.

With the notable exception of *SP* and *Neues hannoverisches Magazin* (1791–1812), the greatest number of inoculation-related articles in the 1790s was published by two successive, short-lived journals established in Schleswig-Holstein (Table 1). Although the articles in those journals were, on average, quite brief, they were nonetheless important for informing the largely rural population of Schleswig-Holstein and the tiny principality of Eutin about inoculation matters in the region. The predominantly local focus of the newer provincial journals was quite a change from the 1750s-60s when the well-established journals paid more attention to inoculation methods, aberrant outcomes, foreign and past inoculation 'events,' high-profile commentators' opinions, and tales of inoculation in foreign lands. Although such articles served the important function of informing doctors and other well-educated readers while piquing public curiosity about various aspects of inoculation, most were of little use to 'average parents' seeking to learn about the inoculation experiences of their local peer group.

3 Regional Influences Come into Play

Several strong influences shaped the regional awareness and general acceptance of inoculation in Germany, one of which was the increasing official recognition of the need to address the population loss from smallpox.[93] The Prussian government may have been influenced in its decision-making on the issue by Johann Peter Sußmilch, the Berlin churchman and pioneer of public-health policymaking who recommended inoculation as a potential solution (1761) to the unacceptably high smallpox mortality: "Is this not an exceedingly important matter that is worthy of attention from the State? Should cost even

92 "Die Inokulation," 520.

93 Karl F.W.A. Vater, *Preussisch-Schlesische Civil Medicinal- and Sanitäts-Verfassung*, part 2 (Breslau: Korn, 1800), 540–3; "Landesfürstliche Aufmunterung an Sachsen, zur Einpfropfung der Pocken," *LI*, no. 21, June, 1963; *Intelligenzblatt der ALZ*, no. 3 (1792): 18–9; Karl W.L.F. von Drais, *Geschichte der Regierung und Bildung von Baden unter Carl Friedrich*, vol. 1 (Karlsruhe: Müller, 1818), 193; Moritz Pistor, "Geschichte der preussischen Medizinalverwaltung," *DVG* 40 (1908): 779.

be considered in making this great benefit well known and bringing it into use?"[94] Six years earlier, Johann Heinrich Gottlob von Justi expressed the view that widespread inoculation would "save a great many people," and wondered why "in the larger German towns there have been no moves to make use of this outstanding measure, since it has been used to such great advantage in England, the Swiss Confederation, and America?"[95] A number of jurisdictions subsequently began to inoculate the orphans in their care, and to encourage inoculation more broadly.[96] Conversely, the realisation that inoculation was causing smallpox outbreaks prompted new regulations in some regions, prohibiting the practice in smallpox-free areas.[97]

The division of Germany into Catholic and Protestant territories turned out to be another factor influencing the regional adoption and spread of inoculation. Many Protestant churchmen were supporters of the practice, and quite a number were prolific contributors of articles that attempted to increase public understanding of the pertinent issues surrounding inoculation, or to promote it more generally.[98] Such publications from Catholic leaders were not so forthcoming, and the advice from the Vatican about how to approach the matter of inoculation was quite inconsistent. Even though Pope Benedict XIV's foreign secretary Cardinal Valenti assured Charles Marie de la Condamine when he visited the Holy See in 1755 that the Church fathers regarded inoculation as "perfectly conformable to principles of Christian charity, to annihilate … the evident risk of death," the Vatican made no effort to publicise the pontiff's

94 Sußmilch, *Ordnung*, 1: 532–3.

95 Apx 2: Justi (1755), 166–7. The foremost German medical policy advocate of the next generation, Johann Peter Frank, first addressed the issue of smallpox prophylaxis after conducting a trial of Jenner's cowpox vaccination in a Vienna hospital in 1801: Bennett, *War*, 131, 230.

96 Apx 2: "Etwas von" (1769), 347–9. "Circulare wegen Einführung der Blatter-Inoculation," *Sammlung aller Ordnungen, Edicte, Mandate, Rescripte, etc. der Regierung Friedrichs II*, vol. 12 (Breslau: Korn, 1770), 48–50; Carl F. Gerstlacher, ed., *Sammlung aller Baden-Durlachischen Anstalten und Verordnungen*, vol. 1 (Karlsruhe: Schmieder, 1773), 527–8; Pistor, "Geschichte," 780.

97 A regulation issued in 1784 limited inoculation in the Bishopric of Münster: Johann C. Scherf, *Archiv der medizinischen Polizey und die gemeinnützigen Arzneikunde*, vol. 6 (Leipzig: Weygand, 1795), 112–17. Such limits were imposed in 1796 in the Rhineland free city, Mühlhausen, the northern principality, Eutin, and the Duchy of Mecklenburg-Schwerin: "Chronik der Reichsstädte," *NZT*, no. 20 (1796), 440–2; Juncker, *Archiv*, 2:229, n. 10; 4:31.

98 Apx 2: Chais (1756, 1770, 1774); Cramer (1759, 1760, 1762); Danneil (1769); Plitt (1768); Wolf (1768); Bock (1770); Eisen (1771); Merkel (1777); Grot (1781); Schwager (1784, 1786, 1790); Klose (1786, 1787); Migula (1786, 1787, 1790); Steiger (1787); Engelmann (1788); Künzel (1788); Sintenis (1790); Michaelis (1792); Piccard (1794); Richter (1799).

stated approval of inoculation.[99] Nor did the situation change under Benedict's successor Clement XIII (incumbent 1758–69), whose *Leibarzt* Cristofano Zanetti declared that "the inoculation of smallpox never would, and never should, be practised."[100] The next pope, Clement XIV, adopted quite the opposite view, though his intention to encourage inoculation in his territories became a casualty of the attempted poisoning that brought on the lingering illness leading to his death in 1774.[101]

In Spain, the dissemination of news and information about inoculation was curbed by censorship influenced by the Church, while in Austria the influential Professor Anton de Haen was an outspoken inoculation opponent and Empress Maria Theresa's *Leibarzt* Gerhard van Swieten was too cautious to recommend the practice. The empress became convinced of the need to test the safety and efficacy of inoculation after several of her children and in-laws had died from smallpox and she suffered badly from the disease herself, leading her to encourage an expansion of the practice.[102] Publications about inoculation that were unrelated to de Haen's opposition began to flow from Austria in 1769 to join the steady stream coming from France and Italy, while the Spanish print media added to the output at much the same time. Yet Catholic regions of Germany published little on the topic compared to the Protestant territories.[103] A rare exception was the intuitive book of advice published in 1789 by Dr. Gottlieb Théophil Ehrhart from Memmingen, which was aimed toward the largely Catholic population of Southern Württemburg and Bavaria.[104] Ehrhart adopted the familiar fatherly style of prose commonly used in Bavaria to address a multitude of issues, and spoke to his readers in a manner

99 Charles-Marie de la Condamine, *Journal of a Tour of Italy* (Dublin, 1763), 107–8; Apx 2: Hensler (1765), 2:276.

100 "Brescia," *Wöchentliche Nachrichten zum hamburgischen unpartheyischen Correspondenten*, no. 26, June 27, 1760.

101 The Marquis Caraccioli, *The Life of Pope Clement XIV (Ganganelli)*, 2nd ed. (London: Johnson, 1778), 164.

102 Jacqueline Gratton, "Smallpox Prevention and the Dissemination of New Ideas in Spain 1725–1775" (MA thesis, University of Tasmania, 2012), 170, 175–80, 190–3; Frank T. Brechka, *Gerard van Swieten and His World 1700–1772* (The Hague: Nijhoff, 1970), 115–8; Antoinette S. Emch-Dériaz, "L' Inoculation Justifiée, or Was it?," *Eighteenth-Century Life* 7 (1982): 69–70.

103 For the first inoculation report from Spain, see Gratton, "Smallpox," 216; for an early report from Vienna: Anton von Störck, *Abhandlung von der Einpfropfung der Kinds-Blattern* (Vienna: Trattner, 1771). Apx 2 lists German reviews of publications from France, Italy, and Austria, as well as translated works. The place of publication of the journals that published 'inoculation articles,' listed at the beginning of Appendix 2, indicates a relative absence of journals based in Catholic regions.

104 Gottlieb T. Ehrhart, *Darstellung der Gründe für und gegen die Blatterneinpfropfung für Leser aus allen Ständen* (Memmingen: Seyler, 1789). Although the book was published anonymously, Ehrhart was identified as the author: *ALZ* 92 (1792), 170.

suggesting a general lack of public awareness of inoculation in the area at that time. He discusses the most common concerns under such straightforward sub-headings as: "Does God permit inoculation?; Inoculated children can also die; Inoculation does not protect against natural smallpox; The more pustules the better;" and "Inoculated children will be unhealthy later." Those topics had all been debated previously in publications from northern Germany prompted by La Condamine's landmark speech (1754) that raised the same perennially vexed concerns.[105] Indeed, Ehrhart cleverly structured his book along the lines that La Condamine had shown to be so effective in reaching a public unfamiliar with inoculation – posing medical and religious questions regarding the pros and contras of the procedure, and providing logical answers.[106]

Dr. Christoph Girtanner commented in 1794 on the greater progress of inoculation in Protestant than in Catholic territories, using Britain and France as his examples. In order to justify his assertion that Catholic leaders tended to question whether inoculation was permitted by religion while Protestant leaders were inclined to support practical experiments, he recalled the time in the 1760s when inoculation was mired in theological objections in France while making considerable progress in Britain.[107] Political considerations may have cautioned him from citing examples closer to home, such as the occasion in 1760 when the Catholic Elector Friedrich August II of the large neighbouring territory of Saxony, concurrently the titular King of Poland, requested an assessment from University of Leipzig theologians as to whether inoculation was justified by divine law. The judgement was in the affirmative.[108]

Whatever the reasons behind inoculation being less common in the mainly Catholic regions of Germany than in predominantly Protestant territories, that was the apparent reality in 1794, as Girtanner asserted.[109] A notable exception was the Catholic Bishopric of Münster where a regulation issued in 1765 prohibited any hindrance of inoculation, and where the inoculation of all children of the poor was officially recommended.[110]

---

105 Ehrhart, *Darstellung*, 24, 41, 44, 48, 52. Apx 2: Justi (1755); Büscher (1755); Matthiä (1756); "Bestätigende Abhandlung" (1756); Chais (1756); Review of *Dissertation* (1757); Cramer (1759).

106 Apx 2: La Condamine, *HAM* (1756), 40–75.

107 Chrisoph Girtanner, *Krankheiten der Kinder und über die physische Erziehung derselben* (Berlin: Rottmann, 1794), 193; Arnold H. Rowbotham, "The 'Philosophes' and the Propaganda for Inoculation of Smallpox in France," *UCP* 18 (1935): 270–84.

108 Apx 2: Heinsius (1780), 24.

109 Lorenz von Westenrieder, *Beschreibung der Haupt-und Residenzstadt München* (*im gegenwärtigen Zustand*) (Munich: Strobel, 1782), 329; Apx 2: Hensler (1765), 1:127.

110 Rolf Gehrmann, *Bevölkerungsgeschichte Norddeutschlands zwischen Aufklärung und Vormärz* (Berlin: Spitz, 2000), 292.

The generally greater inclination toward inoculation in Protestant than in Catholic territories of Germany corresponds with the predominance of Protestant towns in the publication of journals featuring inoculation-related articles (Table 1). Such regional publishing peculiarities tended to be linked to the journal owners' inclination to hold Enlightenment-inspired views commonly shared by academics from the nearby universities, who provided much of the editorial support and readership.[111] Proprietors of the broadly-targeted journals that published inoculation-related articles were usually educated at one of the Protestant universities, and employed as officials of one or other of the territorial governments with a benevolent humanist approach to social issues.[112] Christoph Martin Wieland, the owner and editor of *Der teutsche Merkur* (TM) and tutor to the two princes of Saxe-Weimar during their teenage years, was an ideal fit for that mould. The son of a Lutheran pastor, Wieland was educated at the University of Tübingen (Württemburg) and became a versatile writer inclined to proselytise his views, which were sympathetic to Enlightenment ideology.[113] His embrace of inoculation is clearly evident in an editorial he wrote in TM in response to an anonymous letter to the editor (1774) expressing concern that inoculation in many cases failed to prevent future smallpox. Wieland's advice about the best way to avoid diagnostic errors leading to inoculations that failed to offer protection – choose an experienced inoculator – led to a journal-based discussion of second cases of smallpox.[114] Wieland could well have written the initial anonymous letter to the editor himself, with the aim of

111 Eckhart Hellmuth and Wolfgang Piereth, "Germany, 1760–1815," in *Press, Politics, and the Public Sphere in Europe and North America, 1760–1820*, eds. Hannah Barker and Simon Burrows (Cambridge: Cambridge University Press, 2002), 69–70; Watson, *Genius*, 54–5, 112–3; Blanning, *Power*, 210–11. Protestant universities generally embraced Enlightenment ideology: Johann M. Stroup, *The Struggle for Identity in the Clerical Estate* (Leiden: Brill, 1984), 90. Books about inoculation were also published largely in Protestant towns (Apx 2).

112 Heinrich Christian Boie, the editor of *Deutsches Museum*, studied at Jena and Göttingen: Henri Brunschwig, *Enlightenment and Romanticism in Eighteenth-century Prussia* (Chicago and London: University of Chicago Press, 1974), 34, 37. The founder and owner of the *Hannoverisches Magazin* and its forerunners, Albert Christoph von Wüllen, a lawyer educated at Göttingen in the late-1730s, was later involved in regional government of Calenberg (Hanover): Christoph Starck and Kurt Schönhammer, *Die Geschichte der Akademie der Wissenschaften*, part 1 (Berlin and Boston: de Gruyter, 2013), 117–19. The owners of the *Schlesische Provinzialblätter*, Friedrich Albert Zimmermann and Carl Konrad Streit, were Protestants working for the Silesian branch of the Prussian government: Michael R. Gerber, *Die Schlesische Provinzialblätter* (Sigmaringen: Thorbecke, 1995), 70–1.

113 Watson, *Genius*, 112–13.

114 Apx 2: "Auszug," TM (1773); Wieland, TM (1775); "Nöthige," TM (1775). For other articles referring to smallpox recurring after inoculation, see in Apx 2: Linekogel (1766); Löber (1767); Andreä and Bolten (1769); Elsner (1787), 48. Ploucquet lists sixty publications

prompting a discussion that would allow like-minded contributors, including himself, to allay concerns about a crucial issue that could turn parents away from inoculation. Regardless of who actually did contribute that letter initiating the articles intended to correct misunderstandings damaging the reputation of inoculation, the entire episode underscores the potential for journal owners and editors to shape journal-based discussions.

More stringent censorship in some Catholic states than in Protestant territories was another reason for the preference of certain regions for the establishment of new journals committed to enlightened commentary.[115] Strict censorship by Church authorities even tended to render some regional newspapers bland and boring, or even illegible from being printed on 'blotting paper' using poor quality ink.[116] A popular alternative for readers turned away from such unappealing fare was the variety of generally-targeted journals, which could be accessed for a small membership fee at one of the reading societies that had sprung up in most towns by the 1780s.[117] The allure of the journals and other enticing new kinds of reading material was summed up by the Prussian censor Gottlob Friedrich Hillmer's remark (1797) about "the universal malady, I might almost go so far as to say mania, of reading."[118] Yet in the Catholic territories of Bavaria, Würzburg, and Trier, keen readers had their easy access to journals and books blocked during 1786–89 by the closure of their reading societies by zealous officials suspicious of the influence of the *Illuminati* on the increasing cohort of enthusiastic readers.[119]

Considering the many journal articles and books about inoculation, which of the avid readers with good access to such publications was taking an interest in the topic, apart from doctors, academics, pastors, and others with a professional need to keep up with developments? According to the Jena professor, Christian Gottfried Gruner, businessmen and ladies who wanted to inform themselves about smallpox were among those inclined to read articles on the

---

during 1717–88 dealing with recurrent smallpox: Wilhelm G. Ploucquet, *Initia Bibliothecae Medico-Practicae et Chirurgiae,* vol. 8 (Tübingen: Cotta, 1797), 208–10.

115 Aloys Blumauer, *Beobachtungen über Oesterreichs Aufklärung* (Vienna: Neubacher, 1782), 65–6; Watson, *Genius*, 51.

116 Jospeh Goerres, "Die teutschen Zeitungen," *Rheinische Merkur* 80 (1814): 2.

117 Richard van Dülmen, *The Society of the Enlightenment, the Rise of the Middle Class and Enlightenment Culture in Germany* (Cambridge: Polity, 1992), 83–4, map 3.

118 Brunschwig, *Enlightenment*, 39.

119 Reinhard Wittmann, "Was there a Reading Revolution at the End of the Eighteenth Century?," in *A History of Reading,* eds. Gugliemo Cavallo and Roger Chartier (Oxford: Blackwell, 1999), 310; *Uebersicht des politischen Zustandes Europens im Jahr 1786* (Kempten: Kösel, 1787), 42.

topic, if they were written in a flowing style.[120] Such upper- and middle-class readers tended to be subscribers who read their journals at home and shared them among friends. Journals could also be accessed at public libraries, which were open to all, and men were free to read newspapers in the cafés in Berlin and other towns, where proprietiers supplied reading material to attract customers.[121] Most men could also join reading societies (Figure 12), which became an option for women too in the 1780s when some societies began accepting female members.[122] Surviving membership lists show primarily magistrates, army officers, schoolteachers, government officials, churchmen, merchants, lawyers, doctors, nobles, diplomats, and the occasional businessman.[123] Yet by 1799 reading societies were also accepting traders, craftsmen, economists, and men from many other walks of life, as well as young adolescents, girls, and women of all ages.[124] The uneducated could benefit from a membership too, by listening to others reading aloud, and engaging in the discussions that became an important social function of reading societies and informal reading groups.[125] Inoculation may well have been one of the topics discussed.[126]

While townsfolk, particularly men, could access reading material in several ways, the options were very limited in the countryside where the vast majority of Germans lived. With the notable exception of an informal reading society established in the vicinity of Merseburg (Saxony) in 1786, by a group of pastors aiming to encourage villagers to read newspapers and journals on Sundays and winter evenings, reading societies were rare in rural Germany.[127] Even though the better-educated families of country pastors, village schoolteachers, the occasional rural public official, and the more prosperous landowners would

---

120 Christian G. Gruner, Review of *Mémoire addressé au Congres de Rastadt concernant la petite vérole,* by Johann Christian Wilhelm Juncker, *MCZ* 3 (1798): 278–9.

121 Brunschwig, *Enlightenment,* 36; Wittmann, "Revolution," 299, 307.

122 Ulrich Im Hof, *Das Europa der Aufklärung* (Munich: Beck, 1993), 107; Barbara Becker-Cantarino, "The Scope of German Literature in the Eighteenth Century," in *Literature,* ed. Becker-Cantarino, 17.

123 "Worms im Januar, 1791," *Intelligenzblatt der ALZ,* no. 81 (1791): 670–1: Van Dulmen, *Society,* 88–9; Im Hof, 107.

124 Johann G. Krünitz, *Oekonomisch-technologische Encyclopädie,* part 72 (Berlin: Pauli, 1799), 280.

125 Krünitz, *Encyclopädie,* part 35, 560; Hellmuth and Piereth "Germany," 70, 76; Wittmann, *Revolution,* 309.

126 Ute Frevert, *Krankheit als politisches Problem 1770–1880. Soziale Unterschichten in Preußen zwischen medizinischer Polizei und staatlicher Sozialversicherung* (Göttingen: Vandenhoek & Ruprecht, 1984), 35.

127 "Vermischte Nachrichten," *Deutsche Zeitung für die Jugend und ihre Freunde,* first quarter (1786): 72.

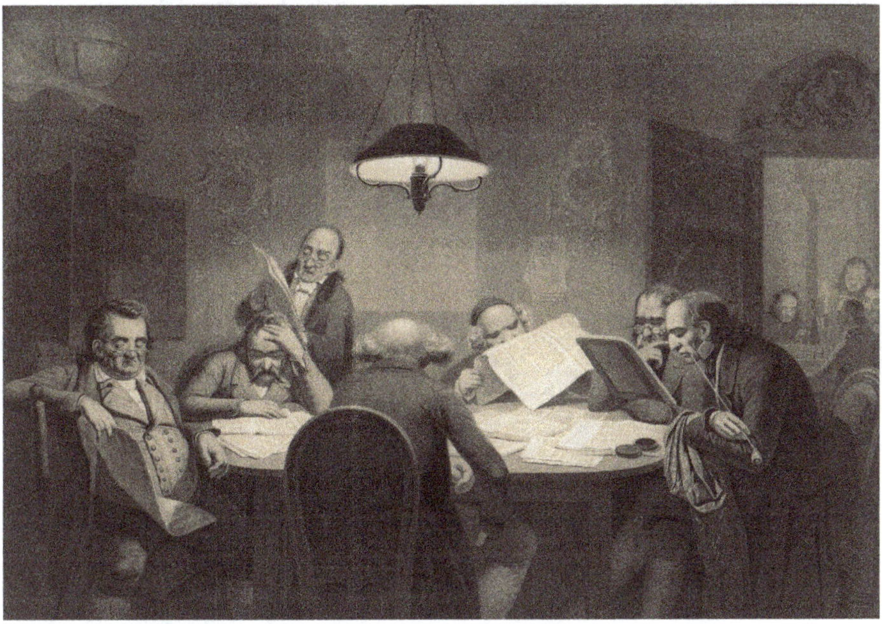

FIGURE 12 Men reading around a table. Lithograph by C. Thielley after J.P. Hasenclever
RIJKSMUSEUM, AMSTERDAM: RP-P-2015-26-2102

have undoubtedly enjoyed the opportunity to read material in addition to the journals to which they subscribed, their numbers were too small and scattered to warrant the establishment of a reading society. Nor was there much likelihood of the cohort of potential readers being augmented by peasants, who generally received a poor education at sub-standard village schools, and showed little inclination to read.[128]

A turnaround in peasant attitudes toward reading occurred in late-1789–90 when the thirst for news of their French counterparts' revolutionary struggle gave villagers a new appreciation for a skill they had previously thought largely redundant. Parents' recognition of the advantage of having at least one child who could read the news caused a marked upturn in attendance at village schools, eventually increasing the cohort of rural readers.[129] The impact of the change was noticeable a decade later when the local demand increased

128 Reinhard Wittmann, *Buchmarkt und Lektüre im 18. und 19. Jahrhundert, Beiträge zum literarischen Leben, 1750–1880* (Tübingen: Niemeyer, 1982), 32; Rudolf Schenda, *Volk ohne Buch; Studien zur Sozialgeschichte der populären Lesestoffe, 1770–1910* (Frankfurt am Main: Klostermann, 1970), 445–7.

129 Wittmann, 37–41.

sufficiently for reading societies to be established in rural Lower-Saxony, Silesia, and East Prussia.[130] The increased literacy and improved access to journals in rural areas provided the impetus for efforts by governments, journal proprietors, pastors, and doctors to enlighten the peasants about matters related to the preservation of good health, and disease prevention, including recommendations of inoculation.[131]

130 Krünitz, *Encyclopädie*, 35:560; 72:280.

131 Mary Lindemann, "'*Aufklärung*' and the Health of the People; '*Volksschriften*' and Medical Advice in Braunschweig-Wolfenbüttel, 1756–1803," in *Das Volk als Objekt obrigkeitlichen Handelns*, ed. Rudolf Vierhaus (Tübingen: Niemeyer, 1992), 111–16; Frevert, *Krankheit*, 52–3.

CHAPTER 5

A Literary Focus on Women

Smallpox shaped the lives of not only the many children it killed, blinded, or crippled but also of the countless women whose beauty it destroyed. Poets found inspiration in such tragedies, which they wove into poetic moral messages and optimistic scenarios of young women choosing inoculation to save their complexions. The value of verse for revealing the social context of smallpox was first highlighted by the Frankfurt doctor Wilhelm Stricker in his lament (1861) over the 'lost' body of German *Pockenpoesie*. 'Smallpox poetry,' as Stricker pointed out, was intrinsically important to the cultural history of smallpox, particularly since Jenner's cowpox vaccination had allowed society to forget the worst impacts of the disease.[1] Much of that 'lost smallpox poetry' has now resurfaced. It shows that German poets and writers, unlike their British and French counterparts, tended to place love-relationships at the core of their 'smallpox and inoculation poetry,' particularly during the so-called literary era of sensibility in the second half of the eighteenth century.[2] They were also inclined to place women in centre-stage as not only smallpox victims but also as decision-makers, with implicit suggestions that women should take control of their own smallpox fate rather than leaving the decision to a male relative. Such a literary focus on women and their capabilities, along with the targeting of inoculation advice to women in recognition that mothers were the primary influence in the inoculation of children, reflects a changing society in which the domestic sphere was gaining increasing attention.[3]

1 Wilhelm Stricker, "Pockenpoesie," *Archiv für pathologische Anatomie und Physiologie und für klinische Medizin* 20 (1861): 394–9.

2 The sensibility genre is explained in Barbara Becker-Cantarino, "The Scope of German Literature in the Eighteenth Century," in *German Literature of the Eighteenth Century: The Enlightenment and Sensibility*, ed. Barbara Becker-Cantarino (Rochester: Camden House, 2005), 10; Rainer Baasner, *Einführung in die Literatur der Aufklärung* (Darmstadt: Wissenschaftliche Buchgesellshaft, 2006), 10–11. For British and French 'smallpox poetry,' see David E. Shuttleton, *Smallpox and the Literary Imagination, 1660–1820* (Cambridge: Cambridge University Press, 2007); Catriona Seth, *Les rois aussi en mouraient. Les Lumières en lutte contre la petite vérole* (Paris: Desjonquères, 2008).

3 Ute Frevert, *Krankheit als politisches Problem 1770–1880* (Göttingen: Vandenhoek & Ruprecht, 1984), 47–8.

 | DOI:10.1163/9789004465374_007

1 Changing Sentiments in Depictions of Disfigurement

'Smallpox poetry' focusing on the terrible consequences of disfigurement, particularly for women, underwent a change in tone as the eighteenth century progressed. Sympathetic poetic depictions of damaged women reveal an increasingly enlightened approach to the issue, firmly dispelling the biblical notion of women being eternally tainted with Eve's original sin that caused God to inflict smallpox on mankind as punishment.[4] Such changing attitudes to disfigured women can be best appreciated in poetry arranged chronologically, beginning with this anonymous cruel satire from a collection of verse by late-seventeenth-century poets well-known in their time:

Mit viel tausend Pocken-narben	With many thousand smallpox scars
Und die Nase samt den Mund …	And her nose joined to the mouth …
Wenn sie Liebe will erwecken,	When she goes to seek out love,
Muß sie seyn darauf bedacht,	She must give consideration
Daß sie gute Anstalt macht,	That, to make a good impression,
Ihr Gesichte zu bedecken,	She ensures her face is covered.
Liesse sie es unbedeckt,	If she should omit the cover,
Würde man nur abgeschreckt.[5]	That would only shock the lover.

By comparison, the author of the two-line epigram "To a Man with Smallpox Pits," from the same mixed collection of verse, does not poke fun at the disfigured man but portrays him in a heroic context of hunting and military imagery:

Wird alle Kugeln gleich Eugenius verschiessen;	If Eugenius were to shoot off all his musket-balls;
Kann man in dein Gesicht doch wieder neue giessen.[6]	In his face, indeed, new ones can again be poured.

4 Theodor G. von Hippel, *Über die bürgerliche Verbesserung der Weiber* (Berlin: Voß, 1792), 13–15 62–3; Johann C.W Juncker, *Gemeinnützige Vorschläge und Nachrichten über das beste verhalten der Menschen in Rücksicht der Pockenkrankheit. Erster Versuch, für die mittlern Stände, nebst einem Anhänge für Aerzte* (Halle and Leipzig, 1792), 138.

5 "Ihre Kleider sind das schönste an ihr," in *Herrn von Hoffmannswaldau und anderer Deutschen auserlesener und bisher ungedruckter Gedichte,* part 2 (Leipzig: Fritsch, 1697), 336–7. The poem's author is not identified.

6 "Auf ein Pocken-grübichte," in *Hoffmannswaldau, Gedichte,* part 6 (Leipzig: Fritsch, 1709), 75. English poets depicted smallpox disfigurement destroying men's as well as women's lives: Shuttleton, *Smallpox*, 137–43.

A sense of compassion for female smallpox victims is more evident in later verse, such as the Lauban (Saxony) schoolmaster Samuel Seidel's heartbroken elegy (1743) to his eighteen-year-old fiancée. Yet Seidel's affirmation of Theodora's unblemished virtue, in his brief allusion to the disastrous impact of smallpox on her appearance, implies a need to correct the common perception that the corruption of Theodora's body could be incorrectly construed as a sign of tainted morality:[7]

Muß dich der heiße Schmerz mit Blattern überstreun?	Must your burning pain be overlain with those pustules,
Da doch die Tugend selbst sonst keine Pockennarbe	Since your still untainted virtue is so pure?
Der Unart an dir fand. Weicht Kraft, Gestalt und Farbe,	Does the sneaking, irritating, sudden danger
Der schleichend reitzenden, der plötzlichen Gefahr?	Sap the strength, as well as changing body shape and colour?
Mein Leben, meine Lust, ach sinkst, ach stirbst du gar?	My life, my delight, you're sinking, is death truly near?
Verhängniß, schone doch, und gieb sie mir, meine Glücke,	Oh Fate, be indulgent, give me back my happiness,
Gieb sie mir gleich verstellt; nur lebend noch zurücke![8]	Give her back to me still living, even with an altered face!

Seidel's appeal to Fate to return his beloved Theodora to him despite her disfigurement is an admission that he first considered her changed appearance before his love for her overrode his concerns over the loss of her beauty. A Saxon contemporary of Seidel during his student years at the University of Leipzig, Pastor Johann Adolf Schlegel, similarly recognised the greater importance of a young woman's personality than her appearance. He had this to say in his lament to Nature about the destruction of his friend's youthful beauty by smallpox (1746):

7 Samuel Seidel, "Schlaf wohl! erblaßte Theodore, schlaf auserwählte Böttnerinn," in *Zeugnisse treuer Liebe nach dem Tode tugendhafter Frauen, von ihren Ehemännern* (Hanover: Försters, 1743), 237. For discussion of the implied immorality of a young woman's body being invaded by smallpox, see Jill Campbell, "Lady Mary Wortely Montagu and the 'Glass Revers'd' of Female Old Age," in *Defects: Engendering the Modern Body,* eds. Helen Deutsch and Felicity Nussbaum (Ann Arbor: University of Michigan Press, 2003), 226.

8 Seidel, 237. Eighteenth-century German elegies to the smallpox dead, in verse, are usually not identifiable as such because of the poets' tendency not to mention the cause of death.

Kannst du dein eignes Werk verwüsten,	Can you destroy your work of sculpture
Das du mit Anmuth auszurüsten,	Whom you endowed with such allure,
Dich, o Natur, mit Luft bemüht;	Since you, oh Nature, made her breathe?
Du magst durch Fieber sie entfärben,	You may have let the fever pale her,
Durch Blattern ganz den Reiz verderben,	And let smallpox destroy the charm
Der überall an Doris blüht;	That bloomed in Doris's demeanour.
Nicht ein Herz wirst du ihr entführen,	Yet you'll not cause one heart to leave her,
Das ihre Schönheit schätzt und preist.	That admired and praised her beauty.
Trotz deiner Wut wird sie noch rühren,	She'll still stir them despite your fury,
So viel vermag ihr Geist.[9]	Because her spirit has such power.

Schlegel's confidence that Doris (Dorothea) had the vibrant personality to attract admirers prepared to overlook her damaged features was affirmed by her subsequent marriage to the writer Johann Christoph Rost. By naming Rost as Doris's husband, in the title of the poem, Schlegel offers implicit praise for his honourable qualities in marrying a woman whose external beauty was no longer in evidence. Quite the contrary attitude to disfigurement was shown by the husband depicted in a humorous poem (1763) by a literary giant of the time, the popular Leipzig poetry professor Christian Furchtegott Gellert:

Ein junges Weib, sie hieß Lisette,	There was a young woman whose name was Lisette,
Dieß Weibchen lag an Blattern blind.	In bed, after smallpox made her go blind.
Nun weiß man wohl, wie junge Weiber sind;	We all know the thoughts in a young woman's mind;
Drum durft ihr Mann nicht von dem Bette,	She would not let her man leave the bed,
So gern er sie verlassen hätte:	Though leaving was just what he wanted.
Denn laßt ein Weib schön, wie Citheren, seyn,	Even Venus, when she's had smallpox,

9 Johann A. Schlegel, "Auf die Schwester meines Freundes, Christiane Dorothea Gärtnern, nachmalige Ehegattin des Dichters Rost, 1746," in *Johann A. Schlegel: Vermischte Gedichte* (Karlsruhe: Schmieder, 1788), 293.

Wenn sie die Blattern hat: so nimmt sie nicht mehr ein.[10]	Is no longer the same, her beauty is lost.

Having shunned his blind, disfigured wife Lisette, the husband chooses the beautiful Lorchen to care for her, leading to his betrayal, the main theme of the poem:

Sie küssen sich recht zärtlich und vertraut;	They kissed with affection and mutual trust,
Allein sie küßten gar zu laut.	But they made too much noise with their kisses.
Wie konnt es anders seyn? Lisette mußt es hören.	How can we avoid it? Lisette must hear it.
Sie hörts, und fragt: was schallt so hell?	She heard it and asked: what's that loud noise?
Madam, Madam! ruft Lorchen schnell,	Madam, Madam, cried Lorchen in haste,
Es ist ihr Herrr: er ächzt vor grossem Schmerz,	It's your husband's groans from the anguish he feels,
Und will sich nicht zufrieden geben.	And he won't allow any relief.
Ach! spricht sie, lieber Mann, wie redlich meynts dein Herz!	My dear husband, she said, your heart's so sincere!
O, gräme dich doch nicht! Ich bin ja noch am Leben.[11]	But I'm here, still alive, you've no need to grieve.

Since Gellert was known for embedding moral truths in humorous fables based on the lives of ordinary people such as Lisette and her husband,[12] the marital situation that gave rise to his moral message about loyalty and fidelity probably represents more truth than fiction.

One of Gellert's former-students and long-time friends, Christian Felix Weiße,[13] followed his mentor's lead in using smallpox-disfigurement as a vehicle for poetic moral messages. Weiße warns about the fragility of beauty and

---

10 Christian F. Gellert, "Lisette," in *Christian F. Gellert: Fabeln und Erzählungen* (Leipzig: Wendler, 1763), 119. Gellert's book was among the most popular of its time: Kevin Hilliard, "Religious and Secular Poetry and Epic (1700–1780)," in *Literature,* ed. Becker-Cantarino, 112.

11 Gellert, 121.

12 Becker-Cantarino, "Scope," 10; Baasner, *Einführung*, 137.

13 Christian E. Weiße and Samuel G. Frisch, *Christian Felix Weißens Selbstbiographie* (Leipzig: Voß, 1806), 12, 132.

the superficiality of narcissistic vanity, in his poem "Vain Beauty," which culminates in the moral judgement that a nobler character emerges when beauty is destroyed:

The brother	
O! ich bin doch ein schöner Knabe!	Oh! I'm such a beautiful boy!
Ja, ja, das ist gewiß:	Yes, yes, that is a fact:
Der Spiegel, den ich vor mir habe,	The mirror before me does not lie,
Sagt augenscheinlich dieß.	It certainly shows just that.
Wie sanft ist mein Gesicht! wie rund!	My face, so soft and so round!
Die blauen Augen schmachten:	With the tantalizing blue eyes:
Und dieser kleine rothe Mund	Nor is this little red mouth
Ist auch nicht zu verachten.	A feature that could be despised.
The sister	
Allein die Schönheit ist vergangen!	Only my beauty was lost to me!
Da kam der Blattern Wuth,	When the wrath of smallpox arrived,
Zerriß mir diese glatten Wangen,	And tore away the lovely smooth cheeks
Löscht' aus der Augen Gluth:	And extinguished the shine in my eyes;
Doch glaube nicht, daß michs verdrußt;	But don't believe that it left me displeased,
Nein; es hat mich gelehret,	No; it taught me a truth,
Daß das nur wahre Schönheit ist,	That the only beauty that's truly real
Was keine Zeit zerstöret.[14]	Is the kind that time cannot ruin.

Christian Gotthold Contius was yet another student at Leipzig during Gellert's tenure who gained the inspiration to express his ideas in verse.[15] He later found so much time to indulge his passion for writing poetry while fulfilling the role of pastor in the small village of Dollenchen (Prussia), that he became known for his copious output. In "The Mirror," Contius follows the pre-eminent Leipzig literary figures Gellert and Weiße in using the theme of smallpox disfigurement as a vehicle for moral messages. He depicts the beautiful fourteen-year-old Selinde often dressing up and preening herself in front of her mother's mirror, encouraged by flattery from admiring adults, until smallpox puts an

14 Christian F. Weiße, "Eitle Schönheit," in *Christian F. Weiße: Kleine lyrische Gedichte*, vol. 3 (Leipzig: Weidmanns Erben und Reich, 1772), 51–3.

15 *Aufgefangener litterarische Briefwechsel der Dodsleyschen Kunstrichter und anderer Gelehrten* (1772), 28–30.

end to her vanity. In the following lines Contius uses Selinde's sad plight to issue some of his social criticisms:

Und kurz, Selinde, die dem Spiegel so getreu,	And soon Selinde, who loved the mirror
Daß sie sich stundenlang ihm gegenüber schmückte,	So much that she'd preen before it for hours,
Ging, seit sie sich verstellt erblickte,	Passed by it in silent haste,
Ganz schnell und still vor ihm vorbey.	When she saw her disfigured face.
So lange wir mit Schmeicheleyen	As long as we use flattery
Der Menschen Eitelkeit erfreuen,	To pander to the human pride,
Nennt man uns höflich und beliebt;	We are loved and called polite:
Doch wenn wir drauf ein Wort der Wahrheit wagen,	But if we dare to say the truth,
So wird ein Jeder selber sagen,	Then they all would criticise,
Was uns die Welt für einen Nahmen giebt.[16]	And soon we would be ostracised.

The reality of poets' representations of the high value that society places on personal appearances was manifest in smallpox-disfigured women's difficulties competing in the marriage market. Dr. Ignaz Joseph Wetsch addressed the issue by recommending the inoculation of women as a patriotic duty, arguing that because young women "often had their entire dowry invested in their appearance," such a move would boost population growth by reducing the number of disfigured women cast into childless spinsterhood. His social appraisal even applied to such a high-ranking bride as Empress Maria Theresa's daughter, Maria Elisabeth, who withdrew from her planned marriage to King Louis XV of France and retreated from public life after smallpox damaged her features.[17] Yet the marriage market was not entirely closed to disfigured women. Peter Skold showed that one-third of smallpox-disfigured women in Sweden married blemished men, though the average bridal age of forty-five left little likelihood of children for a high proportion of those marriages.[18]

---

16 Christian G. Contius, "Der Spiegel, eine Fabel," in *Christian G. Contius: Gedichte* (Dresden: Gerlach, 1782), 86.

17 Ignaz J. Wetsch, *Das bestrittene Vorurtheil in zweyen Abhandlungen: die Einpfropfung der Kindspocken und die Beerdigung der Toten in den Kirchen und Städten betreffend* (Vienna: Krauß, 1764), 20 (quote) –22; Donald R. Hopkins, *The Greatest Killer: Smallpox in History* (Chicago: University of Chicago Press, 2002), 64.

18 Peter Skold, "The Beauty and the Beast – Smallpox and Marriage in Eighteenth- and Nineteenth-Century Sweden," *Historical Social Research* 28 (2003): 157–61.

2 Poets and Writers Focus on Young Women

In a society that prevented women from studying at university and disapproved of female participation in the public sphere, the male literary elite tended to act as mouthpieces for women-in-general.[19] Christian Felix Weiße (Figure 13) and Moritz August von Thümmel (Figure 14) adopted such a role with their respective explorations of links between smallpox disfigurement, inoculation, and young women's love-relationships. A comic opera by Weiße and a verse-story by Thümmel similarly advertise the benefits of inoculation through the fictional young female characters choosing to have themselves inoculated for the sake of their future happiness and marital security.[20] Both depictions are subtly critical of a paternalistic society that misunderstands the fragility of women's social position, which was then limited largely to marriage with an

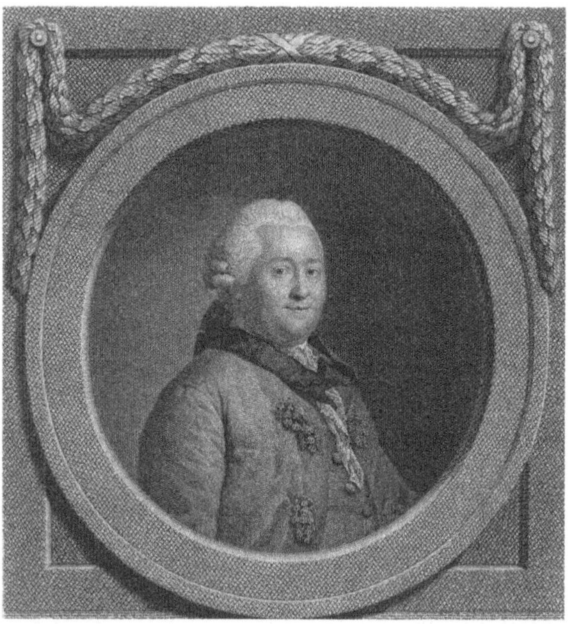

FIGURE 13
Christian Felix Weiße. Engraving by J.F. Bause after A. Graff, 1771
RIJKSMUSEUM, AMSTERDAM: RP-P-1937-925

19 W. Daniel Wilson, "Eighteenth-century Germany in its Historical Context," in *Literature,* ed. Becker-Cantarino, 276. Dorothea Christiane Leporin was able to complete her doctorate in medicine at Halle in 1753 only because Friedrich II of Prussia gave her special permission to study. Doctors in Leporin's home town, Quedlinburg, disapproved of her practising medicine: Elisabeth Poeter, "Gender, Religion, and Medicine in Enlightenment Germany: Dorothea Christiane Leporin's Treatise on the Education of Women," NWSA *Journal* 20 (2008): 106–7.

20 Moritz A. Von Thümmel, *Die Inoculation der Liebe. Eine Erzählung* (Leipzig: Weidmann's Erben und Reich, 1771); Christian F. Weiße, *Der Aerndtekranz. Eine komische Oper, in drey Aufzügen* (Leipzig: Dyck, 1771).

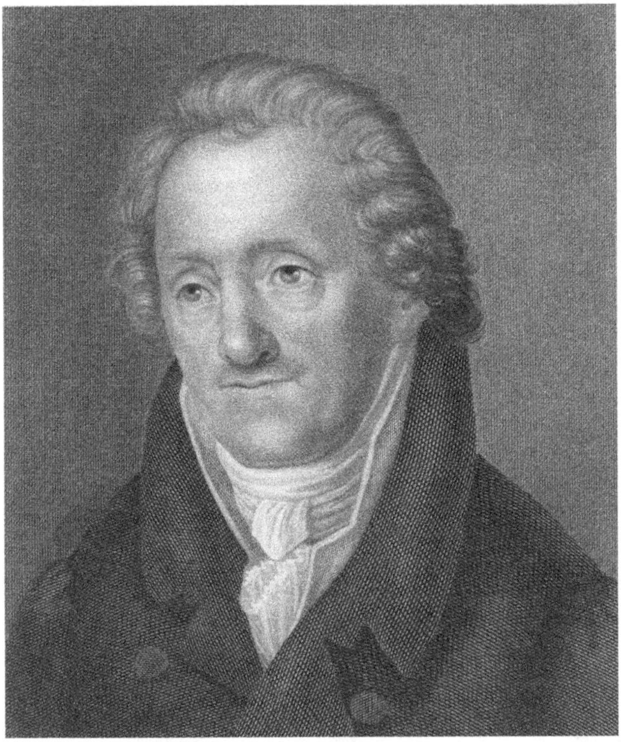

FIGURE 14
Moritz August von Thümmel. Engraving by F.W. Müller after L.C. Seideler
RIJKSMUSEUM, AMSTERDAM: RP-P-1914-531

'approved' man who may value his wife mainly for her appearance.[21] A strong social conscience and support for inoculation were indeed typical of men such as Weiße, a Leipzig tax official, and Thümmel, a Saxe-Coburg privy counsellor, both of whom belonged to an enlightened intelligentsia peculiar to Germany at that time, which included many influential public officials.[22]

Amalia, the heroine in Weiße's comic opera "The Harvest Wreath," shows the foresight and confidence to have herself inoculated before her marriage, albeit without the knowledge or approval of her fiancé or a male guardian. Yet, when she tells her friend Thomas of her bold move, he has scant knowledge of inoculation and shows little interest. This scene perhaps reflects Weiße's awareness of a general ignorance or indifference about inoculation among young men, compared to their female counterparts. Amalia's delight over her inoculation is enhanced by not only the realisation that she has become

21 Almut Spalding, *Elise Reimarus (1735–1805): The Muse of Hamburg: A Woman of the German Enlightenment* (Würzburg: Königshausen and Neumann, 2005), 328–31.

22 Tim C.W. Blanning, *The Culture of Power and the Power of Culture; Old-Regime Europe, 1660–1789* (Oxford: Oxford University Press, 2002), 207–11.

more self-assertive after the experience but also by the many compliments she receives on the improvement in her looks since her 'self-inflicted illness.' Amalia's glowing complexion sends an obvious message to female readers that inoculation offers benefits over and above smallpox prophylaxis, and that women who decide to have themselves inoculated should be sure to go ahead with it.[23] Inoculation was actually very likely to produce a healthy glow to the skin, considering doctors' recommendations of a largely vegetarian diet, mild non-alcoholic drinks, avoidance of chocolate, and abundant fresh air, during recovery.[24]

Weiße points out that women would benefit from inoculation through the preservation or even enhancement of their good looks, because most had a man in their life who placed a high value on his partner's appearance. He addresses that theme through Amalia's pretence in a letter to her husband while he was away for an extended period, that she was disfigured by smallpox. Although the aim of her deception was to re-kindle Lindford's love by giving him a pleasant surprise with her improved appearance, on his return, rumours of his loose behaviour after receiving her 'bad news' made her realise that her dishonesty had the opposite effect of threatening her marriage.[25] Lindford's claim after his eventual reconciliation with Amalia that he loves her dearly, in the light of his previous lack of courage confronting their future together after her 'disfigurement,' seems to be an appeal to husbands to pay attention to their wives' many endearing and enduring qualities, rather than focusing on their appearance.[26] The issue of a husband shunning and betraying his smallpox-disfigured wife had been raised almost a decade earlier by Weiße's former teacher and long-standing friend Professor Gellert in his poem "Lisette" (1763).[27]

The lengthy verse-story, "The Inoculation of Love" (1771), by Weiße's close friend Moritz August von Thümmel is another work rooted firmly in the literature linking inoculation to romance and marriage. Although Thümmel plagiarised his title from Hubert François Gravelot's classic illustration captioned *L'inoculation de l'amour,* in Jean-Jacques Rousseau's epistolary novel *Julie,* or *La nouvelle Héloïse,* Thümmel's work bears no relation to either that illustration

---

23 Christian F. Weiße, *Komische Opern* (Leipzig: Dyck, 1773), 259–61. From the 1770s, German women were enthusiastic readers of novels and plays: Reinhard Wittmann, "Was There a Reading Revolution at the End of the Eighteenth Century?," in *A History of Reading,* eds. Gugliemo Cavallo and Roger Chartier (Oxford: Blackwell, 1999), 297–300.

24 Thomas Dimsdale, *Neue Methode für die Einpfropfung der Pocken, auch Anhang* (Zürich: Füssli, 1768), 11–12.

25 Weiße, *Opern,* 254–8.

26 Weiße, *Opern,* 382–7, 405–7.

27 Weiße and Frisch, *Selbstbiographie,* 132, 152; Gellert, "Lisette," 119–21 (see pp. 134–5 above).

or that novel. Nor did Rousseau's 'inoculation of love' scene have anything to do with inoculation as a prophylactic measure. On the contrary, Rousseau's depiction of a young man kissing the arm of his beloved while she lies in bed suffering from smallpox suggests his desire to be infected by her disease.[28] Thümmel's verse-story *Die Inoculation der Liebe* has the very different theme of a beautiful young woman seeking an inoculation to preserve her complexion from smallpox, and falling in love with the young man who agrees to inoculate her but merely pretends to do so while seducing her.[29]

Thümmel's poem is set in a village where the beautiful teenage Karoline lives in a poor farmhouse with an elderly spinster who loves her dearly. Karoline has been in the woman's care ever since her miserly father, a wealthy aristocrat who lives nearby, placed her with the woman after his wife died during her birth. When Karoline is fifteen and aware of the importance of her beauty to her future prospects, the following events unfold that alert her to the promise offered by an inoculation using Dr. Thomas Dimsdale's method:

Einst las sie Zeitungen, und fieng von Frankfurt an,	That time reading the newspapers, at Frankfurt she began,
Die seltne Neuigkeit zu lesen:	Intending to read about what was new and rare:
"Es sey Dimsdal, der große Mann,	It says here that that Dimsdale, that now famous man,
Der Blatternimpfer, da gewesen." –	The smallpox inoculator, had recently been there.
Drauf, wie man denken kann, drauf fuhr	As you can believe, the newspaper was sure
Die Zeitung fort, die Leser zu belehren,	To instruct its readers and to be quite clear,
Wie viele Mädchen schon mit Hülfe seiner Kur	How many girls already helped by his cure
Vor dem Verlust der Reize der Natur	Had been left consoled, as well as quite secure
Zu ihrem Trost' gesichert wären ...	That losing their beauty was no longer to be feared ...

28 Jean-Jacques Rousseau, *Julie, ou la nouvelle Héloïse*, vol. 2 (Amsterdam: Rey, 1772), plate 5; Mary McAlpin, *Female Sexuality and Cultural Degradation in Enlightenment France: Medicine and Literature* (Routledge: Oxford and New York, 2016), 96.

29 Christian C.L. Hirschfeld, Review of *Die Inoculation der Liebe. Eine Erzählung*, by Moritz A. von Thümmel, *ADB*, no. 2 (1771): 352–6.

Auch unser Mütterchen, das doch sonst eben nicht	Yet, our dear old mother, who was in other cases
Schwergläubig war, fieng an dabey das Maul zu rümpfen. –	Not so hard to convince, showed distaste in her expression –
Die Blattern? schrie sie, was? die Blattern einzuimpfen? –	Smallpox? She cried, inoculate smallpox?
Unmöglich ist das gut: doch wollt' ich, der Bericht	It can't be any good, though I wish the news were true,
Wär' wahr! Ich weis, was sie mir einst verdarben.	I know that the disease once ruined my complexion.
Auch ich war einstens schön. – Da sah mich jedermann	I was a beauty at one time, and as I went by
Mit freundlichen und güt'gen Augen an:	Everyone looked with approving, friendly eyes
Doch itzt! – Wie bald ist es um uns gethan!	But now! How soon it messes with our lives!
Bey diese Larve voller Narben	This scarred, misshapen lump that did arise
Denkt weiter keine Seele dran. –	No longer rates a thought in anybody's mind.
Das junge Fräulein hört zum erstenmal' erschrocken	When the girl first heard this, she was really shocked,
Der Alten zu, und sieht zugleich in ihr,	Yet, in old the woman she could clearly see,
Mit angstvoll stiller Neubegier	With a new-found inner fear and quiet curiosity,
Ein traurig Monument der fürchterlichen Pocken.[30]	A tragic monument to the dreadful scourge of smallpox.

Karoline's path to securing an inoculation for herself was littered with obstacles:

So wäre, rief sie aus mit traurigen Geberden,	So, she cried out, with a sad demeanour,
Dieß Alles nur auf kurze Zeit so schön?	All of this beauty could vanish in an instant?
Dieß Alles könnte noch ein Raub der Blattern werden?	Smallpox could come and take it, like a robber?

30 Moritz A. von Thümmel, *Die Inoculation der Liebe. Eine Erzählung* (Biel: Heilmann, 1773), 14–15.

Und gäb' es denn kein Mittel auf der Erden	Is there no earthly way that anyone can counter
Der Schönheit Feinden zu entgehn? –	And can defeat such an enemy of beauty?
Dürft' ich nur meinen Vater fragen!	If I could only ask my father what to do!
Allein ich weiß es schon, es rühren meine Klagen	Yet I know already, my worries never move
Ihn niemals: denn sein Kopf ist nur von Zahlen voll,	Him in any way at all; his head is full of numbers,
Und stets schmählt er auf mich ... Es sey! –Man kann ja wohl	And he always scolds me ... yet should it not be up to us
Für seine Schönheit etwas wagen? –	To dare to take a risk that can save our beauty?
Der väterliche Trost war der Erwartung werth,	The fatherly comfort lived up to expectation,
So heuchlerisch, so schriftgelehrt,	So cold, like an official explanation,
Als ob er ihn in *** studieret: –	As if he'd found it in some scholarly oration –
"Das ist ein Thor, wer seine Schmerzen häuft,	That's foolish, one who gives himself such pain,
Ein Sünder, welcher Gott in seine Rechte greift,	Is none other than a sinner fighting God in His domains,
Ein Bösewicht, – wer sich inoculiret." –	A villain – to choose inoculation. –
Damit entließ er sie. – Die junge Schöne schlich	With that he let her go. The lovely young one crept away,
Zu ihrer Fee, und fieng so weinerlich,	Back her good fairy, and then began to cry,
So rührend an, ihr Herz dem Mitleid zu Entfalten,	Touching the woman's heart brimming with compassion.
Daß jeder Laut der guten Alten	Each tone pounding on the old one's soul
Bis in die Seele drang; und gleich entschloß sie sich	Prompted her decision to take immediate action.
Die Zeitung in der Hand, im Dorfe öffentlich	With newspaper in hand, in the village, openly,
Mit ihren Nachbarn Rath zu halten.	She went to her neighbours asking for advice.

Sie lief von Haus zu Haus und fieng zu fragen an,	As she walked from house to house, she began to find,
Vom Schulzen bis zum Leyermann:	That from the mayor to the organ-grinder,
Doch keiner war, der sie belehrte.	No one could advise her there.
Der Küster selbst, so klug er war, erklärte,	Even the verger, smart as he was, declared,
Daß eine Kur, wie die, noch nie erfunden sey.	That a cure such as that had never been discovered.
Indem sie nun betrübt nach ihrer Hütte kehrte,	Returning to her hut, depressed at how she'd fared,
Ritt ein geputzter Herr vorbey: …[31]	A well-turned out young man rode past …
Wagt' er es einst zu Mergentheim	At Mergentheim he had first taken on the risk
Das Kreuz der Keuschheit umzubinden,	To attach the cross upon his breast, binding him to chastity,
Schwur Haß und Tod (das gieng zur Noth noch an)	Swearing hatred and death (a vow still made in an emergency)
Den Türken und den Sarazenen. …[32]	To the Turks and Saracens. …
Ich bin ein deutscher Herr, der in der Nachbarschaft	I'm a German from this neighbourhood who lives upon his lands
Auf seinen Güthern lebt; doch misch' ich mich zuweilen	And on occasion too, I involve myself in medicine,
Gern in die Medecin, und kann so meisterhaft,	I can indeed cure with my skilful hands,
Als Dimsdale nimmermehr, ein hübsches Mädchen heilen.[33]	Just as well as Dimsdale, a beautiful young maiden.

The knight persuades the old woman to allow him to perform the 'inoculation cure' on the lovely Karoline, and the girl agrees.[34] The rest of the story revolves

31 Thümmel, 16–18.

32 Thümmel, 19.

33 Thümmel, 25. As a celibate knight from Mergentheim boasting traditional medical skills, the young man clearly belonged to the Order of Teutonic Knights, which was founded in the thirteenth century to force Christianity onto Slavic peoples of East Prussia and Livonia, and had its headquarters at Mergentheim in the eighteenth century: Hartmut Brockmann, *Der Deutsche Orden* (Munich: Beck, 1999), 11–12, 22–3, 31–7, 223.

34 Thümmel, 33–6.

around his ministrations. He convinces the naïve teenager and old woman that his kisses are the actual 'cure,' and Karoline's elevated pulse, hot cheeks, and listlessness after the knight's visits seem to indicate 'smallpox symptoms.' Yet even after several days the old woman could still see none of the characteristic spots.[35] By then, the knight realises that he cannot keep up the pretence, and that he is hopelessly in love and wishes to abandon his oath of celibacy. He asks Karoline's father for her hand in marriage, the old man agrees, and the happy couple soon have matters other than inoculation to occupy their time.[36]

Thümmel's character portrayals, which one reviewer praised for their close approximation to reality, suggest that a generational change in attitudes to inoculation was occurring.[37] The teenage Karoline reading about the benefits of the procedure in a newspaper marks her as one of the generation whose social outlook was broadened by reading, a pastime gaining in popularity at the time. Karoline also represents the young women with the courage and determination to make their own decisions. Even though she adheres to the ingrained obedience in asking her father for advice, she is not only well-aware that the staid, cold-hearted old man is unlikely to understand her desire to save her beauty, but she is also quite willing to disobey his advice on the issue. Thümmel suggests with his portrayal of the father's diatribe that older men failed to recognise the impact smallpox could have on their vulnerable daughters' futures, and that girls should be permitted to have themselves inoculated to protect their own future security, if they chose to.

Thümmel portrays the women – the beautiful teenage girl quite ignorant about smallpox, and her smallpox-disfigured old carer – as much more open-minded than Karoline's elderly father. Yet the old woman's horrific personal experience of smallpox prevents her from sharing Karoline's enthusiasm about the report of Dimsdale's 'new cure' that could preserve her beauty, which involved the inoculation of the feared disease. Nonetheless, she is prepared to trust the newspaper report and help Karoline secure her inoculation. Thümmel's implicit advice to young women lies in the smallpox-disfigured old spinster warning of complacency regarding smallpox, while Karoline 'advises' young women that inoculation using Dimsdale's new method offers them a choice, and that they should inform themselves before passing judgement about inoculation, even if their parents are sceptical.[38] The old woman and

---

35 Thümmel, 38–40.

36 Thümmel, 42, 52–6.

37 Hirschfeld, review of *Die Inoculation*, 357.

38 Two German translations of Dimsdale's book were published in 1768, three years before Thümmel's poem: Dimsdale, *Neue Methode* (Zürich: Füssli, 1768); Apx 2: Dimsdale (1768).

the old man are the most sharply contrasting characters: Karoline's old carer is not only compassionate but also willing to help the girl secure an inoculation to preserve her beauty, while her elderly father is hard-hearted, bigoted, and indifferent to his daughter's needs, perhaps reflecting a common reality of the time. Thümmel's depiction of Karoline's father ranting about the practice of inoculation "fighting God in his domains" may indeed have been a parody of his older Saxon acquaintances, considering the many pronouncements along the same lines by the elderly Saxon Professor Triller, in his poem *Geprüfte Pockeninoculation*.[39]

Thümmel's choice of the inoculation theme for a verse-story may have been inspired by Christian Felix Weiße, with whom he stayed for three months in 1768. Thümmel's dedication of "The Inoculation of Love" to Weiße suggests that his friend influenced the work in a significant way, perhaps through their discussion of ideas for new compositions. It is probably no coincidence that Thümmel's verse-story and Weiße's comic opera "The Harvest Wreath" are both about inoculation, and were both published three years after that prolonged visit. Other notable similarities between the two works lie in the principal characters. In each case, a young women is enthusiastic about inoculation, and self-assertive in choosing to have herself inoculated for the preservation of her beauty, without the approval of the relevant male authority in her life. The male characters in each work, by contrast, are either ignorant about inoculation or opposed to it.[40] An alternative source of Thümmel's inspiration for a verse-story about inoculation was perhaps his work as a privy counsellor in Duke Ernst Friedrich's enlightened government of Saxe-Coburg-Saalfeld.[41] Top-level discussions may have included inoculation, which was very topical in 1768 when both the Austrian and the Russian empress publicly embraced the practice themselves and offered parents free inoculation for their children, in response to widespread virulent smallpox.[42]

3 Real and Fictional Women as Inoculation Promoters

The image of self-assertive young women embracing inoculation to save their beauty, and of prominent mothers having their children inoculated to save

39 Apx 2: Triller (1766), 1–2, 12, 107–8. See also ch. 1, n. 48; ch. 4, n. 80.

40 Weiße and Frisch, *Selbstbiographie*, 132, 152; Thümmel, *Die Inoculation*, 3; Ernst von Gruner, *Leben MA von Thümmels* (Leipzig: Göschen, 1819), 29–33, 77.

41 Gruner, 76–7.

42 Apx 2: Heinsius (1780), 137–8, 144–5.

them from smallpox display the sensibility trademark of the 1770s-1800 literary works representing the private sphere.[43] Yet 'sensibility' was not always at the forefront in men's depictions of women who involved themselves in inoculation. A meaningful starting point for works of literature indicating men's attitudes to not only fictional women who publicly embraced inoculation but also to prominent real women who did so, is the opinion expressed in 1766 by an old scholar with a pre-Enlightenment mindset – Professor Triller:

Frau Worthley hat sie erst, zu London eingeführet,	Mrs. Wortley was the first to bring it into London,
Daher ihr allerdings, ein Ehrenlohn gebühret:	She should indeed be honoured for her contribution:
Vielleicht wird ihr nicht weit von Even Platz gemacht:	Perhaps not far from Eve is where she should be placed:
Denn wie dieselbe Gift den Seelen beygebracht:	Since that one put poison in the soul of our race:
So hat auch die hernach, den Leib mit Gift beflecket:	The later woman's poison acts to taint the the flesh:
Zwey Weiber haben nun zwey Gifte hier erwecket.[44]	Two women have now brought two poisons to afflict us.

Triller's disdain for Lady Montagu's leadership role in the promotion of inoculation in 1720s Britain is quite the opposite of the empathy shown by Weiße, Thümmel, and other younger poets and writers toward women asserting their independence by making their own decisions about inoculation. The use of the biblical allusion that all women are inherently sinful, as daughters of Eve, to disparage Lady Montagu was indeed quite out of step with other poets' praise for 'Montagu' as an 'inoculation heroine.'[45] Triller's disapproval was likely directed at both Lady Montagu's prominent role in promoting a practice he abhorred, and at her audacity in moving outside prescribed gender-roles by publicly pioneering and recommending a medical procedure. Yet his advanced age does not entirely explain Triller's medieval attitudes to women, since his five-years-younger friend from Leipzig, the poetry professor Johann Christoph

43 Becker-Cantarino, "Scope," 10.

44 Apx 2: Triller (1766), 196.

45 Many British and European poets and writers praised 'Montagu:' Shuttleton, *Smallpox*, 45–103, 137–57; 163–7; M.L.R., *L'inoculation, poème en quatre chants* (Amsterdam: Lacombe, 1773), 10, 11, 24, 27, 31 (the author was Abbé Jean-Joseph-Thérèse Roman); Francesco Zacchiroli, "La Inoculazione," in *Francesco Zacchiroli: Versi* (Lausanne, 1778), 31–2.

Gottsched, actually assisted women's endeavours to participate in the German intellectual milieu in the 1730s.[46] The pious Triller's negativity toward women having a role in the public sphere reflects St. Augustine's teaching that women were assigned the role of a husband's 'helpmate' because they were subordinate to men.[47] Rousseau's reinforcement of the idea that women lacked the capacity for profound thought and reasoning, in his bestselling novel *Julie, ou La nouvelle Héloïse* (1761), helped to keep women's activities restricted to the private sphere.[48] The more enlightened German poets' and writers' depictions of women as capable decision-makers, choosing inoculation, were so at odds with the notion of female intellectual inferiority that it seems they were following a deliberate agenda to emancipate women from their prescribed subservience and gender-roles.

Empress Catherine II of Russia was another woman for whom English and European poets were inclined to use 'inoculation heroine' imagery.[49] Catherine was well-known for not only having herself and her son inoculated in 1768 but also for her annual thanksgiving festivities celebrating the imperial pair's survival, which were intended to remind the public about inoculation and inspire others to follow her lead. An additional incentive for parents to adopt the procedure was her offer of monetary rewards for each child inoculated at the specialised centres she established in several towns.[50] Catherine's support for public inoculation contributed to her proudly-held status as one of the more enlightened European leaders of the time.[51] One overt admirer was the Königsberg-educated Prussian poet Johann Gottlieb Willamov, the director of a private school in St. Petersburg, who was so inspired by Catherine's leadership that he dedicated a number of panegyrics to her.[52] Willamov even sang

---

46 Spalding, *Reimarus*, 34; Wilson, "Germany," 278.

47 Poeter, "Gender," 103.

48 Spalding, *Reimarus*, 56.

49 Zacchiroli, "Inoculazione," 36–40; Seth, *Rois*, 234–7. Abbé Romans dedicated his panegyric about inoculation to Catherine: M.L.R., *L'Inoculation*, 1.

50 Apx 2: Review of "Petersburgische Kanzelvorträge von Joachim Christian Grot, Pastor bey der evangelischen Katharinenkirche auf Wasiley-Ostrow," *JP* 13 (1782): 223; Apx 2: "Die Geschichte" (1787), 174–5.

51 Apx 2: "Empfehlung der Blattereinimpfung" (1783), 63–5, 72; Hippel, *Verbesserung*, 59–62.

52 Johann G. Willamov, "Auf Ihro Russischkaiserlichen Majestät und des Durchlauigsten Großfürsten Wiedergenesung von Einimpfung der Blattern, im November 1768," in *Johann Gottlieb Willamov's Sämmtliche poetische Schriften* (Leipzig: Schwickert, 1779), 88–95; Christian H. Schmid, *Nekrolog, oder Nachrichten von dem Leben und den Schriften der vornehmsten verstorbenen teutschen Dichter* (Berlin: Mylius, 1785), 691–5.

his Pindaric ode rejoicing over the imperial inoculation success, in Catherine's presence, at the first annual celebration (1769) of the significant 'event.'[53]

Willamov's ode begins with an emotive poetic account of the smallpox 'monster' decimating the Russian people, a threat Catherine avoids by retreating to her palace. There she is visited by a distinctly female saviour, Hygeia, the goddess of health in ancient Greek mythology. The goddess informs Catherine that she and her precious son can be protected from deadly smallpox through inoculation, and that she herself trained an English descendant of Aesculapius in the technique. That is, of course, a reference to Dr. Thomas Dimsdale who made his name by inoculating the imperial pair.[54] Willamov proceeds to paint the empress as a benevolent, all-powerful mother whose only thoughts during the contemplative hours recovering from her inoculation are focused on the benefits of the practice for her people. To highlight Catherine's courage, strength of determination, and heroic selflessness in offering herself in that way, he uses the powerful simile of a soldier in the army of ancient Rome who earns a laurel wreath for his bravery in battle. Willamov also reminds his readers that Catherine is not only the mother of her people but also of the heir to the imperial crown, whose life she protected through inoculation as well as her own:

6. *Antistrophe*

Gleich öffnet der geschäftge Geist	In a short time, her active mind gazed
Zum Wohlthun neue Aussicht Ihr. Vergebens	On potential new vistas for doing good deeds.
Nimmt nicht ein Gott die Sorge meines Lebens,	A god would not bear my cares without reason,
So dachte sie, vielleicht mein Beyspiel reitzt	She mused. Through my example I could perhaps save
Aus schon gewisser Gruft viel tausend meiner Kinder.	Thousands of children from certain disaster.
Da wallt empfindungsvoll Ihr Blut geschwinder.	Compassion caused her blood to pulse faster.

53 Peter Drews, "Johann Gottlieb Willamov – ein deutscher Dichter im Russland Katharinas II," *Germanoslavica* 3 (1996): 210–11. A Pindaric ode consists of eight triple rhyming stanzas: strophes, antistrophes, and epodes: Sara de Ford and Clarinda H. Lott, *Forms of Verse* (New York: Meredith, 1971), 258–64.

54 Willamov, "Majestät," 91–3; Aesculapius was the God of Medicine and Hygeia's husband, in Greek mythology: Barry Powell, *Classical Myth* (Englewood Cliffs, NJ: Prentice Hall, 1995), 344.

6. *Epode*	
Ans Mutterherz, das für des Volkes Wohl	In that heart of a mother, the people's welfare
Mehr als für eigne Rettung wagte,	Was more important than saving herself,
Und des erhabensten Gedankens voll	And filled with the noblest thoughts and cares,
Nicht vor des Ausgangs Mißglück zagte. …	She'd not flinch for fear of a failed result. …
7. *Strophe*	
Entschloßner warf nicht Decius	Decius was no more determined when he charged
Sich in der Feinde dicht gedrängte Haufen,	Right into the enemy's closely-packed lines,
Um tausend Bürgerleben zu erkaufen …	To buy a thousand citizen's lives …
7. *Antistrophe*	
Genesen ist Sie: heil dir, Volk!	She has recovered: you people are saved!
Ihr menschenfreundlich Auge glänzet wieder,	Her compassionate eyes are sparkling again,
Vom Thron auf dich huldlächelnd nieder.	Paying smiling homage to you from her throne.
Genesen ist auch Er. – Heil Dir, o Volk! –	He has also recovered – what joy today! –
Der seiner Mutter Ruhm auf deine Nachwelt führet,	He'll bring his mother's fame down through generations,
Wenn Ihn, wie Sie, dein Diadem einst zieret.[55]	When he, like her, wears the crown of your nation.

The widely-circulated *Hamburgischen unpartheyischen Correspondenten* (HUC), with many readers in northern Germany where Catherine was born and raised, published Willamov's ode in 1769.[56] Those who had followed Catherine's rising fortunes since she left her home in Stettin (modern Szczecin, Poland) in 1744

55 Willamov, 93–5. Decius was fighting the Gauls at Sentinum in 295BC: Livy, *History of Rome*, 10.27–30 (London: Bell, 1892), 664–5.

56 The HUC had a circulation of 58,000 in 1750: Baasner, *Einführung*, 47.

to marry the Kiel-born heir to the throne of imperial Russia may have taken particular interest in the sycophantic poem about the empress's inoculation experience. Willamov's praise of the Russian imperial 'inoculation heroine' would also have interested readers with an inclination toward inoculation, who would undoubtedly have found the poem more inspiring than the often verbose opinion pieces and reports that had brought news of such matters for some years.

Another panegyric along the lines of Willamov's work was Pastor Johann Friedrich Danneil's preface to his book (1769) comparing inoculated and naturally-acquired smallpox, that he dedicated to the Royal Princess Anna Amalia, Margravine of Brandenburg and Abbess of Quedlinburg.[57] Danneil's conclusion that inoculation was a far preferable course of action than anxiously awaiting the arrival of potentially fatal smallpox is encapsulated in his homage to the Hohenzollern princess, whom he credits with 'taming' smallpox by encouraging inoculation. Having highlighted in the first two verses of the poem the imperatives of curbing the impact of the disease, in the last two verses Danneil praises Anna Amalia and her brother, the Prussian king Friedrich II, for promoting inoculation for the Prussian people's benefit:

Wie viele sehn noch, statt das Wüthen	How many watch the monster's rage,
Des Ungeheuers zu verhüten,	With sad indifference to the ways
Mit traurigträgem Kaltsinn zu!	They could avoid it when it's due?
Wer warnt, mit Friedrich, seinen Schaaren	Who, with Friedrich, gave the warning
Vor künftig drohenden Gefahren?	To the folk, of dangers dawning,
Wer? Königliche Fürstinn, Du!	Who? Oh Royal Princess, you!
Dein Blick wird diese Hyder zähmen,	Your glance will make this hydra tame,
Und ihr durch Kunst den Gift benehmen.	Your powers will take its poison away.
O Vorsicht, laß es benedeyn!	Let it be jealous, but please stay alert!
Frohlockend solls die Nachwelt hören,	Future folk should cheer your contribution,
Und ihrer Kinder Herzen lehren,	And teach their children of your action,
Noch dankbar, wie Dein Knecht, zu seyn.[58]	Still thankful just like me, your servant.

57 Apx 2: Danneil (1769), preface. Danneil identifies himself as consistorial adviser, inspector of the grammar school for the high nobility, and pastor of the St. Aegidius church in Quedlinburg.

58 Danneil, preface.

By depicting both the king and his sister as far-sighted visionaries for recommending inoculation before smallpox claimed many more lives, Danneil underscores the support for inoculation at the highest level in Prussia. He reinforces that message in the introduction to his book, stating that "the best and wisest monarchs, princes, and administrators are enthusiastically making known the benefits of this curative and blessed inoculation for their state and their people."[59] That reminder, along with Danneil's maternal imagery of the princess caring for Prussian children's futures by encouraging inoculation, was a recommendation to mothers, in particular, that they could accept inoculation with confidence.

Danneil (1740–71), Willamov (1736–77), and Johann Timotheus Hermes (1738–1821) who also created a literary 'inoculation heroine' to urge the adoption of inoculation, were all students in Prussia at the time the spirit of the Enlightenment encouraged by Friedrich II swept through the Protestant universities.[60] Hermes, as a Breslau church official, would have shared Pastor Danneil's awareness of the king's inoculation promotion efforts.[61] Hermes lent his own support to the royal initiative by transforming the fictional young mother from his popular novel "Sophie's Journey from Memel to Saxony," into a 'maternal inoculation heroine.' Sophie's account of her supposed journey in 1762 from Memel on the Baltic coast of East Prussia to Dresden (Saxony), during the Seven Years War, with its intrigues involving espionage, Sophie's kidnap, her rescue, and a series of love affairs, made Sophie one of the most popular fictional characters of the time.[62] Hermes capitalises on her popularity as a way of promoting inoculation, by inserting new text depicting her as an inoculation enthusiast. In that passage in volume two of the revised edition (1778), Sophie states in reply to the question of her son's smallpox status: "naturally he is inoculated, here is my doctor," and produces a copy of Professor Wagler's book (1772) describing the famously simple, so-called Gatti-Wagler inoculation method. She reinforces her recommendation by remarking that a female companion had already purchased the book for all their young women friends.[63] Hermes even cites the details of Wagler's book in a footnote, along with an apology for referring to a book that the fictional Sophie could not have known about in 1762 when she made her journey. He justifies its mention with the

59 Danneil, 1.

60 Johann M. Stroup, *The Struggle for Identity in the Clerical Estate* (Leiden: Brill, 1984), 90.

61 F.A. Pischon, *Denkmäler der deutschen Sprache, von Haller bis jetzt* (Berlin, 1845), 635–6.

62 Johann T. Hermes, *Sophiens Reise von Memel nach Sachsen* (Leipzig: Junius, 1771); Köpke, "Aus dem Leben des Johann Timotheus Hermes," in *Zeitschrift für das Gymnasialwesen*, ed. J. Mützell, 16th year (Berlin, 1862), 657.

63 Hermes, vol. 2 (Leipzig: Junius, 1778), 542–3; Apx 2: Gatti and Wagler (1772).

comment that "if this novel has no other value, then at least it has served to recommend that excellent book for the benefit of loyal fathers' and mothers' hearts."[64]

By depicting Sophie's nonchalant attitude to inoculation, Hermes takes the mystique out of the procedure and encourages readers to accept inoculation in the same relaxed manner as their heroine. Sophie's recommendation of Wagler's book as an ideal gift for women issues a similarly subtle message that women, not just men, should be making decisions about inoculation. The popularity of Hermes's novel would have ensured that a wide audience of both men and women received his overarching message that women should be in control of their own lives, advice already issued loudly and clearly in the very act of the fictional Sophie undertaking long-distance travel without an 'approved' male chaperone. Sophie's well-informed approach to inoculation also reinforces the image of an 'average mother' as a responsible decision-maker.

Works of literature depicting not just empresses adopting inoculation but also 'average mothers' were a way of boosting confidence in the practice and encouraging the perception that inoculation was for everyone, not just for the aristocracy and upper-class. More subtle nuances are evident in depictions of real and fictional women embracing not only inoculation *per se* but the newer, simpler procedures: Thümmel pinpoints Dimsdale's new method as the best chance for his poetic heroine, the teenage Karoline, to save her beauty, while Willamov alludes to Dimsdale as the highly-skilled inoculator of the Russian Empress and her son. A few years later, Hermes's fictional heroine Sophie recommends the equally effective, more recent, Gatti-Wagler method. Such portrayals of female role-models adopting up-to-date inoculation procedures paint women as modern, self-assertive, and capable of making good choices. Poets and writers, perhaps more than other men, were acquainted with independent-minded women through their involvement in the literary milieu where the women were known for resisting the constraints that society of the time selectively placed on womankind.[65]

4 Women as Authors, and as Targets of Advice

Through their roles as the primary carers in the household, many more women than men were confronted with the agonising day-by-day ordeal of smallpox.

64 Hermes, 543, n.

65 Spalding, *Reimarus*, 130–1; Ruth Finckh, ed., *Das Universitätsmamsellen-Lesebuch*, (Göttingen: Göttingen University Press, 2015), 14, 18.

Yet the exclusion of women from the public discourse left the commentary about smallpox treatments and the benefits of inoculation largely to the men. On the other hand, the occasional mother had put pen to paper by the 1790s to write about the impact of smallpox, and at least one managed to have her work published. Philippine Engelhard (Gatterer), a mother and poet well-known for turning ordinary experiences into compelling verse, conveys in poignant clarity the dreadful smallpox experience of a fictional noble family, which may well have been based in reality:[66]

Wohl keinem Brauch, ich anzudeuten,	I really have no need to mention,
Wie sehr die Aeltern der lieben Kinder sich freuten.	That the parents doted on their lovely children.
Allein ein Blättchen ward bald aus diesen Kleeblatt gepflückt;	Soon one leaflet was plucked out from that clover plant;
Auch Fränzchen ward vom Tod entrückt!	When death carried off the toddler Franz!
Ihn faßten die Pocken – die kleinen Schwestern nicht minder.	Smallpox attacked him – no less his little sisters.
Es nahm die Krankheit ihn weg! Die Feindinn Erwachsner und Kinder;	The sickness took him! That foe of children and adults;
Die im Gesicht der schönen Margaris,	Which left its marks imprinted clearly on the face
Nach schwerem Lager, Spuren hinterließ;	Of lovely Margaris, after her bad case;
Doch unbeschadet der Füßen, lieblichen Mine.	Yet did no damage to her feet, a charming plot.
Hingegen die kleine Adeline,	Little Adeline was cast the other lot,
Die schmauste und zechte im Bett – wie ein Abt!	She drank and feasted like an abbot, in her bed!
Man sah es ihr nachher nicht an, daß sie die Blattern gehabt. –	She showed no traces of it after she recovered.
Ach aber der Junker war tod![67]	But, alas, the young nobleman was dead!

Published female poets were rare enough at that time. Even rarer were women with the courage to engage in the public discourse in the print media. One

66 Engelhard was inspired to write by the student-poets she met at Göttingen university where her father, Johann Christoph Gatterer, was a history professor: Finckh, 33–4.

67 Philippine Engelhard, "Eine wahrscheinliche Historia," in *Philippine Engelhard: Gedichte* (Göttingen, Dieterich, 1782), 121–2.

woman, who disguised her identity by calling herself Hlodowich, was bold enough to write (1789) to Justin Bertuch, the editor of a prominent fashion journal, appealing to him and to the exclusively male editors of other fashion journals to recommend inoculation forcefully to their readers. Accompanying her letter, Hlodowich provided a well-written submission from a female counterpart explaining a woman's view of the importance of inoculation, and appealed for its insertion in Bertuch's fashion journal. To his credit, Bertuch published the anonymous woman's submission:

> Has this beneficial discovery not earned a place in your magazine of advice for the common good? ... You, my men, should show your female readers that this discovery is not just a slight benefit for beauty ... The most normal facial features are often altered by smallpox, the most beautiful eyes are darkened by it, or lost completely, the mouth is distorted, the straightest nose is made crooked, and the whole face becomes pocks and seams ... Try to make inoculation fashionable! Assure your female readers that there is no more trustworthy means of preventing a tragic outcome, than inoculation.[68]

The writer goes on to assert that beauty is more important to women than their general health that doctors were so busily promoting.

Bertuch sought, and received, an opinion from Dr. Christoph Wilhelm Hufeland (see Figure 8 on p. 88) who was at that time practising in Weimar before being appointed to a professorship at Jena. Bertuch published Hufeland's response alongside Hlodowich's letter and the anonymous woman's assertions, adding his own introduction to each item. Hufeland not only agreed with the contributor's sentiments but also praised her admirable intentions in advising women-in-general to do their children the favour of having them inoculated to ensure lifelong protection from smallpox-disfigurement:

> Inoculation would be ... the simplest, surest and most enduring beauty treatment by which a mother can secure the advantage of a good external appearance for the lifetime of her child... In Georgia and Circassia it is the mothers' general duty... Recently, Pastor Eisen in Livonia introduced the inoculation of children by their mother, through word and example, so that many hundreds of average mothers successfully inoculated their children, with the best of outcomes. A sewing needle was the instrument

68 Apx 2: Hufeland et al., "Empfehlung" (1789), 79–80.

> used for the operation, and fresh air, water, and finally a laxative were the only medicines. I recommend to all caring and sensible mothers his small instruction leaflet, to raise awareness, and as the best advice in this matter.[69]

Hufeland extended his praise to Swiss mothers and to a German mother who inoculated their own children, though he fell short of overtly recommending that course of action to all German mothers.[70] His mention of Pastor Eisen in Livonia teaching mothers to inoculate their children is pertinent to the Königsberg (East Prussia) doctor J.C. Moritzfeldt's observation in 1797 that women were "very keen for advice about inoculation," and that "inoculation is very widespread here." Moritzfeldt's additional comment: "I know of many private individuals and pastors in rural areas who are doing it successfully, as in Lithuania and Kurland," strongly suggests influences coming from the Russian Baltic states linked to East Prussia through coastal shipping.[71] Inoculation in the Baltic region to the north-east of Prussia had greatly expanded during the previous two decades under the influence of a number of Lutheran pastors enticed to the region by the needs of the peasant population on the extensive farming estates, which were owned largely by German landlords. One of the most recognised of those pastors, Johann Georg Eisen von Schwarzenberg, conducted a campaign in the 1770s to teach peasant mothers in Livonia to inoculate their own children, in which he was strongly supported by Pastor Joachim Christian Grot, originally from Holstein.[72]

Hufeland brought the combined recommendations of inoculation in the fashion magazine article to a later group of young mothers, by re-utilising the article as a chapter in his (1797) book: "Beneficial Essays for the Promotion of Health and Well-Being."[73] His move was part of a trend in the 1790s for doctors to target women with health advice, in recognition of women's importance

---

69 Hufeland et al., 82–3, 85–6. Pastor Eisen's publication, cited by Hufeland: Johann G. Eisen, *Die erleichterten und den Müttern selbst übertragenen Blatternimpfung* (Riga: Hartnoch, 1774). For further discussion of Hufeland and his career, see pp. 87–8.

70 Hufeland et al., 86.

71 Johann C.W. Juncker, *Archiv der Aerzte und Seelsorger wider die Pockennoth,* vol. 5 (Leipzig: Weygand, 1798), 197; Neil MacGregor, *Germany. Memories of a Nation* (London: Allen Lane, 2014), 237–44.

72 Arnold C. Klebs, *Die Variolation im achtzehnten Jahrhundert: ein historischer Beitrag zur Immunitätsforschung* (Gießen: Töpelmann, 1914), 55. Rural landlords in Livonia tended to heed the pastors' advice to adopt inoculation to protect their peasant work-force: Apx 2: Elsner (1787), 38.

73 Christoph W. Hufeland, *Gemeinnützige Aufsätze zur Beförderung der Gesundheit und das Wohlseyns* (Vienna: Schmidbauer and Kemp, 1797), 29–47.

as the usual decision-makers on family dietary and health matters. Friedrich Benjamin Osiander from Göttingen was another high-profile professor who recognised that women were the most appropriate targets for certain kinds of medical advice. He not only directed his book about midwifery (1796) to "practising midwives … and every mother" but also advised midwives and mothers to learn the inoculation procedure. Osiander points out to his female readers that farmers, tailors, and other non-medically-trained people had already inoculated their own children successfully.[74] Ten years earlier, Pastor Christian Gottfried Klose from Domanze (Silesia) issued a similar message to women, albeit much more forcefully, in his article "To Silesia's Mothers," which appeared in a 1786 issue of the *Schlesische Provinzialblätter*. Klose not only exhorted mothers to inoculate their own children if a medical man was unavailable but also provided them with a specialist doctor's step-by-step inoculation procedure.[75]

Samuel Gottlieb Bürde, a high-ranking Silesian government official and poet of some repute, adopted quite a different mode of delivery for 'messages' to women about inoculation. He issued his implicit advice in a romantic verse-novel (1794), clearly indicating the subject-matter and target audience by giving the work the title: "The Inoculated Bride." While romantic love and inoculation do take centre-stage, the lengthy poem is by no means a simple romance. It is more of an exploration of loyalty, trust, and betrayal in love- and family-relationships, based on an inoculation experience. Bürde's choice of the foremost monthly magazine of the very large region of Silesia, the *Schlesische Provinzialblätter*, for the publication of "The Inoculated Bride" ensured that the story reached a wide audience. Moreover, the serialisation of the work in four consecutive issues, forcing readers to wait a month for the next instalment, not only helped to maintain suspense about the progress of the inoculated heroine's romance but also ensured that smallpox prophylaxis captured the readers' attention for quite some time.[76]

Bürde's main 'message' to his target audience of young women was that inoculation was the best way to avoid being disfigured by smallpox, and that wives and fiancées risked being shunned or abandonded by their partners if their complexions were badly damaged. Bürde's implicit advice about the urgent need for young women to protect themselves from such an eventuality was made even more compelling by its mode of delivery: in a fictional romance. The problem of men's inability to tolerate a partner's loss of beauty,

---

74 Friedrich B. Osiander, *Lehrbuch der Hebammenkunst* (Göttingen: Rosenbusch, 1796), title page (quote), 607.

75 Apx 2: Klose (1786), 405, 408–10.

76 Apx 2: Bürde (1794), 21–36, 120–35, 234–52, 497–514.

because men placed paramount importance on a woman's appearance, was very real according to the poets and writers.[77] Contemporary commentators were otherwise largely silent on the issue, which is not surprising considering the implied slur on men-in-general, and the exclusively male prerogative to issue the published social commentary.

Bürde's poem revolves around the Italian violin virtuoso Philidor falling in love with the beautiful teenage Mathilde while she accompanies him on the piano at a private concert at her old uncle's house, where she lives. The young couple's betrothal and the events surrounding Mathilde's inoculation to preserve her beauty for her marriage are the underlying theme of the remainder of the work. Importantly, Philidor knows nothing of Mathilde's inoculation, which is timed to coincide with his absence on a business-trip. The recommendation of inoculation by Mathilde's Aunt Ursula, the unnamed old uncle's sister, was a warning from Bürde aimed directly at young women:

Schön bist du jetzt! allein, mein Kind, du hast	You're beautiful now! But, my child,
Die Blattern noch zu überstehen.	You've yet to withstand smallpox.
Ach! wenn einst dieser fürchterliche Gast	Alas! When this awful guest finds you,
Dich heimsucht, deinen Reiz in Häßlichkeit verwandelt, –	Ugliness can transform beauty –
Wer weiß, ob Philidor alsdann so edel handelt,	Who knows if Philidor would act honourably,
Was er der Rahel war der Lea noch zu seyn,	And regard Leah as fondly as Rachel,
Gelassen den Verlust der Schönheit zu verschmerzen.	If he has to endure the loss of her beauty.
Und seiner Gattin Werth allein,	Would he value his wife for her true worth,
Vom Körper abgesehn, nach ihrem Geist und Herzen	Her mind and heart, apart from her body?
Zu schätzen? – Ich behaupte – nein![78]	Weighing it up – I believe – no!

77 Gellert, "Lisette," 119–21; Weiße, *Aerndtekranz*, 382–7; Apx 2: "Die Inokulation" (1799), 518–9.

78 Apx 2: Bürde (1794), 236. Rachel and Leah were biblical women, the daughters of Laban. Jacob fell in love with Rachel who was more beautiful than Leah, and agreed to work for Laban for seven years in exchange for marrying her. After that time Laban deceived Jacob into marrying Leah: 29 Genesis 15–28 (King James Version, New York, 1974).

In an apparent attempt to assure his female readers that the inoculation procedure was tried and proven, Bürde has Ursula issue this haughty pronouncement:

Mein Bruder hat ja den Versuch	My brother, indeed, has already tried
Schon oft mit Glück gemacht – die Blattern einzuimpfen,	To inoculate smallpox, often with luck,
Und über diese Cur" (setzt sie mit Naserümpfen	And (she states with her nose in the air),
Hinzu), so gar ein dickes Buch	He has even written a thick book on this cure.
Geschrieben. Würd' er sich nicht öffentlich beschimpfen,	Would he not publicly blame himself
Ein Mittel, das er als bewährt	If a means that he recommends
Empfiehlt, nicht selber anzuwenden? [79]	As protection, he did not employ himself?

Mathilde's uncle gives a defensive explanation for not having inoculated his niece at a younger age, which was a reminder that early childhood was the best age for the procedure:

Der Alte nickt, und spricht: dein Rath ist Beyfalls werth,	The old man nods, and speaks: your advice deserves acclamation,
Auch gab ich ihn schon längst; du, Schwester, warst dagegen.[80]	I said just that a long time ago, but sister, you were against it.

At this point, the malevolent Ursula's ulterior motive in advising Mathilde's inoculation is about to be revealed: Philidor's purchase of a large farm with his earnings as a violin virtuoso that inspires her to dream of her own elevated status if she were Philidor's wife instead of Mathilde. Ursula actually hopes that the inoculation will cause either Mathilde's death or disfigurement, removing her from contention as Philidor's bride. Her alternative plan if the inoculation succeeds is to convince the unsuspecting Mathilde to wear a veil when Philidor returns for their wedding, as a test of his loyalty. Crucial to Ursula's strategy is her plan to waylay Philidor before he reaches Mathilde so that she can bemoan the tragic destruction of his bride's beauty, fully expecting him to reject the veiled Mathilde. In Ursula's fantasy world, Philidor would turn to her when she convinces him of her own impeccable credentials as a wife for a wealthy farmer.[81]

79 Bürde, 237–8.
80 Bürde, 238.
81 Bürde, 239–40, 244–7.

As it turns out, the inoculated smallpox leaves no trace on Mathilde's blooming complexion.[82] With these lines, Bürde presents a clear advertisement for inoculation:

Die, ihr durch Kunst gegebne, Krankheit brach	The illness produced by the new art
In wenig Tagen aus; ein kleiner Fieberschauer,	Showed itself in a few days; just a mild fever,
Ohn' alle Heftigkeit und nur von kurzer Dauer,	Not too severe and only short-lived,
Geht ihr voran, die Wangen glühn	Her cheeks then glow a bright purple-red.
Vom höherm Purpurroth. Nicht lange drauf erschien	Not much later came the first sign
Der vorgelockte Feind, — ein Heer von kleinen Flecken,	Of the enticed foe – a mass of small spots,
Die rothen Perlen gleich der Kranken Haut bedecken,	The red pearls soon cover the patient's skin –
Doch die, – so schnell wie auf der Flur	Yet just as quickly as out in the fields
Die frühsten Kinderchen des jungen Mays verblühen,	The first corn-sprouts finish their flowering,
Dank der vereinten Macht der Kunst und der Natur!	The technique and nature's power, combined,
Allmählich wieder sich verziehen.[83]	Cause them to vanish forever.

The simplicity of Mathilde's inoculation and the mildness of her disease would have impressed anyone who had witnessed a case of severe smallpox. Moreover, the described method seemed simple enough for any competent doctor to carry out safely. At that time many Silesians knew little about inoculation, which only began to receive much publicity in the region in 1786 when smallpox was claiming many lives.[84] Bürde's line that the "technique and nature's power, combined" caused inoculated smallpox to vanish without a trace reflects the contemporary focus on nature ensuring the well-being of people who chose a healthy lifestyle. Prussia was indeed one of the regions where doctors,

82 Bürde, 243.

83 Bürde, 242–3.

84 A number of articles in *SP* pointed to the unfamiliarity of inoculation: Apx 2: Migula, "Noch etwas" (1787), 428; "Bericht" (1788), 294; "Waldenburg" (1790), 166.

government officials, and pastors pursued an agenda to improve the people's health by providing them with advice about diet and other health-related matters, including inoculation.[85]

No young woman keenly anticipating the next issue of the *Schlesische Provinzialblätter* to find out how the plot was unfolding could have missed Bürde's depiction of Mathilde's beauty being protected by inoculation, with no adverse consequences. Nor could readers miss his message that smallpox disfigurement could destroy a young woman's marriage prospects. Although smallpox was in abeyance in most of Silesia in 1794 when *Die inoculierte Braut* was published, Bürde clearly recognised the need to raise the topic of inoculation and highlight the risk of smallpox for teens who had not contracted the disease naturally.[86] He was also warning parents to protect their children, and young women to protect themselves, before the inevitable return of the disease.

Another of Bürde's powerful messages was the high value of loyalty and trust. He makes that point through Philidor's rush to reiterate his vows to the veiled Mathilde after the contemptible Aunt Ursula told him when he returned for the wedding that his bride's beauty was lost to smallpox. The failure of Ursula's treacherous plot not only aroused Philidor's disdain and shattered her fantasy but also caused her to be shunned by the guests attending the nuptials when they learned of her lies and betrayal. Ursula's disloyalty to Mathilde, and her cynical wish for her niece to succumb to the inoculation she herself convinced her to adopt were reminders that women would often go to great lengths to raise their own status at the expense of others they regarded as rivals. Joachim Christian Blum, another Prussian poet, touched on that theme too, with these 'thoughts' (1771) of a jealous 'wallflower' at a local festival where an attractive, vivacious counterpart was receiving all the attention. Smallpox is once again depicted as a woman's 'weapon:'

Mit hohlem Aug' indeß sieht auf die Königin	With her jealous, vengeful eyes
Des Bals, die neidische Gespielin hin,	She gazes at the party queen,

85 Mary Lindemann, "'*Aufklärung*' and the Health of the People; '*Volksschriften*' and Medical Advice in Braunschweig-Wolfenbüttel, 1756–1803," in *Das Volk als Objekt obrigkeitlichen Handelns,* ed. Rudolf Vierhaus (Tübingen: Niemeyer, 1992), 11–13; Ute Frevert, *Krankheit als politisches Problem 1770–1880* (Göttingen: Vandenhoek & Ruprecht, 1984), 32–3.

86 Articles about inoculation appeared in the *Schlesische Provinzialblätter* in the smallpox-epidemic years 1790–91, but not in 1792–3 (Apx 2). Periods when smallpox was epidemic in various parts of Silesia are indicated in Heinrich A. Gins, *Krankheit wider den Tod* (Stuttgart: Fischer, 1963), 68–70.

Die ihr, dafern sie sich durch ihren Fall erhöbe,	To whom she'd love to give smallpox,
Die Blattern allenfalls zum andermale gäbe.[87]	To bring her down and raise herself.

Notably, "The Inoculated Bride" is absent from all volumes of Bürde's extant published works, leaving only the original serialised journal publication. Yet Bürde published a similar verse-story two years later with essentially the same plot and characters, though it was more simply structured and lacked the erudite classical references in the earlier work. "The Bridegroom's Test" follows the already familiar path toward the bridegroom learning of his bride's bout of smallpox, shortly before encountering her wearing a veil. As in the earlier poem, the disease was inoculated by the bride's uncle, and the outcome is the same happy reaffirmation of the young couple's love in spite of the bride's concealment of her features.[88] An obvious difference is Bürde's toned-down 'message' about inoculation, which is mentioned just once, by the uncle, thirty-one lines from the end of the long verse-story:

Und durch die Blattern (die, von meiner eignen Hand	As you can see, from the smallpox (that I inoculated
Ihr eingeimpft, sie längst schon überstand),	With my own hand, from which she recovered
Ward, wie du siehst, die glatte Aussenwand	Quite long ago), the walls that were smooth
Des niedlichen Gebäudchens nicht verschlimmert.[89]	In that cute little house are still the same.

Bürde's mere passing mention of inoculation in "The Bridegroom's Test," in the light of his overt, prolonged pro-inoculation 'message' in "The Inoculated Bride" just two years earlier, suggests compliance with changes in official policy. As an inoculation enthusiast and as a high-ranking secretary in the Silesian government, Bürde may have been aware of the official policies about inoculation.[90] His depiction in "The Inoculated Bride" (1794) of inoculation being

87 Joachim C. Blum, "An den Komates, 1771," in *Joachim Christian Blum's Sämmtliche Gedichte* (Karlsruhe: Schmieder, 1781), 286.

88 Samuel G. Bürde, "Die Bräutigamsprobe. Eine Erzählung," in *Samuel Gottlieb Bürde: Erzählungen* (Berlin, 1796), 57–140.

89 Bürde, 134.

90 "Nekrolog, Samuel Gottlieb Bürde," *SP* 93 (1831): 445–6.

carried out by a doctor who had written a book about the methodology was consistent with a directive from the Prussian *Ober-collegium medicum* to the Silesian Medical Board requiring doctors to be properly trained in inoculation procedures.[91] Similarly, Bürde's understatement of inoculation in "The Bridegroom's Test" (1796) corresponds with a Prussian Medical Board directive at the end of 1794 recommending a cautious approach, owing to concerns that an unregulated expansion of the practice could increase the spread of smallpox.[92]

The targeting of women with advice about smallpox and inoculation reflects a growing recognition that women were best-placed to effect changes consistent with the medical and health Enlightenment, through their supremacy in domestic matters.[93] The Königsberg mayor Theodor Gottlieb Von Hippel, in his book "On the Civil Advancement of Women" (1792), made a confident assessment of women's ability to contribute to the public as well as the domestic sphere when given the opportunity. He even goes as far as recommending a wider leadership role for women, naming Queens Margaretha from Denmark, Christina from Sweden, and Sophie Charlotte from Prussia as women whose great deeds were largely ignored but would have been praised if they were accomplished by men. He reserves special praise for the Russian Empress Catherine II, listing many of her achievements in all spheres of government, including her inoculation initiatives.[94]

Long before doctors began directing advice to women on matters of inoculation and family health, enlightened poets and writers were championing women's decision-making capabilities on those matters. The literary elite were also ahead of their time in using smallpox and inoculation as themes to criticise society's fixation on beauty as the measure of a woman's true worth. The 'smallpox poetry and literature' indeed paints a broad picture of a vision of social progress, with its contrasting imagery of elderly men pontificating that inoculation was dangerous, innovative nonsense while women were casting off the paternalistic shackles and making their own decisions on the matter. It seems that by the end of the eighteenth century, the enlightened cohort of the broader society had caught up with the literary elite in perceiving women as strong-willed decision-makers and not always mere followers of men's advice.

91 Karl F.W.A. Vater, *Preussisch-Schlesische Civil Medicinal- and Sanitäts-Verfassung*, part 2 (Breslau: Korn, 1800), 544–5.

92 Moritz Pistor, "Geschichte der preussischen Medizinalverwaltung," *DVG* 40 (1908): 780–1.

93 Johann G. Kühn, *Medicinischer Briefwechsel eines Arztes mit einigen Frauenzimmern* (Breslau: Korn, 1796); Johann P. Frank, *Abhandlung über eine gesunde Kindererziehung, besonders für Mütter, denen ihre und ihre Kinder Gesundheit am Herzen liegt* (Leipzig: Baumgärtner, 1794); Friedrich W. Hennig, *Abhandlung über das Selbstsäugen der Kinder* (Breslau: Korn, 1797).

94 Hippel, *Verbesserung*, 67–8.

CHAPTER 6

Pastors and Peasants

Parish clergymen who conducted the funerals and recorded details of the deaths in church registers were acutely aware of the carnage wrought by smallpox. The more progressive churchmen tended to embrace inoculation, in many cases encouraged by reports of their more high-profile counterparts' dismissal of objections to the practice. Isaac Maddox, the Bishop of Worcester, led the way in that regard with his widely-publicised sermon (1753) that inspired a number of European churchmen to speak out in support of inoculation too.[1] Clergymen keen to promote inoculation tended to underpin their stance with simple examples based on the principle that the preservation of life was the paramount consideration, which had replaced the earlier doctrine of predestination that was conceptually inconsistent with any form of disease prophylaxis.[2]

Many German pastors promoted inoculation from the pulpit, and some extended the reach of their words by publishing their sermons or by submitting promotional articles to provincial journals.[3] Pastors also arranged group inoculations carried out by local medical men with the requisite experience.[4] Others tended to inoculate their children themselves if suitably skilled practitioners were unavailable, which was often the case in rural areas.[5] A successful outcome sometimes encouraged those pastors to offer to inoculate their parishioners' children too, as some of their counterparts in areas of rural Scotland, Sweden, Denmark, and Russia were doing.[6] Pastors also wrote books about inoculation. Johann Friedrich Danneil from the St. Aegidius Church in

1 Apx 2: Bishop of Worcester (1753), 346–52; Chais (1756); Cramer (1759); Wolf (1768); Löber (1769).

2 Johann P. Süßmilch, *Die göttliche Ordnung in den Veränderungen des menschlichen Geschlechts, aus der Geburt, dem Tode und der Fortpflanzung desselben erwiesen*, 2nd ed., vol. 2 (Berlin: Buchhandlung der Realschule, 1762), 441–2; Apx 2: Cramer (1760), 327–8; Chais (1756), 51–2, 55.

3 Apx 2: Löber (1769); Merkel (1777); Klose (1786); Schwager, "Patriotische" (1786); Migula, "Inokulation" (1787); Künzel (1788); Vasmer (1795).

4 Apx 2: "Pokkeneinimpfung" (1796), 160–67; Brinckmann (1797), 125–27; Christian S. Ungnad, "Nachricht von einer zahlreichen Blatter-Impfung auf dem Lande," *Jahrbücher der preußischen Monarchie unter der Regierung Friedrich Wilhelms des Dritten*, vol. 3 (Berlin: Unger, 1800), 304–5.

5 Johann C.W. Juncker, *Archiv der Aerzte und Seelsorger wider die Pockkenoth*, vol. 5 (Leipzig: Weygand, 1796–99), 83, 118, 173, 197; Apx 2: Migula (1786), 208–9.

6 Apx 2: Migula (1786), 208–10; Piccard (1794), 673–6; "Die Geschichte" (1787), 179. Deborah C. Brunton, "Smallpox Inoculation and Demographic Trends in Eighteenth-Century Scotland,"

 | DOI:10.1163/9789004465374_008

Quedlinburg was so weary of seeing lives damaged by smallpox that he outlined in some detail the many advantages of adopting inoculation rather than awaiting the arrival of the disease that he described in this way:

Noch würget, gleich Lernäens Hyder,	Smallpox, just like Lerna's hydra,
Die Blatternkrankheit Menschen nieder,	Murders and casts down mankind;
Und schlachtet Hekatomben ab.	Leaves slaughtered millions in its wake.
Die Länder mit den Fürsten zittern,	While people and their leaders shudder,
Und tausend Väter mit den Müttern	Countless fathers with the mothers
Beweinen ihrer Kinder Grab.	Grieve beside their children's graves.
Die nicht von ihrem Gifte starben,	The ones its poison did not kill
Sind krank und ungestalt von Narben,	Are left disfigured, scarred, and ill,
Und tragen heimlich ihre Schmach.	As social outcasts doomed to hide.
Was noch vom Biße dieser Schlange	Those who escape the deadly bite
Verschont ist, bleibt vor Anfall bange,	Live in fear this snake will strike,
Und diese Furcht läßt nimmer nach.[7]	And never will this fear subside.

Governments keen to curb the smallpox mortality generally recruited the country pastors to distribute their medical advice circulars, in line with a longstanding tendency to view the pastors as strategically-placed rural helpmates ready and willing to do their bidding.[8] The pastor would usually deliver the advice from the pulpit and discuss the matter with interested churchgoers before distributing the circulars more widely. In their journal articles and reports, pastors would in some cases bemoan their parishioners' resistance to not only the government's smallpox treatment recommendations but also to other kinds of official advice.[9] The strong adherence of country folk to their traditional beliefs and practices, and the widespread belief that smallpox outcomes were

---

Medical History 36 (1992): 409, 413; Peter Skold, "From Inoculation to Vaccination: Smallpox in Sweden in the Eighteenth and Nineteenth Centuries," *Population Studies* 50 (1996): 250.

7 Apx 2: Danneil (1769), preface.

8 Ute Frevert, *Krankheit als politisches Problem 1770–1880* (Göttingen: Vandenhoek & Ruprecht, 1984), 54–6; Mary Lindemann, "'*Aufklärung*' and the Health of the People; '*Volksschriften*' and Medical Advice in Braunschweig-Wolfenbüttel, 1756–1803," in *Das Volk als Objekt obrigkeitlichen Handelns,* ed. Rudolf Vierhaus (Tübingen: Niemeyer, 1992), 104–5.

9 Juncker, *Archiv*, 5:237; 7:223; "Glücklicher Erfolg der Bemühungen eines Predigers, der seine Kirchkinder anzuweisen suchte, wie sie sich bei herrschenden Pocken in Ansehung ihrer kranken Kinder zu benehmen hätten," *SP* 25 (1797): 148; Apx 2: Schwager, "Patriotische" (1786), 230.

determined by God's will were problems that some pastors tried to counter with intuitive strategies aimed toward convincing parents to change their usual smallpox treatment approach.[10] Other pastors recommended inoculation as the best course of action.[11] Pastors' accounts of their interactions with their parishioners on the matter of smallpox treatment and inoculation are the only sources from many eighteenth-century rural parishes that describe peasants' ways of dealing with the disease.

In many villages across the countryside the pastor was the only person sufficiently well educated to write with a high degree of fluency. Aware that most townsfolk were quite unfamiliar with the rhythms of rural life, certain country pastors used their writing skills to inform the wider society about day-to-day village living, and the ways in which local country folk approached various issues.[12] Collectively, the country pastors provided most of the lasting eighteenth-century accounts of the lifestyle and ideas about myriad matters among the peasantry in various regions. Those reports provide an understanding of the rural social issues pertinent to not only the problem of smallpox but also to the efforts to curb the impact of the disease at that time.

1 The Problem of Smallpox in Rural Areas

German peasants in the eighteenth-century had a reputation for being quite backward compared to the townsfolk, which had much to do the generally poor education offered at village schools.[13] Although the standard should have improved in the second half of the eighteenth century, at least in Prussia after Friedrich II issued his edict (1763) requiring all children aged between five and thirteen to attend school for six hours per day except in rural areas during the harvest, several factors compromised that initiative.[14] The appointment of inadequate

10 Juncker, 3:127, 131–2; 5:212; 6:130–1; 7:226.

11 Juncker, 2:261; 3:8; Apx 2: Schwager (1784).

12 L.F.A. von Coelln, "Beytrag zur Charakteristik des Lippeschen, Ritbergischen und Paderbornischen Bauern," *WM* 1 (1784): 104–16; "Etwas zur Characteristik des Landmanns in der westphälischen Grafschaft Mark," *Neues WM* 3 (1792): 185–202; Johann M. Schwager, "Ueber die Ravensburger Bauer," *WM* 2 (1786):49–74. See also pastors' reports in the seven volumes of 'Juncker's Archive,' such as those cited in notes 10 and 11 above.

13 Juncker, *Archiv*, 4:69; R.Z. Becker, "Versuch über die Aufklärung des Landmannes," *TM* 3 (1785): 120–6; "Warum man mit der Aufklärung der Bürger und Bauern noch so weit zurück, und wie weit man gleichwohl gekommen ist," *Beyträge zur vaterländischen Historie, Geographie, Statistik* 3 (1790): 336–9.

14 Eduard Clausnitzer, *Die Volksschulpädagogik Friedrichs des Grossen und der preussischen Unterrichtsverwaltung seiner Zeit* (Halle: Schroedel, 1902), 65–86; James van Horn Melton, *Absolutism and the Eighteenth-Century Origins of Compulsory Schooling in Prussia*

teachers to village schools, the burden of children's farm-duties, peasants' general scepticism about the very need for schooling, and landlords' concerns about potential unrest from educated peasants all contributed to a continuation of the generally poor standard of teaching, which limited the peasants' ability to understand material written with any complexity.[15] The villagers' inclination to adhere to traditions handed down from their forefathers, which was ingrained through many generations of survival without outside assistance, was another characteristic that hampered the personal, social, and economic advancement of the peasantry.[16] In the context of smallpox and inoculation, pastors were confronted with quite a challenge in convincing peasants to abandon their harmful traditional remedies in favour of newer treatments, and to consider inoculation.

Reforming the annual *Kalender* (Figure 15) that many of the common folk used as their guide for daily life was recommended as a way to not only modernise the peasants' approach to farming but also to improve the well-being of the population more generally. Reformers regarded the traditional *Kalender* as not only misleading, in its designation of auspicious days for attending to personal matters and agricultural tasks, but also sadly lacking in useful information about matters such as diet, health, and appropriate nutrition for livestock.[17] One commentator made his point by citing a local farmer's admission that the recently-cut hay rotting in the wet fields "is my hay, my *Kalender* advised me ... this year it showed the hay-harvest during eight days of rain."[18] Another reform advocate remarked that "sensible people ... cut the hair when it becomes too long, and smart mothers wean their children when the child is strong enough to digest other foods," rather than choosing an auspicious day designated in their *Kalender*.[19] Yet when revised versions of the *Kalender* were published without the usual prophesies and planetary aspects, not only the peasants were disappointed but also some of the townsfolk who had welcomed *Kalender* reform.

---

and Austria (Cambridge: Cambridge University Press, 1988), 174–5. Jonathan Israel suggests that Friedrich II deliberately undermined his own education initiative, in relation to peasants: Jonathan I. Israel, *Democratic Enlightenment. Philosophy, Revolution and Human Rights 1750–1790* (Oxford: Oxford University Press, 2011), 275.

15 Melton, 177, 181, 194–7; Reinhard Wittmann, *Buchmarkt und Lektüre im 18. und 19. Jahrhundert* (Tübingen: Niemeyer, 1982), 4–8, 13.

16 Juncker, *Archiv*, 3:125–6; 7:222; Schwager, "Bauer," 71–3. Eberhard Wolff, *Einschneidende Maßnahmen: Pockenschutzimpfung und traditionale Gesellschaft im Württemberg des frühen 19. Jahrhunderts* (Stuttgart: Steiner, 1998), 59–60.

17 "Von den Calender-Prophezeihungen," *HM* 5 (1767): 92–3; Johann G. Krünitz, *Oekonomisch-technologische Encyclopädie*, part 32 (Berlin: Pauli, 1784), 563–6. For a typical old-style *Kalender*, see: *Neuer katholischer Schreib-Kalender* (Augsburg: Labhart, 1737).

18 "Prophezeihungen," 93–4.

19 "Kalenderlegenden," in *Almanach für Aerzte und Nichtärzte auf das Jahr 1782*, ed. Christian G. Gruner (Jena: Cuno's Erben, 1782), 231–2.

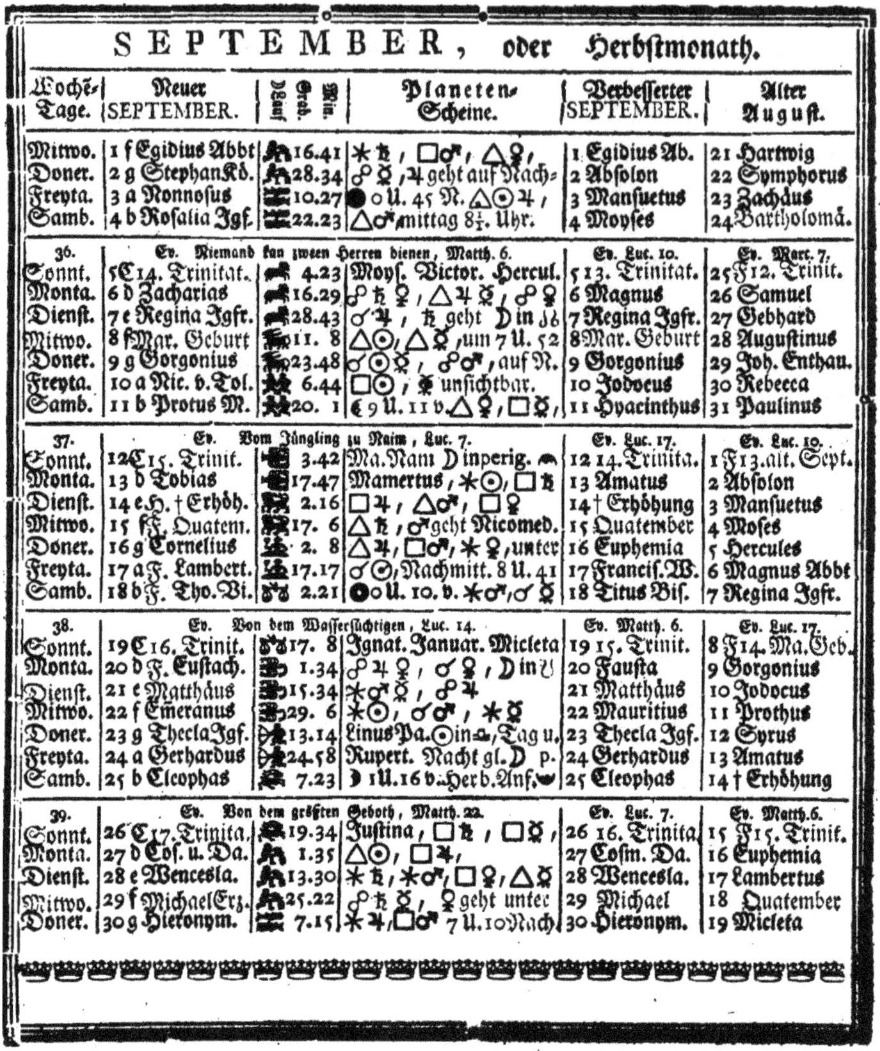

SEPTEMBER, oder Herbstmonath.

Woche-Tage.	Neuer SEPTEMBER.	Lauf Grad. Min.	Planeten-Scheine.	Verbesserter SEPTEMBER.	Alter August.
Mittwo.	1 f Egidius Abbt	16.41	✶♄, □♂, △♀,	1 Egidius Ab.	21 Hartwig
Doner.	2 g Stephan Kö.	28.34	☍☿, ♃ geht auf Nach-	2 Absolon	22 Symphorus
Freyta.	3 a Nonnosus	10.27	● o U. 45 M. △☉♃,	3 Mansuetus	23 Zachäus
Samb.	4 b Rosalia Jgf.	22.23	△♂ mittag 8½. Uhr.	4 Moyses	24 Bartholomä.
36.	Ev. Niemand kan zween Herren dienen, Matth. 6.			Ev. Luc. 10.	Ev. Marc. 7.
Sonnt.	5 C 14. Trinitat.	4.23	Moys. Victor. Hercul.	5 13. Trinitat.	25 F 12. Trinit.
Monta.	6 d Zacharias	16.29	☍♄♀, △♃☿, ☍♀	6 Magnus	26 Samuel
Dienst.	7 e Regina Jgfr.	28.43	☌♃, ♄ geht ☽ in ♎	7 Regina Jgfr.	27 Gebhard
Mittwo.	8 f Mar. Geburt	11. 8	△☉, △☿, um 7 U. 52	8 Mar. Geburt	28 Augustinus
Doner.	9 g Gorgonius	23.48	☌☉☿, ☍♂, auf M.	9 Gorgonius	29 Joh. Enthau.
Freyta.	10 a Nic. v. Tol.	6.44	□☉, ✱ unsichtbar.	10 Jodocus	30 Rebecca
Samb.	11 b Protus M.	20. 1	☾ 9 U. 11 v. △♀, □☿,	11 Hyacinthus	31 Paulinus
37.	Ev. Vom Jüngling zu Naim, Luc. 7.			Ev. Luc. 17.	Ev. Luc. 10.
Sonnt.	12 C 15. Trinit.	3.42	Ma. Nam ☽ inperig.	12 14. Trinita.	1 F 13. alt. Sept.
Monta.	13 d Tobias	17.47	Mamertus, ✶☉, □♄	13 Amatus	2 Absolon
Dienst.	14 e H. † Erhöh.	2.16	□♃, △♂, □♀	14 † Erhöhung	3 Mansuetus
Mittwo.	15 f Q. Quatem.	17. 6	△♄, ♂ geht Nicomed.	15 Quatember	4 Moses
Doner.	16 g Cornelius	2. 8	△♃, □♂, ✶♀, unter	16 Euphemia	5 Hercules
Freyta.	17 a F. Lambert.	17.17	☌☉, Nachmitt. 8 U. 41	17 Francisc. W.	6 Magnus Abbt
Samb.	18 b F. Tho. Vi.	2.21	● o U. 10. v. ✶♂, ☌☿	18 Titus Bis.	7 Regina Jgfr.
38.	Ev. Von dem Wassersüchtigen, Luc. 14.			Ev. Matth. 6.	Ev. Luc. 17.
Sonnt.	19 C 16. Trinit.	17. 8	Ignat. Januar. Micleta	19 15. Trinit.	8 F 14. Ma. Geb.
Monta.	20 d F. Eustach.	1.34	☍♃♀, ☌♀, ☽ in ♉	20 Fausta	9 Gorgonius
Dienst.	21 e Matthäus	15.34	✶♂☿, ☍♃	21 Matthäus	10 Jodocus
Mittwo.	22 f Emeranus	29. 6	✶☉, ☌♂, ✶☿	22 Mauritius	11 Prothus
Doner.	23 g Thecla Jgf.	13.14	Linus Pa. ☉ in ♎, Tag u.	23 Thecla Jgf.	12 Syrus
Freyta.	24 a Gerhardus	24.58	Rupert. Nacht gl. ☽ p.	24 Gerhardus	13 Amatus
Samb.	25 b Cleophas	7.23	☽ 1 U. 16 v. Herb. Anf.	25 Cleophas	14 † Erhöhung
39.	Ev. Von dem größten Geboth, Matth. 22.			Ev. Luc. 7.	Ev. Matth. 6.
Sonnt.	26 C 17. Trinita.	19.34	Justina, □♄, □☿,	26 16. Trinita.	15 F 15. Trinit.
Monta.	27 d Cos. u. Da.	1.35	△☉, □♃,	27 Cosm. Da.	16 Euphemia
Dienst.	28 e Wencesla.	13.30	✶♄, ✶♂, □♀, △☿	28 Wencesla.	17 Lambertus
Mittwo.	29 f Michael Erz.	25.22	☍♄☿, ♀ geht unter	29 Michael	18 Quatember
Doner.	30 g Hieronym.	7.15	✶♃, □♂ 7 U. 10 Nach.	30 Hieronym.	19 Micleta

FIGURE 15 *Kalender* for September 1762. From the *Astronomische-Physicalischer Kalender* (Munich, 1762)

As one well-educated Prussian lamented: "Is there a letter in red anywhere in the whole *Kalender*? ... Now we have a black *Kalender*. Who will buy it? The feast-days of the saints, all in black ... no heavenly signs, no planets."[20] Custom-

20 "Geheime Nachricht, von der wahre Ursache, warum der königliche Preussische Kalender des 1780sten Jahres wieder auf den alten Fuß gesetz worden," *DM* 1 (1781): 275–9, 276–7 (quote).

ers indeed refused to purchase the revised *Kalender*, forcing the restoration of some of the traditional content, though not the superstitious prophesies.[21] A revised *Kalender* from Hanover in 1793 even contained added information about smallpox treatment and inoculation.[22]

Smallpox tended to spread across the countryside every four to seven years.[23] The disease was usually carried to rural areas by infected children coming from one of the larger towns where the disease was endemic, to visit relatives, or by infected children of travelling gypsies, beggars, or army troops. Travellers wearing smallpox-contaminated clothing into country inns were another common source of disease transmission, as were the cottage industries that disseminated smallpox scabs on flax, wool, or cloth that was spun, woven, or sewn in the presence of afflicted children. Extended families spread smallpox through their own ranks by the tradional sharing of the garments and bedclothes of dead relatives.[24] Parents helped to spread the disease through their village in other ways too, particularly by deliberately exposing their children to a mild case of smallpox in the hope that the mild symptoms would be transmitted, or by engaging in the 'smallpox-buying' ritual whereby a child would 'purchase' scabs to be rubbed into the skin to induce smallpox.[25] Inoculation was a source of contagion as well, though to a greater extent in the towns, where it was more commonly practised than in rural households.[26]

Funeral traditions often disseminated smallpox of a potentially fatal kind, particularly the customary open-coffin that could spread the disease to the church village through the display of smallpox victims from outlying areas. Children in the church choir were placed at very high risk from the traditional practice of accompanying the coffin to the graveside, where the deceased was often displayed once again.[27] The Prussian government responded to warnings that the smallpox dead remained infectious, by issuing a regulation in 1769 requiring smallpox victims' coffins to remain closed and to be buried at twice

---

21 Wittman, *Buchmarkt*, 33; *Haushaltungs-Kalender* (Berlin, 1792).

22 Georg C. Conradi, "Unterricht über die Behandlung der Blattern und Empfehlung der Inoculation, dem Landmanne bestimmt," *Neuer Volkskalender* (Hanover: Hahn, 1795), 242.

23 Juncker, *Archiv*, 1:169; 5:12, 31, 48; 6:21.

24 Juncker, 4:89, 91–3, 106–7; 5:179; 6:28 (transmission by visits to relatives); 4:95 (by gypsies); 3:86, 96, 133–4; 4:12–13, 156; 6:28 (by beggars); 3:96, 134; 4:98 (by army troops); 4:11, 13 (at the tavern); 3:135; 4:5, 100; 5:5, 28, 48–9, 204–5; 6:49 (by scabs); 4:87, 5:203; 6:28 (through inherited goods); see also Apx 2: Möhsen (1775), 166.

25 Juncker, 3:140–1; 4:100–1, 156; 6:28, 49.

26 Juncker, 3:9; 4:76; 5:9, 83, 157, 200.

27 Juncker, 3:134–5; "Einige Nachrichten und Beobachtungen, den Zustand der Bevölkerung hiesiger Lande, und der öffentlichen Gesundheit im Jahre 1790 betreffend," *Neues HM*, no. 37 (1791): 601.

the usual depth in churchyards located outside the towns. That regulation was reiterated during the severe 1787 smallpox epidemic, and a new rule issued in the 1790–91 outbreak required pastors to ensure that smallpox victims' coffins were sealed.[28] Yet the old traditions died hard. *Landphysikus* Schäffer reported (1798) that people in Felsberg (Hesse-Kassel) recited the motto: "a dead dog cannot bite" in response to his warnings of the dangers of displaying smallpox victims' bodies.[29] Dr. Bechner from Unruhstadt (Prussia) reiterated the local saying: "some take home with them the nail to their coffin," in offering this description of smallpox victims' funerals (1797):[30]

> In most of this area, the smallpox dead will be displayed before burial; whole gangs of children move around the body and breathe in the foul smallpox vapours, and when the body is shaken around all the way to the churchyard, it will be shown again before burial.[31]

Pastor Theinemann from Altendorf (Saxony) lamented the clergymen's lack of authority over funeral-related events beyond the church, citing an instance where a boy caught smallpox by looking into a coffin awaiting transport to the church village, causing the disease to spread to the school.[32] Very shallow graves and small graveyards that necessitated the recycling of burial plots every eight to ten years also spread smallpox, according to *Stadtphysikus* Ludwig from Hirschberg (Silesia) who blamed such inadequacies for the return of smallpox to his region in the mid-1790s.[33] An overarching difficulty in bringing about changed public attitudes to the burial of the smallpox dead seemed to be the inconsistency between the notion of contagion, and the widespread belief that smallpox was innate or was 'sent' by God to each individual.[34] Countering the misconceptions and the behavioural and structural issues spreading smallpox were among the many challenges confronting pastors and other officials on the front line of efforts to curb the disease in rural areas.

Much of the rural smallpox mortality was blamed on treatments recommended by the unauthorised practitioners who plied their trade in the towns

---

28 Juncker, 1:281–2; 3:134–5; Moritz Pistor, "Geschichte der preußischen Medizinalverwaltung," *DVG* 40 (1908): 242, 780; Apx 2: Wolf (1768), 31.

29 Juncker, 6:92.

30 Juncker, 4:79.

31 Juncker, 4:79.

32 Juncker, *Archiv*, 5:208–9.

33 Juncker, 5:164–5; 6:54.

34 Apx 2: Schwager, "Patriotische" (1786), 202–3. Wolff, *Maßnahmen*, 228–9, 238–9.

and villages, who were known variously as *Quacksalber*, *Pfuscher*, or *After-Aerzte*.[35] Some of those participants in the so-called 'medical marketplace' of 'healers' who made a living from selling home-made medicines undoubtedly did some good by offering beneficial herbal remedies. Patients dosed up with inocuous substances may have also been helped in some instances by having faith in the prescribed 'cure.'[36] Yet that was not always the case. Many unauthorised practitioners preyed on the vulnerable, such as the self-confessed *Quacksalber* who reported having dispensed "many tons" of a "white powder," which he identified as *Cremor tartari*, as "a cure for everything." He admitted that "I hung on the purses of the truly dizzy people until they had custody of their graves … I kept away from educated sick people … because they asked for expansive explanations about the cause, nature, and course of the illness."[37] He also confessed that the idea of making a living by posing as a 'country doctor' came to him through a social encounter with a charlatan who disclosed:

> his entire rip-off, his ignorance, and his greedy deception. He … laughed about the gullibility and blindness of the people who trust with complete confidence … a man who does not understand the least about the condition, structure, and workings of the human body; …even admitting that merely his advice made him a murderer of his fellow-man.[38]

Believing that villagers turned to the *Quacksalber* because of a dearth of competent medical care in rural areas, government officials saw the solution in a wider distribution of doctors.[39] Yet mistrust of doctors was actually a cause of the tendency for the common man to deal with illness by either doing nothing or seeking out a relative, a neighbour, the pastor, the blacksmith, the forester, or some other local willing to offer medical advice, even if a town and its

---

35 Juncker, 4:103, 143, 150, 155, 179–80, 198; 6:93, 133; 7:225; G.B. Schäffer, "Ueber medizinisches Aufklärung," *Neues HM* 2 (1792): 1397.

36 "Beantwortung der Frage: Welches sind die gewöhnlichen Ursachen, warum der gemeine Landmann bey vorfallenden Krankheiten seine Zuflucht lieber zum Pfuscher, als zu einem ordentlichen Arzt, nimmt?," *Neue MM* 4 (1795): 134; *Parabeln oder Gleichnißreden für Junge und Alte*, book 3 (Vienna: Deutschen Schulanstalt St. Anna, 1794), 72; "Wohlgemeinte Vorschläge zur Abschaffung der Quacksalberey in Schlesien," *SP* 34 (1801): 215–6; J.U. Günther, "Anleiting, gesund zu werden," *VSH* 4 (1797): 451–2.

37 "Schreiben eines Quacksalbers aufm Lande an seinen Herrn Gevatter in der Stadt," *BMN* 3 (1776): 78, 80 (quote).

38 "Schreiben," 76.

39 Frevert, *Krankheit*, 50, 56–61; Robert Heller, "Johann Christian Reil's Training Scheme for Medical Auxiliaries," *Medical History* 19 (1975): 324.

resident *Physikus* were as close as two or three miles.[40] Moreover, landlords' or public officials' offers to pay for a doctor's services were often rejected, and even if a doctor were consulted, in many cases the patient failed to follow the proffered advice and take the prescribed medicines.[41] Mistrust of doctors, and the harm from treatments administered by *Quacksalber* were longstanding concerns that prompted many regulations, proposals, and initiatives aimed at the extirpation of harmful quackery.[42] Yet the plethora of reports in the 1790s lamenting unauthorised practitioners' advice to apply the 'heating treatment' for smallpox, and to recommend other harmful remedies suggests that little had changed.[43]

Efforts to curb the impact of smallpox were hampered by a general belief in the overriding principle of God's will that gave rise to the motto "what should live will live, what should die, will die," according to many of the vast collection of reports about smallpox submitted to Professor Juncker.[44] Parents who did make an effort to help their children often packed them in bedclothes in over-heated, stuffy rooms, and gave them alcoholic drinks sometimes laced with pepper to increase the heating effect.[45] The alcoholic beverage commonly offered in poor rural households was a concoction made from the strained broth from fermented sheep or goose faeces, known as *Ulandwein*.[46] Warnings against the use of both *Ulandwein* and the 'heating treatment' were included in the smallpox advice circulars issued in 1768 by Margrave Carl Friedrich of Baden and by the Prussian *Obercollegium medicum*, both of which strongly

40 Juncker, *Archiv*, 3:90; 4:103, 198; 5:34–7; "Beantwortung der Frage," 133–5.

41 Juncker, 5:109, 137, 145.

42 Ernst Schwabe, *Pflichten und Geschäften eines Stadt-oder Land-Physikus*, vol. 1 (Erfurt: Keyser, 1786), 260–7; Karl F.W.A. Vater, *Preussisch-Schlesische Civil Medicinal- and Sanitäts-Verfassung*, part 2 (Breslau: Korn, 1800), 264, 268–72; Christian G. Gruner, *Gedanken von der Arzneiwissenschaft und den Aerzten* (Breslau: Korn, 1772), 491–2.

43 Juncker, *Archiv*, 3:90, 92; 4:98, 143, 179–80, 182, 198; 5:35–6, 108–9, 136–7, 182, 210, 230; Johann J.W. Dedekind, "Ueber Königslutters angenehme und gesunde Lage," *Curart der natürlichen Pocken*, no. 2 (1791): 25–6; F.L. Lüders, "Ueber die gefährlichen Folgen der Quacksalberei," *Neues HM* 2 (1792): 1268–72.

44 *Was lebe soll leben, was sterbe soll sterben*: Juncker, *Archiv*, 3:127 (quote); 3:70, 90; 4:69; 5:119, 211–2; 6:130–1; 7:221; "Einige Gedanken bey dem Vorschläge: die Blattern auszurotten," *Neue MM* 5 (1796):109.

45 Juncker, 5:35, 229; 6:50, 131; 7:22, 226; Johann G. Otto, *Medicinische und chirurgische Bemerkungen* (Leipzig: Böhme, 1793), 65–6.

46 Juncker, 1:194; 4:19, 98, 111; 5:64; 6:56; Johann P. Rüling, "Einige bey den Pocken zu beobachtende Vorschriften," *HM* 16 (1778): 468–9. Faeces from various animals were part of the traditional pharmacopoeia: Kristian F. Paulini, *Neu-Vermehrte heylsame Dreck-Apotheke*, part 1 (Frankfurt: Köllner, 1714), 311–6; part 2, 191.

recommended cool conditions and water-based drinks for smallpox patients.[47] In Baden the circulars were delivered directly to families dealing with the illness, while in Prussia the circulars intended for "country-folk and others unable to access a doctor" were sent to the country pastors for distribution. The advice appeared in a Hanover-based journal too, ensuring a wider audience.[48]

Pastor Johann Moritz Schwager from Joellenbeck remarked on his parishioners' difficulties in trying to understand the Prussian Medical Board's circular, including the more literate among them. He also noted his congregation's inattention when he read the circular aloud from the pulpit.[49] Schwager and other pastors highlight the added communication difficulties for peasants with a poor understanding of the high-German in which official advice was delivered.[50] On the other hand, as Pastor Johann Carl Migula from Weigwitz (Upper Silesia) lamented, rural congregations were so wedded to their traditions that they would ignore any advice delivered by their pastor, even if it were about increasing crop yields.[51] Another Silesian country pastor who read the Prussian Medical Board's circular from the pulpit remarked on his pleasant discussion with parishioners afterwards, when they agreed to pass copies to their absent friends. Yet he found when he visited households with smallpox-afflicted children that the official advice had little impact. Even parents who had shown an interest in the circular were persuaded by their neighbours and friends to ignore the new recommendations and adhere to the traditional treatments. As a way of convincing his parishioners to accept the Board's advice, the pastor and his wife adopted a strategy of raising the matter of smallpox in conversation, and expressing their delight that their own three children came through the disease so well, pointedly attributing that good recovery to the helpful treatment advice in the Board's circular. The pastor credits those conversations with the wider adoption of the official advice when smallpox reappeared in 1791, and fatalities fell to just 2 per cent of total births, from the 1786 level of 19

47 Carl F. Gerstlacher, ed., *Sammlung aller Baden-Durlachischen Anstalten und Verordnungen*, vol. 1 (Karlsruhe: Schmieder, 1773), 529–32; Prussian Medical Board, "Kurze Anleitung wie der Landmann und diejenigen, die keinen Arzt erlangen können, bei der grassirenden Pocken sich zu verhalten haben," *HM* 7 (1769): 568–75.

48 Gerstlacher, ed., *Sammlung*, 1:528; Prussian Medical Board, "Kurze Anleitung," 561–76; Apx 2: Schwager, "Patriotische" (1786), 220, 230.

49 Schwager, 230–1.

50 Johann M. Schwager, "Wie kann der Prediger sich das Zutrauen des gemeinen Mannes erwerben?," *JP* 2 (1789): 380; Coelln, "Beytrag," 115; Johann C. Tode, "Etwas von der medizinischen Aufkärung des Volks," *Der unterhaltende Arzt* 4 (1789): 145.

51 Apx 2: Migula (1786), 211.

per cent.[52] That unnamed pastor's wife was one of many clergymen's helpful partners whose collective contribution to their respective community's welfare is largely unacknowledged in the historical record.

The Prussian Medical Board's revised treatment advice circular issued during the 1796 smallpox epidemic gained more traction than the earlier version, apparently because of its mode of delivery. In the Breslau region and elsewhere in Prussia, the new circular was not only widely distributed and read from the pulpit but also copied in school classrooms.[53] The effectiveness of teaching the Board's smallpox treatment advice to schoolchildren was noted particularly by Pastor Kern from Mittelshofen (Bayreuth).[54] Teachers and pastors in other territories too were passing on advice about smallpox to children, in many cases from Dr. Bernard Christoph Faust's "Catechism of Health," while in Schwarzburg-Rudolstadt the schoolchildren copied the treatment recommendations compiled by *Landphysikus* Johann Gottfried Otto at the request of the church superintendent.[55] It was one of few strategies with the rare potential to counter the tendency lamented by the Prussian *Stadtphysikus* Jungken from Burg, that the common man in his region neither read nor understood medical advice.[56]

Pastor Christian Ernst Bergler from Hummelshagen (Saxony) used his own intuitive approach, born of long experience, to convince his parishioners to change the way they treated smallpox (1789). Having achieved some success while traversing his parish advising parents to abandon the 'heating treatment' in favour of cooler conditions, he held a special thanksgiving service after the smallpox epidemic had passed as a way of driving home his treatment advice. Before the service, he positioned in front of the altar the children who had come through the disease, alongside the mothers with babies who had survived, so they were all under the gaze of the congregation bereaved by the loss of their own children and relatives in the epidemic. In that way, the pastor gained his audience's attention for the delivery of his message that God helped the sick by the sensible use of good treatment. Bergler's congratulations to the parents of those fortunate children at the front for heeding his advice to keep them cool, in well-ventilated rooms, and to give them cool drinks during their illness was a reminder to the congregation that those survivors were not

---

52 "Glücklicher Erfolg," 147–9.

53 Juncker, *Archiv*, 4:162; 6:34; Pistor, "Geschichte," 781.

54 Juncker, 7:229.

55 Juncker, 7:226, 228; Samuel C. Wagener, "Der Schulmeister vom Haina," *PAD* 1 (1799), 156–9; Otto, *Bemerkungen*, 65.

56 Juncker, 5:156; 7:229.

treated using the traditional remedies.[57] Other country pastors, too, reported a local reduction in the smallpox death-toll after convincing parents to adopt up-to-date treatments, as did several doctors.[58] Yet many Germans remained sceptical of the new recommendations, to the extent that the 'heating treatment' was still being applied well into the nineteenth century in some rural areas and towns.[59]

2 Challenges for Country Pastors

German pastors who began promoting inoculation in the 1770s were sometimes inspired to do so by the sermons reported in the "Journal for Pastors." At that time, when word was spreading about the Bavarian pastor Johann Georg Eisen von Schwarzenberg teaching the inoculation procedure to peasants in the Russian Baltic region, other pastors became quite active in encouraging inoculation as well.[60] Johann Gottfried Merkel from Torgau and Christian Gottlieb Klüge from Meißen (Saxony) both made a point of recommending the practice in their sermons, though Pastor Klüge went a step further and inoculated a number of children using a sewing needle, according to Eisen's method. The thanksgiving service he conducted to publicise the children's recovery reportedly had the desired effect of inspiring attending parents to have their own children inoculated.[61] Another Saxon pastor, Johann Wilhelm Frotscher from Drognitz, began inoculating his parishioners' children in 1778 after successfully testing the procedure on his own offspring. By 1791 he had gained such a high reputation for his skill that he was called upon to help the medical men inoculating in the villages of Probstelle, in the neighbouring territory of Schwarzburg-Rudolstadt. By the time he died in 1797, Frotscher's tally of inoculations reputedly exceeded one thousand.[62]

57 "Nachricht von einem in Hummelshayn gefeierten Blatternfest," *JP* 22 (1790): 289–95.

58 Juncker, 1:190–1; 3:70; 4:93; 5:3; 6:35, 7:226–9.

59 Wolff, *Maßnahmen*, 248–53.

60 J.C. Grot, "Kanzelrede von der Rechtmäßigkeit der Blatter-Einimpfung aus allgemeinen Gründen, am ersten Nov. 1769," *JP* 3 (1770): 349–50; "Vermischte Nachrichten," *JP* 3 (1773): 462–3; "Nachrichten und Urtheile von den neuesten Predigten und andern dahin gehörigen Schriften," *JP* 8 (1777): 239–41; "Schreiben aus Liefland vom 20.Mai," *Augspurgische Extra-Zeitung*, no. 141 (Augsburg), June 14, 1774.

61 "Pastoralkorrespondenz," *JP* 8 (1777): 135; "Nachrichten und Urtheile," 235.

62 Otto, *Bemerkungen*, 68; Friedrich Schlichtegroll, ed., *Nekrolog auf das Jahr 1797*, vol. 8, part 2 (Gotha: Perthes, 1801), 341.

Pastor G.F. Piccard from Lachem (Hanover) was another rural clergyman who gained a local reputation as a successful inoculator. When he first carried out the procedure on his own children and followed up with fourteen more inoculations during a smallpox outbreak in 1783, he encountered much scepticism. Yet the community's doubts about his action turned to amazement when virulent smallpox was wreaking havoc on their families, and the inoculated children remained unaffected. This evidence that 'superficial smallpox,' as the locals referred disparagingly to inoculation, was indeed protective, encouraged many parents to overcome their prejudice and ask the pastor to inoculate their children too, adding a further 73 to his tally. The one death following Piccard's inoculations, in a region where the smallpox case fatality rate was one-in-five, offered a persuasive argument in favour of inoculation.[63]

While parents were legally permitted to inoculate their own children, laymen engaging in the practice outside their own family transgressed the regulation limiting inoculation to doctors and surgeons. Pastors were thus at risk of official reprimands or accusations of quackery if they inoculated their parishioners' children.[64] As self-protection, pastors enthusiastic about inoculation were inclined to publish articles extolling the simplicity and success of procedures carried out by doctors or surgeons, even if they may have been successful inoculators themselves.[65] Sometimes a pastor would begin such an article with a lament over past loss of life from smallpox in his parish, then provide a village-by-village account of recent deaths from the disease, and conclude with rejoicing over the lives saved through inoculation. In that way, the pastors hoped to encourage wavering parents to overcome their fears and adopt the procedure for the sake of their children.[66]

While pastors in some country areas were publicising the advantages of inoculation, reports from other rural areas suggest that the procedure was still unknown, even as late as the mid-1790s.[67] Pastor Johann Carl Migula and his wife, from Upper Silesia, inoculated their own children in 1786 because no

---

63 Apx 2: Piccard (1794), 665–72, 673–4.

64 Juncker, *Archiv*, 5:83, 118, 173, 197; "Warnung gegen die medizinische Pfuscherey eines Geistlichen," *JD* 7 (1790): 287–8; Pistor, "Geschichte," 781.

65 Apx 2: Steiger (1787), 161–3; Migula, "Inokulation" (1787), 244; Engelmann (1788), 70; Künzel (1788), 76–7; Sintenis (1790), 47; "Blattern Einimpfung" (1796), 190–2; Richter (1799), 244–6.

66 Apx 2: "Tödlichkeit der Blattern" (1787), 91; Steiger (1787), 160; Migula (1790), 41, 50; "Blattern-Einimpfung" (1791), 261–2; Richter (1799), 246. A pastor's duties included the compilation of figures on causes of death: G.W. Block and J. Müller, "Beitrag zur Entscheidung der Frage: 'Sollen die Landprediger auch Aerzte seyn?,'" *Neues HM* 7 (1797): 342.

67 Juncker, *Archiv*, 3:136; 4:80; 5:120; Apx 2: Piccard (1794), 665; Richter (1799), 244.

skilled practitioners were in the area. Migula describes their use of "an ordinary sewing needle somewhat broadened at the point by grinding," and praises "the humane Gatti and Wagler who so simply and vividly described the beneficial method of inoculation of smallpox in their excellent written work." Mothers living nearby were so impressed on seeing the Migula children recover so rapidly that they asked the pastor to inoculate their children too, which he did successfully.[68] Migula also agreed to inoculate the children of the bailiff in nearby Gaulau where smallpox was claiming the life of one in four of its victims. When he entered the village he found several mothers keenly awaiting his arrival, and inoculated an additional eleven children on that occasion. He was greatly moved by the gratitude of "those poor people, largely of the Catholic religion" who thanked the Lutheran Pastor for saving their children, offering their handshakes and prayers for God to reward him.[69] For such parents unable to afford a doctor, even if one were nearby, Migula recommended self-help inoculation using the Gatti-Wagler method, also highlighting an article by Pastor Klose from Lower Silesia that provided advice to mothers about inoculating their own children.[70]

Unlike the Catholic mothers in Gaulau who were so enthusiastic about inoculation, Migula's Lutheran congregation was largely indifferent to their pastor's overt promotion of the practice. Even after conducting a funeral for four smallpox victims at which he reiterated the lifesaving benefits of inoculation, Migula received just one request for the procedure. When he went to inoculate those children in Kauer, where smallpox had cast many families into mourning, several additional mothers beseeched him to save their remaining children too, bringing his tally that day to seventeen.[71] Curious about the reasons behind the widely differing attitudes to inoculation that he encountered, Migula investigated by asking various people around the district for their opinions. He found that inoculation was commonly regarded as a matter for the upper-class and wealthy, and that many were turned off the procedure by hearsay about past suffering during the time when pre-inoculation 'preparation' and incisions were used. Parents were also concerned by the common belief that inoculated children would die from the first disease they encountered, though no-one could give an example of such an occurrence.[72] Collectively,

68 Apx 2: Migula (1786), 207–8 (quotes), 209–10. For further discussion of Gatti and Wagler's book, see p. 84 above.

69 Apx 2: Migula, "Noch Etwas" (1787), 414, 417–8, 419 (quote).

70 Apx 2: Migula, 411, 421–2; Klose (1786), 405–11; Gatti and Wagler (1772, 1782).

71 Apx 2: Migula, "Inokulation" (1787), 244–5.

72 Apx 2: Migula, "Noch etwas" (1787), 411–2; 422–3, 427. See Juncker, *Archiv*, 4:20–1; 5:213, for instances of poor technique causing children's deaths.

Migula's experiences suggest that mothers with no knowledge of either inoculation or the surrounding polemic were likely to embrace inoculation at times of high local smallpox mortality, while the parents aware of the arguments for and against the procedure were more likely to reject it than to accept it.

Pastors reacted in various ways to suggestions that inoculation may become one of their official duties, which were included in proposals for country pastors to provide not only spiritual guidance but also practical assistance to their parishioners, particularly basic medical advice.[73] Such proposals arose from the pressure for a more utilitarian rural pastorate, prompted to some extent by the Enlightenment-inspired abandonment of religious studies by droves of theology students at Protestant universities, who had become convinced that the clerical estate was a "plot against humanity."[74] Theologians and educators considering ways to counter accusations of clerical parasitism and to regain lost prestige for the clergy saw the solution in an expanded role for the rural pastorate, which was already known for performing 'useful' extra functions. High on the list of recommendations was the provision of targeted medical training to theology students that would enable them, as pastors, to provide a basic medical service if appointed to a rural parish.[75] Pastor Müller from Gaffel (Hanover) was one country pastor who made known his opposition to the proposed changes, making particular mention of his abhorrence of any requirement to carry out inoculations.[76]

Not only theologians and educators saw pastors in rural parishes as a potential medical resource but also the authors of 'self-help' medical books. Dr. Samuel-Auguste Tissot was one such author who had long been targeting his advice to pastors rather than toward the relatively poorly-educated peasants.[77] Inspired by the broad discussion generated by a number of serious proposals during the 1760s-90s for formal medical training for theology students, some students made their own moves in that direction.[78] Pastor Johann Moritz Schwager (Figure 16) wrote of his attendance at medical lectures while

73 G.W. Block, "Sollen die Landprediger auch Aerzte seyn?," *Neues HM* 6 (1796): 1559–60; Anthony J. La Vopa, *Grace, Talent, and Merit. Poor Students, Clerical Careers, and Professional Ideology in Eighteenth-Century Germany* (Cambridge: Cambridge University Press, 1988), 342–3.

74 Johann M. Stroup, *The Struggle for Identity in the Clerical Estate* (Leiden: Brill, 1984), 90.

75 Stroup, 109, 112–19; Schäffer, "Aufklärung," 1410–11; Frevert, *Krankheit*, 55–6.

76 Block and Müller, "Beitrag," 348.

77 Juncker, *Archiv*, 5:36, 118; 6:70; Samuel-Auguste D. Tissot, *Anleitung für das Landvolk in Absicht auf seine Gesundheit*, trans. H.C. Hirzel (Zürich: Heidegger, 1762), 19, translated from *Avis au peuple sur sa santé* (Lausanne: Grasset, 1761), 20–21, which was first published in 1753. The book went to many editions as well as being published in several languages.

78 La Vopa, *Grace*, 342; Stroup, *Struggle*, 104–5.

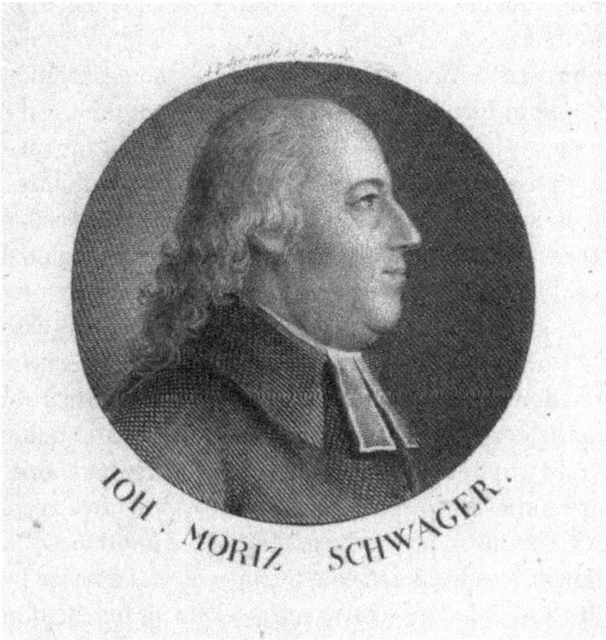

FIGURE 16
Johann Moritz Schwager. Engraving by J.G. Schmidt, 1794
ÖSTERREICHISCHES NATIONALBIBLOTHEK: PORT_00111369_01

undertaking his theology studies at the University of Halle, where he graduated in 1762. He also admitted that although he was satisfied with being a pastor, he had yearned to become a doctor but the family finances would not stretch that far.[79] While making a living as a tutor in Bremen during his wait for a pastoral appointment that suited him, Schwager became involved in Freemasonry, which was then an association of men inclined to embrace the ideas of the Enlightenment.[80] That ideological direction is evident in Schwager's approach to his ministry during 1768–1804 as the pastor at the Marienkirche in Joellenbeck, in the Prussian county of Minden-Ravensburg, where he stands out as a multi-skilled visionary who not only embraced progressive ideology but forged those ideas into a course of action aimed toward social improvement.[81] Not just in his local pastoral work but also in his many publications he made every effort to eradicate the social blights of prejudice, superstition, and

79 Johann M. Schwager, "Johann Moritz Schwager, Prediger zu Joellenbeck in der Grafschaft Ravensburg," *NB* 1 (1801): 50–51.

80 Schwager, 60–62, 68; Ulrich Im Hof, *Das Europa der Aufklärung* (Munich: Beck, 1993), 220; Christopher Clark, *Iron Kingdom. The Rise and Downfall of Prussia, 1600–1947* (London: Allen Lane, 2006), 252.

81 Udo Halama, ed., *Ein + verbindet. 150 Jahre Marienkirche Jöllenbeck* (Bielefeld: Anzeigen & mehr, 2004), 61–3; La Vopa, *Grace*, 338, n. 23.

harmful quackery while encouraging Germans to consider social issues from an enlightened perspective.[82]

Like many of his counterparts, Schwager was appalled at the destruction caused by smallpox, and tried to turn his parishioners away from their usual home-remedies toward better treatment choices. He also promoted inoculation, which he practised with considerable skill.[83] To modern sensibilities, country pastors acting as inoculation practitioners may seem irresponsible considering doctors' increasing concerns that the movement of inoculated children was spreading smallpox. Yet when Schwager and other country pastors began inoculating in the 1780s, they tended to do so only when the disease was an imminent threat.[84] During the deadly 1786 smallpox epidemic Schwager repeatedly recommended inoculation from the pulpit. That his entreaties were largely ignored is consistent with the Prussian Medical Board's finding that inoculation was generally unpopular in rural areas.[85] Schwager had nonetheless managed to inspire sufficient interest during the previous five years to have fifty successful inoculations to his credit, and he added another 110 in 1789–90.[86] Having been taught by a local surgeon, Eichmeyer, and advised by Dr. Rudolph Christian Opitz from Minden, Schwager backed up his inoculation activity with a thorough knowledge of specialist books.[87] His initial efforts to teach his parishioners about inoculation were centred on his own seventeen-page circular, "Is Inoculation a Duty, or Not?" (1784), in which he stresses the point that smallpox commonly claimed the life of at least one in four or five afflicted children, compared to the death of just one or two in every thousand from a competent inoculation. He urges parents to reject the untruths peddled by inoculation opponents, advises them that local surgeons offered inoculation at no cost, and reminds them that he himself had inoculated many parishioners' children for free, and would continue to do so if asked.[88] What he seemed not to consider was parents' reluctance to lose not only their own work

82 Schwager, "Prediger," 90–2; Holger Böning, "Johann Moritz Schwager als Volkskundler und Volksaufklärer," in *Er War ein Licht in Westfalen. Johann Moritz Schwager (1738–1804), ein Westfälische Aufklärer*, eds. Walter Gödden, Peter Hesselmann, and Frank Stückemann (Bielefeld: Aisthesis, 2013), 53–78.

83 Schwager, "Prediger," 49–51, 62, 68; Apx 2: Schwager, "Patriotische" (1786), 202.

84 Juncker, *Archiv*, 2:260; 5:9, 157, 200; Apx 2: Henschel (1795), 78–9; Schwager, "Patriotische" (1786), 203; Migula, "Inokulation" (1787), 244–5.

85 Pistor, "Geschichte," 780; Apx 2: Schwager, "Patriotische" (1786), 202–8.

86 Schwager, "Prediger," 77; Apx 2: Schwager, "Noch etwas" (1786), 550; Schwager, "Patriotische" (1786), 204, 207, 213, 235–7.

87 Apx 2: Schwager, "Noch etwas" (1786), 547, 550; Schwager, "Patriotische" (1786), 223, 229, 236.

88 Apx 2: Schwager, "Patriotische" (1786), 201–16; 219–20. For other discussion of Schwager's circular, see pp. 35–6 above.

time in caring for children with inoculated smallpox, but also the loss of the sick children's contribution to routine farm duties. On the other hand, children were very likely to catch smallpox anyway, and inoculation at least offered an opportunity to choose a season of lighter work-load for the illness.

Schwager recalled with sadness the grief of parents who considered inoculation and lost their treasured children because they dithered and delayed. He observed, too, that parents opposed to inoculation tended to change their mind and have their remaining children inoculated after losing others to smallpox. *Stadtphysikus* P.D. Rosenbach from Münden (Hanover) and several other commentators agreed that the greatest motivation for parents' adoption of inoculation was the previous death of some of their children at the hands of "this murdering angel, smallpox."[89] Schwager was well-aware that many parents rejected inoculation owing to the fear that their child may die from the disease they themselves had caused. In order to counter those fears, he stressed that the procedure was rarely fatal and was carried out only when smallpox was an imminent threat. He also reminded parents that the disease had killed large numbers of un-inoculated children in recent years.[90]

Scepticism about whether inoculation produced 'true' smallpox that would protect against the disease in future, and the notion that God 'sent' smallpox to each individual were other reasons Schwager cites for his parishioners' rejection of inoculation. He was aware that some mothers lived in hope that their child would be somehow 'overlooked' for smallpox, just like an occasional person they had heard about.[91] According to his account, beliefs that inoculation caused ill-health and premature death, and that smallpox could be contracted more than once were other reasons for his parishioners' rejection of inoculation. Although he agreed that smallpox occasionally returned to the same individual, citing a few cases that mystified his doctor friends in nearby Bielefeld, he vehemently disagreed with the premise that inoculation predisposed to premature death.[92] He also battled against the fatalistic ideas coming from nearby Minden, where the pastors adhered to the literal interpretation of predestination, and were opposed to inoculation. Those pastors were apparently unaware that the Lutheran church had replaced the doctrine of predestination

89 Juncker, *Archiv*, 2:288; Apx 2: Rosenbach (1771), 1303 (quote); "Waldenburg" (1790), 169; Richter (1799), 244–5; Schwager, "Patriotische" (1786), 207.

90 Schwager, 203–4, 216.

91 Schwager, 202, 206–7.

92 Schwager, 206–8. Many instances of second cases of smallpox were reported over several decades: Johann G. Krünitz, *Verzeichniß der vornehmsten Schriften von der Kinderpocken und deren Einpfropfung* (Leipzig: Hilscher, 1768), 78–81.

with the principle that each person has a duty to preserve life in the best way possible.[93]

Prepared to defend inoculation against all detractors, Schwager engaged in a war of words with the Leipzig professor Ernst Platner. At issue was Platner's presumptive assertion that the much higher rates of inoculation among the young elite than in other social groups caused the lassitude, infertility and stupidity supposedly exhibited by upper-class youth, in particular.[94] Schwager's outrage at such unfounded claims that cast doubt on the value of inoculation prompted him to issue an open challenge to Platner's assertions. Without hiding behind the cloak of anonymity as many contemporary commentators were inclined to do when criticising eminent persons, Schwager argued that any notable weaknesses among the wealthier classes were more likely caused by an unhealthy lifestyle of indulgence and excess than by inoculation. To support his arguments, he affirmed that neither his own children, inoculated twelve years previously, nor any other acquaintances inoculated some time ago showed the kinds of failings that Platner linked to inoculation, and demanded the evidence for such presumptuous claims.[95] The like-minded Pastor Klose from Silesia raised similar criticisms of Platner's arguments, as did more high-profile critics: the Rostock medical faculty professor Samuel Gottlieb Vogel, and Johann Ulrich Schäffer, *Leibarzt* to the Count of Oettingen-Wallerstein.[96]

Pastor Klose, from Domanze (Lower Silesia), like many of his counterparts, was so dismayed at the high rates of death and disability from smallpox in 1786 that he urged parents to adopt inoculation. Having himself been disfigured during childhood when he lost two of his siblings to the disease, and having recently feared losing his daughter as well, Klose points out in his article "To Silesia's Mothers" that even the best doctors lacked the ability to save patients with severe smallpox, and that the only alternative was to curb the severity of the illness through inoculation. He regarded the Prussian Medical Board's treatment advice circular as not only insufficient but of no use at all to the many people with a poor understanding of such complex written material.[97] Klose also warns of the dangers of 'buying smallpox,' which had led to a recent local death, and exhorts mothers to either have their children inoculated by a doctor or surgeon, or do it themselves. He reminds Silesian mothers that their

93 Gehrmann, *Bevölkerungsgeschichte*, 293; Apx 2: Opitz (1774), 107.

94 Von Haen and Platner, *Heilungsmethode*, 437–8.

95 Apx 2: Schwager, "Noch etwas" (1786), 35–7; 545–51.

96 Samuel G. Vogel, *Handbuch der practischen Arzneywissenschaft zum Gebrauche angehende Aerzte* (Vienna: Trattner, 1789), 123–4; Johann U.G. Schäffer, *Versuche aus der theoretischen Arzneykunde* (Nuremberg: Grattenauer, 1784), 296, 316; Apx 2: Klose (1786), 414.

97 Klose, 394, 400.

counterparts in nearby Russia inoculated their own children, and urges the hesitant ones to join with other mothers prepared to inoculate their children as a group.[98]

Klose's article was more of a self-help instruction manual than an inoculation promotion *per se*. To assist mothers willing to take his advice, he describes in great detail a simple method well within their capabilities, which was provided to him by a specialist doctor.[99] Klose recounts the events leading up to his meeting in 1781 with Dr. Johann Friedrich Cloß, who was invited to Silesia by Count von Hochberg von Fürstenstein. When the count informed the pastor of his invitation to the specialist, to inoculate his son, Klose quickly recognised the potential for wider benefits from Cloß's visit. He gained the count's agreement for Cloß to teach the inoculation procedure to the local surgeon, "our very talented Herr John," and for surgeon John to inoculate Klose's two sons under Cloß's supervision, in exchange for surgeon John's assistance in the after-care of all three boys.[100] Having himself learned the finer points of inoculation on that occasion, Klose passed the specialist's method to friends and neighbours, leading to several successful inoculations that convinced him to disseminate the method more widely. Klose indicates that the recent reports by Pastors Schwager and Migula, describing their many successful inoculations using simple methods without any 'preparation' of the candidate, provided him with additional inspiration to publicise the detailed description of Dr. Cloß's procedure that was equally simple and successful.[101]

Pastors Schwager, Migula, and Klose all pointed to the pervasiveness of the misguided belief that inoculated children would die from the next disease they encountered.[102] Klose himself was even targeted with the kind of mob derision observed by Schwager where a jeering crowd mocked parents for having their children inoculated. A group of Klose's own parishioners assailed him with smug, cruel taunts accusing him of causing his son's death by having him inoculated, after his boy died in an outbreak of dysentery three months after the procedure. Yet some kinder, more logical members of his congregation, albeit inoculation opponents too, offered condolences to their bereaved pastor, admitting that the dysentery outbreak killed many un-inoculated people as well as his son. According to Klose, those groups claimed that even a successful inoculation was not protective, and that inoculation interfered with

98 Klose, 393, 400–1, 405, 418.

99 Klose, 404–5, 408–11.

100 Klose, 408 (quote) –13.

101 Klose, 395–6.

102 Apx 2: Migula, "Noch etwas," 411–2; Schwager, "Patriotische" (1786), 207–8, 212–13.

Providence, though he suspected that a general scepticism about anything new was behind their stance.[103] Many such comments from that time, including a report claiming that country folk were inclined to regard not only inoculation but also lightning rods as frivolous, suggest that a general mistrust of innovation was a common, yet understated, reason for the widespread rejection of inoculation in rural Germany.[104]

Objections to pastors promoting inoculation were raised by inoculation supporters as well as the detractors unable to reconcile the practice with their religious beliefs and traditional practices. Among the latter, Professor Triller made known his opposition to clergymen making proclamations about not only inoculation but medical matters in-general, while the Saxon pastor Christian Gotthelf Hauck criticised publicly his counterparts' tendency to promote inoculation in their sermons, attracting a scathing review of the tract in which he issued his complaints.[105] Friedrich Erhard also questioned the wisdom of pastors giving advice about inoculation from the pulpit (1784), though his concerns were from the viewpoint of an inoculation supporter who had noted that the common man was more likely to reject than to accept advice delivered in such an official way. The Berlin doctor Johann Georg Krünitz echoed Erhard's disquiet, pointing out that inoculation rates fell when pastors promoted inoculation too enthusiastically in their sermons.[106] Instances of overbearing inoculation opponents bullying parents into abandoning their plans to adopt the procedure, noted by Pastor Schwager, offer one explanation for falling inoculation rates following pastors' encouragement of inoculation from the pulpit.[107]

Schwager was so convinced that the benefits of inoculation should be spread as widely as possible that in 1785 he sent a copy of his circular promoting inoculation to the Prussian king, Friedrich II, with a recommendation that the advice be widely distributed.[108] Yet his initiative was rejected by not only the *Ober-collegium medicum* but also by the General Directorate, owing to concerns about the contagiousness of inoculation:

103 Klose (1786), 412–5, 419.

104 Juncker, *Archiv*, 3:22, 127–9, 136; 5:237; 7:223; Apx 2: Bail (1796), 223.

105 Apx 2: Triller (1766), 81, 91–2, 156–8; Hauck (1778); review of Hauck (1779).

106 Friedrich Erhard, "Anfrage, die medicinischen und ökonomischen Predigten betreffend, *NMI* 20 (1785): 193–4; Johann G. Krünitz, *Oekonomisch-technologische Encyclopädie*, part 35 (Berlin: Pauli, 1793), 406.

107 Apx 2: Schwager, "Patriotische" (1786), 207, 211–13.

108 Apx 2: Schwager (1784); Schwager, "Patriotische," 201–25. For earlier discussion of Schwager's circular, see pp. 35–8 and 180 above.

> (inoculation would) spread smallpox to all places ... everyone unprepared would be struck down ... through ruined foodstuffs and poor conditions the greatest disaster would surely be precipitated ... so this matter could not in good conscience be left to the ignorant peasants themselves, necessitating trained doctors and surgeons being put in place everywhere to carry out the inoculations.[109]

The Medical Board advised Schwager to seek out the Bishop of Worcester's and Pastor Eisen's sermons about inoculation, which it regarded as more informative than his own circular. The Board was apparently unaware that Eisen was best known for teaching peasants to inoculate their own children, and for exhorting them to show the procedure to their neighbours so that it would become more widely-known and commonly practised in their villages. Such 'self-help' inoculations were exactly what the Board stated that it was trying to avoid.[110] The Prussian General Directorate, in its letter, asked Schwager to do it the favour of "promoting by all means the recently printed instructions to peasants about dealing with epidemic smallpox, of which two hundred will be sent to him," rather than continuing to promote inoculation. Yet Schwager had already issued the government's advice about smallpox treatments to his parishioners from the pulpit, as well as distributing its printed intructions, with little effect.[111] Notably, the negative official attitude to his inoculation initiatives gave way to more positive responses from the Medical Board appointed by King Friedrich Wilhelm II, who succeeded his uncle Friedrich II in August 1786.

3 Inoculation Makes Inroads

The Prussian *Ober-collegium medicum* appointed by the incoming king adopted a new approach to tackling the problem of smallpox, led by the royal example.

---

109 Schwager, "Patriotische," 203, 218 (quote). Three known inoculation opponents were among the four signatories to the Board's letter: the director Christian Andreas Cothenius, the Berlin *Physikus* Christian Ludwig Roloff, and the king's *Leibarzt* Johann Karl Wilhelm Möhsen: Gotthold L. Mamlock, "Friedrich der Grosse und die Einführung der Impfung in Berlin," *ASZ* 10 (1904): 39; Review of "On the most efficacious preservative against the contagion of the small-pox," by Christian A. Cothenius, *The Monthly Review, or Literary Journal* 43 (London, 1771): 521–2. The stance of the fourth signatory, Dr. Kurella, is unknown.

110 Johann G. Eisen, *Die erleichterten und den Müttern selbst übertragenen Blatternimpfung* (Riga: Hartnoch, 1774), 8–13; Schwager, 217–8.

111 Schwager, 220 (quote), 230–1.

With regard to inoculation, Friedrich Wilhelm II had a distinct advantage over his childless predecessor in having seven legitimate children who could potentially be inoculated to highlight the king's confidence in the practice. The good news of the royal children's recovery from their inoculation in late-1789 was indeed officially publicised as widely as possible, by means of thanksgiving services held in churches throughout Prussia.[112] Pastor Schwager turned his own enthusiastic sermon to celebrate the happy outcome into an overt inoculation promotion that he delivered not only from the pulpit but also to a publisher, then he sent a copy to the king.[113] Officials in Berlin were so impressed with Schwager's oratory that they delivered further copies to their counterparts in the provinces and to provincial magistrates, along with "instructions to familiarise themselves with the content, in order to counter the ongoing prejudices against inoculation and alert the less-enlightened folk to the good examples."[114]

Before the reverberations from the royal thanksgiving services had faded, provincial officials received another government directive demanding a special effort to encourage inoculation.[115] Minden-Ravensburg officials took additional action by arranging with the provincial medical board for pastors to be notified of the new requirement to recommend inoculation from the pulpit. Schwager, whose church was in that administrative area, clearly recalled the time in 1790 when parents from neighbouring parishes began streaming to his door with their children, expecting a free inoculation, after their pastors had suddenly begun promoting the practice after previously pronouncing their strident opposition to it. He promptly directed the parents to take their children to the local medical men who carried out competent inoculations without charge.[116]

A Prussian *Ober-collegium medicum* review of the government's approach to smallpox resulted in a revised treatment advice circular for country-folk unable to access a doctor (1796), to which was added a notification that smallpox mortality rates fell in areas where inoculation was common. The Board nonetheless rejected proposals for compulsory inoculation, owing to concerns about restricting personal decision-making, and about the potential spread of smallpox from such a move. It also rejected any extension of the inoculation authorisation to include midwives and other 'healers.'[117] Yet various reports

---

112 Review of "Deutsche Monatsschrift," *ALZ*, no. 182 (1790): 734.

113 Apx 2: Schwager, *Zur Beherzigung* (1790).

114 *Intelligenzblatt der ALZ*, no. 3 (1792): 18–19.

115 Apx 2: Schwager, "Inoculationsgeschichte" (1790), 26–7.

116 Schwager, 27–30.

117 Prussian Medical Board, *Kurze Anweisung, wie der Landmann bei grassirenden Pocken und Scharlachfieber sich zu verhalten habe* (Berlin: Decker, 1796); Pistor, "Geschichte," 781. The

(1796) that inoculations were being carried out by midwives and apothecaries as well as "quacks, blacksmiths, old women, etc.," in addition to many pastors, indicate that the longstanding restriction of inoculation authorisation to doctors and surgeons had little effect.[118] Professor Juncker called for all doctors to work against so-called lay inoculations, which he regarded as a direct threat to not only the health of those inoculated but also the wider community through the spread of the smallpox contagion. He made special mention of pastors' inoculations needing to be curbed, which perhaps reflects the sheer number of pastors engaging in the practice.[119] Yet doctors were more inclined to encourage country pastors' involvement in medical matters and inoculation than to oppose it, since the pastors tended to be great promoters of their advice. Having seen first-hand the damage that harmful quackery was wreaking on their communities, country pastors tried hard to convince their parishioners to call in a doctor, or at least to follow advice compiled by a doctor.[120] Pastors occasionally reported that such efforts had been successful.[121]

Medical men in towns adjacent to rural areas derived considerable benefit from country pastors' entreaties to parents to have their childen inoculated, which encouraged wealthy farmers and other country-folk to take their children to the nearest town for the procedure.[122] Medical men, in their turn, agreed to country pastors' requests to teach them the inoculation method, knowing that pastors would only inoculate children of parents who were unlikely to seek out a doctor or surgeon for the procedure. Pastor Schwager acknowledges (1786) the willing assistance he received from the two medical men who taught him the finer points of inoculation. One of those instructors, Dr. Rudolph Carl Opitz, praised Schwager for setting a positive example to his parishioners by having his children inoculated by a doctor, a course of action he regarded as far preferable to pastors merely proclaiming that God permitted inoculation.[123] Pastors in some cases reciprocated the assistance

---

principality of Kleve and the town of Leer in East Friesland reported a low incidence of smallpox, owing to inoculation: Juncker, *Archiv*, 4:82; 6:227.

118 Juncker, 5:112–3, 197; Otto, *Bemerkungen*, 68, 71; Apx 2: "Pokkeneinimpfung" (1796), 161, n. (quote).

119 Johann C.W. Juncker, *Gemeinnützige Vorschläge wider die Pockenkrankheit. Dritter Versuch, für möglichst alle Aerzte, die der deutschen Sprache kundig sind; zur Sammlung ihrer Gutachten hierüber* (Halle: Hemmerde and Schwetscke, 1796), 33, 47–50.

120 Juncker, *Archiv*, 3:130–2; 4:93; 5:36, 212; 6:38–9; 7:222–30.

121 Juncker, 3:130; 4:93; 5:212; 6:39; 7:229–30.

122 Juncker, 5:8, 49, 83, 87, 89–91, 111, 235; 6:79, 101.

123 Apx 2: Schwager, "Patriotische" (1786), 226; Schwager, "Noch etwas" (1786), 550; Opitz (1774), 104, 108–9.

they received from doctors, by identifying suitable smallpox cases as potential donors for inoculation. Even more help were those with the acuity to recognise pustules at the correct stage of 'ripeness,' particularly the pastors with the ability and willingness to respond to a doctor's request to collect such material.[124] Pastors also helped the local medical men by convincing villagers of the benefits of inoculation, then arranging for a doctor or surgeon to come to the village to undertake a group inoculation for which the cost would be borne by a landlord or other benefactor.[125] Schwager delivered such a favour in 1785 to Dr. Hartog, from Herford, after his circular recommending inoculation convinced a large leaseholder in the district to follow his advice. On that occasion, Meier Johann called in the experienced Hartog to inoculate thirty-three children on two farms after gaining the agreement of his tenants and a neighbour to join him in having their children inoculated.[126]

In many instances of group inoculations on farming estates, the local pastor was the primary influence in gaining the peasants' agreement. Pastor Rältig from Radlingen (Prussia) was spurred into taking such action by a report indicating that smallpox mortality in his parish was worse than elsewhere in the region. He set about teaching the peasants the best treatments for smallpox and explaining the benefits of inoculation, gaining the parents' agreement to have their children inoculated. When he approached the estate owner Count von Reuß, to make the arrangements, the count not only agreed to Rältig's request for the use of an isolated forest house for carrying out the procedure and caring for the children while they remained contagious, but also funded the inoculation of the thirty-one peasant children when smallpox arrived in the area in 1800.[127] Pastor Rältig's initiative had the broader impact of inspiring the owner of a large estate in the neighbouring parish to follow suit. Count Feldreich initially set an example for the peasants by having his own child inoculated, then followed up by offering the procedure for free to all of the children in the villages and small towns on his lands. When Dr. Christian Samuel Ungnad from nearby Züllichau was called in to carry out the 114 inoculations, five local noblewomen generously volunteered to help the peasant mothers care for the children. The noblewomen co-ordinated their caring activities with

124 Apx 2: Klose (1786), 416; Klose (1787), 457; Sintenis (1790), 141.

125 Juncker, *Archiv*, 5:38, 84, 234–5; Ungnad, "Nachricht," 304–5; Apx 2: Brinckmann (1797), 125–7.

126 Schwager, "Patriotische" (1786), 230–1. For earlier discussion of Schwager's circular, see pp. 35–6, 180, and 184–5 above.

127 Ungnad, "Nachricht," 304–5.

Pastor Poeler and his wife, who supervised the children's recovery and kept the inoculator informed.[128] In a similar spirit of co-operation in the Brandenburg village of Rathenow, Pastor Lympius and a group of local noblewomen helped the peasant mothers care for thirty-four children inoculated in 1797 by Dr. Johann Christian Meier.[129]

Another kind of inspirational leadership by a wealthy landholder was reported from the tiny principality of Eutin. That remarkable landlord's tireless efforts to introduce enlightened ideas to the village of Thürk eventually succeeded in fostering a positive attitude to innovation, to the extent that the villagers chose to accept inoculation when smallpox threatened the area in 1796. Their collective agreement to invite a doctor to undertake the procedure was well-supported by the wealthier farmers, who offered to fund the inoculation of the poor. That initiative had a wider influence by making such an impression on the pastor in nearby Bosau that he worked toward a collective agreement for a mass inoculation involving all of the surrounding communities.[130] A similar joint initiative among a group of villages in neighbouring Holstein in 1797, arranged by another local pastor, was perhaps influenced by the events in Thürk and Bosau.[131] Such instances of voluntary inoculation among peasant groups underscore not only the often crucial efforts of country pastors in bringing inoculation to rural communities but also the importance of cooperation between wider groups of influential locals.

By the mid-1790s, the inoculation of peasants on some large farming estates had been carried out for decades, particularly in Mecklenburg and Brandenburg. According to Pastor Christian Schmidt from Prillwitz (Mecklenburg), the von Bredow estate in Neustrelitz was smallpox-free in 1796 owing to the landlord's action in calling in a doctor to inoculate the children on four occasions in the past thirty years. He noted that 123 inoculations had been carried out since the tenants first agreed to have their children inoculated every ten years, or whenever smallpox threatened.[132] Pastor Kronis suggests similarly that the village of Ihlenfeld on *Klosterhauptmann* von Rieben's estate, further to the north, had been smallpox-free for the past twenty years because

128 Ungnad, 305–8. For more details of the ladies involved, see ch. 2, n. 167.

129 "Nachricht von der Pockeninokulation zu Nennhausen bei Rathenow," *Jahrbücher der preußischen Monarchie* (1798), 2:97–9. For more details of the ladies involved. See ch. 2, n. 166.

130 Apx 2: "Pokkeneinimpfung" (1796), 164–5.

131 Apx 2: Brinckmann (1797), 125–7.

132 Juncker, *Archiv*, 4:13–14.

of a similar long-term strategy of inoculating the children when smallpox was approaching.[133] The tendency for landlords in the Mecklenburg region to undertake regular group inoculations may explain the comparatively high tally of 500 inoculations attributed in the 1780s to *Landchirurgus* Burmeister from Lauenburg.[134]

Group inoculations of peasants in Mecklenburg reached a high-point when smallpox was spreading through the region during 1796–97. On a notable earlier occasion, in 1791, *Kammerherr* von Lepel, the leaseholder of a large farm in the Güstrow region, informed his tenants, "both free and serf," of the benefits of inoculation, and gained their agreement to have their children inoculated at his cost. Having spread the word to his neighbours and called in *Kreisphysikus* Westendorff and *Kreischirurgus* Richter, 105 inoculations were carried out on the *Kammerherr's* estate and an additional 130 on two neighbouring farms.[135] Impressive though those numbers may seem in the context of other inoculation activity in Germany, the ongoing serfdom in Mecklenburg at that time may have involved a degree of coercion that would be unacceptable to free tenants.[136] In the instances where peasants were actually given a choice of whether or not to agree to the inoculation of their children, the offer was sometimes rejected for one reason or another. Pastor Maywan from Polkwitz (Silesia) points to an occasion when the successful inoculation of the landowner's children in 1796 convinced only two tenants to accept the owner's free inoculation offer.[137]

Rolf Gehrmann, in his study of the impact of cowpox vaccination on smallpox mortality in nineteenth-century Germany, shows a set of figures which suggest that rural mass inoculations may have had a measurable impact in lowering mortality-rates in some regions. His graph showing the collective smallpox fatalities per 4,000 individuals for Mecklenburg, Kurmark (West Brandenburg), and the much smaller principality of Lippe indicate that the smallpox mortality rate fell from 12 per cent in 1788, to 10 per cent in 1796, to 8 percent in 1797, and to 6 per cent in 1800, which amounts to a halving of the smallpox mortality rate during the twelve years (1788–1800) before cowpox vaccination was first introduced. Professor Gehrmann noted that the anomalous fall in smallpox mortality before the introduction of cowpox vaccination

---

133 Juncker, 4:10.

134 Vogel, *Handbuch*, 116. Lauenburg was a small territory on the western border of Mecklenburg.

135 Apx 2: "Nachricht" (1791), 515–6.

136 von Coelln, "Beytrag," 106; Schwager, "Bauer," 69; Clark, *Kingdom*, 164–7.

137 Juncker, *Archiv*, 4:87.

in 1800 was yet to be explained.[138] That explanation may lie in the sizeable group inoculations and the smallpox-free zones created by the regular inoculation of children in the two largest of the regions examined: Mecklenburg and Kurmark. Perhaps those territories can be tentatively added to Kleve and East Friesland as areas in Germany where inoculation was shown to have a noticeable impact in lowering local smallpox mortality rates.[139]

A long history of peasants having to rely on traditional ways of dealing with illness, because competent medical care was sparse in rural areas, proved to be a considerable obstacle to the penetration of new ideas. The country pastors deserve recognition for their innovative strategies aimed toward convincing their parishioners to adopt new approaches to smallpox, which usually began with gentle persuasion to abandon the traditional harmful treatments, and sometimes progressed to the encouragement of inoculation. Pastors who achieved the feat of allaying parents' fears about inoculation probably managed to save more lives than they would have realised at the time, by paving the way for easier acceptance of cowpox vaccination.

138 Rolf Gehrmann, "The impact of smallpox and vaccination in Northern Germany in the 18th and 19th centuries," *Przeszlość Demograficzna Polski* 36 (2014): 48–9. Mecklenburg in the 1790s comprised Mecklenburg-Schwerin and Mecklenburg-Strelitz.

139 Juncker, *Archiv*, 4:82; 6:227.

CHAPTER 7

To Inoculate, or Aim to Eradicate Smallpox

By the mid-1780s smallpox was increasingly being recognised as a problem in urgent need of a solution, and the contagiousness of inoculation as part of the problem. A new approach based on the isolation and containment of the disease seemed feasible in the light of the recent consensus among doctors that the longstanding theory of innate smallpox was incorrect and that smallpox spread only through contagion.[1] Germans were well-aware that quarantine and isolation measures had been used successfully in the past to keep bubonic plague at bay, and were optimistic that another deadly pestilence, smallpox, could be defeated in the same way.[2] Inspiration came particularly from the successful containment strategy used in the English town of Chester by Dr. John Haygarth and his colleagues, who prevented severe epidemic smallpox from wreaking havoc in 1784.[3] That achievement prompted even some of the most ardent German inoculation supporters to agree that isolating smallpox cases was more likely to reduce overall mortality than inoculation.[4] Ideas for preventing the spread of smallpox turned into two campaigns for the actual eradication of the disease, both of which attracted followers. The main point of difference was inoculation, which was an integral part of one campaign and was omitted from the other.[5]

The very aim of eradicating smallpox by the proposed means generated lively debates in the print media, raising the broader question of whether eradicating smallpox was a realistic objective or merely a utopian dream. A variety

1 Christoph W. Hufeland, "Neue Aussicht zur Vertilgung der Blattern," *TM* 4 (1786): 170–3, 179–81.

2 "Ueber die Ausrottung der Blattern," *Münchner Intelligenzblatt*, no. 23 (1797): 280–3; Apx 2: Bolten (1774), 5, 59–76.

3 John Haygarth, *An Inquiry How to Prevent the Small-Pox and Proceedings of a Society for Promoting General Inoculation at Stated Periods and Preventing the Natural Small-Pox, in Chester* (Chester: Monk, 1784), 169–73.

4 Hufeland, "Vertilgung," 167–81, 258; Ernst B.G. Hebenstreit, *Lehrsätze der medicinischen Policeywissenschaft* (Leipzig: Dyck, 1791), 175–9.

5 Bernhard C. Faust, "Versuch über die Pflicht der Menschen, jeden Blatternkranken der Gesunden abzusondern; und dadurch zugleich in Städten und Ländern und in Europa die Ausrottung der Blatternpest zu bewirken," *PJ* 4 (1794): 40–95; Johann C.W. Juncker, *Gemeinnützige Vorschläge wider die Pockenkrankheit. Dritter Versuch, für möglichst alle Aerzte, die der deutschen Sprache kundig sind; zur Sammlung ihrer Gutachten hierüber* (Halle: Hemmerde and Schwetscke, 1796), 1–22.

 | DOI:10.1163/9789004465374_009

of foreign and local influences intersected in the 1790s to inspire those hopes of a smallpox-free future, even before the first reviews (1798–99) of Edward Jenner's report of his promising new experiments with cowpox upgraded those hopes into the realm of possibility. At that time of the Coalition Wars ensuing from the French Revolution, the more optimistic and nationalistic Germans saw smallpox as yet another enemy that could be defeated by a united effort. The realists thought otherwise.[6]

1 Inoculation versus Containment Strategies

The Rostock (Mecklenburg-Schwerin) professor Georg Christoph Detharding and the Swiss physician Samuel-Auguste Tissot issued the first public denials (1754) of the theory of innate smallpox originally proposed by the ninth-century Arabic physician known as Rhazes. Their respective conclusions that an external agent caused the disease, and that the isolation of patients could contain the contagion was a watershed in ideas about smallpox prevention.[7] The Leipzig professor Carl Christian Krause expanded that concept eight years later with a comparison of smallpox and bubonic plague. His conclusion that both diseases were contagious fevers led him to suggest that smallpox could potentially be eradicated using the same measures that succeeded in banishing the plague from German communities.[8] Dr. Friedrich Casimir Medicus from Mannheim agreed, congratulating Krause on his courage in publicly presenting such a novel concept, considering that the educated elite usually greeted new ideas as they would a "hostile invasion by a great prince into a neighbouring state."[9]

Medicus pointed out that if smallpox were indeed an essential part of human biology, as the innate smallpox theory suggested, the disease would have been mentioned in ancient times by Hippocrates or Galen, and would have been known in the Caribbean, America, Greenland, and other colonial

---

6 Friedrich B. Osiander, "Urtheil über die vergebliche leichte Möglichkeit der Blatternausrottung in Europa," *Neues HM* 8 (1798): 1274–5; "Abgedrungene Erklärung über die Pockenangelegenheit, besonders in Rücksicht des Junckerschen Ausrottungsplans," *JE* 21 (1799): 140–1.

7 Georg C. Detharding, *De facie a variolarum insultibus praeservanda* (Rostock: Adler, 1754), 12–14; Samuel-Auguste D. Tissot, *L'Inoculation justifiée, ou dissertation pratique et apologétique sur cette méthode* (Lausanne: Bousquet, 1754), 138–9; Miller, *Adoption,* 264–5. For an explanation of Rhazes's theory, see pp. 32–3 above.

8 Apx 1: Krause (1762), 40–3.

9 Friedrich C. Medicus, *Send-Schreiben von der Ausrottung der Kinder-Blattern* (Frankfurt and Leipzig, 1763), 2.

outposts before the arrival of Europeans. Yet neither was the case.[10] The medical fraternity gave Krause and Medicus widespread recognition for their novel idea. Their suggestion that smallpox could potentially be eradicated 'like bubonic plague' resonated not only in Britain, the Netherlands, and Germany, where it was highlighted by reviewers for various journals, but also in France where Antoine le Camus repeated it in 1768, without attribution.[11]

Increasing acceptance of the idea that smallpox could actually be eradicated 'like the plague' prompted a variety of strategies to achieve that objective, though there was little agreement on what regulations may be effective or whether inoculation should have a part. The Berlin doctor, Leon Elias Hirschel, pointed out (1770) that the effectiveness of implementing past containment strategies would be negated by fundamental differences in contemporary public attitudes to smallpox compared to earlier attitudes to bubonic plague epidemics. He reasoned that the minority of people who survived a bout of the plague had no idea why they 'escaped' death or whether they could catch the plague again, so they avoided contact with the disease. Smallpox survivors, by comparison, were sufficiently confident of their immunity to visit afflicted relatives and friends, causing the inadvertent spread of the contagion around their community. Hirschel called for consideration of such behaviour in the design of measures for isolating smallpox. He also recommended an expansion of inoculation "through good public institutions."[12] *Stadtphysikus* Johann Friedrich Bolten from Hamburg adopted the opposite view, expressing his confidence that the quarantine rules used against the plague would keep smallpox at bay, and condemning inoculation because of its contagiousness (1774).[13] The high-ranking Berlin physician, Johann Karl Wilhelm Möhsen, made his own assessment of past quarantine and containment measures, perhaps hoping to offer the king a valid alternative to an expansion of inoculation, which he

---

10 Medicus, 1–4, 17, 67–74.

11 Review of *De divers ouvrages pour l'inoculation de la petite vérole*, by Carl C. Krause and Friedrich G. Beer (Leipzig, 1762), *Journal de médecine, chirurgie, pharmacie* 19 (1763): 389–90; "Account of a Letter on the Extirpation of the Small Pox, Lately Published in Germany by Dr. Frederic Casimir, Physician at Mannheim," *The Gentleman's Magazine* 34 (1764): 290–1, and *The Scots Magazine* 26 (1764): 293–6; "Friederich Casimir, Send-Schreiben," *The Monthly Review, or Literary Journal* 23 (1764): 545–6; Review of *Send-Schreiben*, by Friedrich C. Medicus, *Natuur-en Genees-kundige Bibliotheek*, ed. Eduard Sandifort (The Hague: Tersier, 1765), 697. Six other, mainly German, reviews of Krause and Medicus are listed in Johann G. Krünitz, *Verzeichniß der vornehmsten Schriften von der Kinderpocken und deren Einpfropfung* (Leipzig: Hilscher, 1768), 37–8.

12 Leon E. Hirschel, *Abhandlung von den Vorbauungs-und Vorbereitungs-Mitteln bey den Pocken* (Berlin: Bosse, 1770), 4 (quote) –10.

13 Apx 2: Bolten (1774), 59–76.

personally opposed. Yet he reached the unwelcome conclusion that the movement of foreigners and traders across the open country would thwart any such measures put in place around Berlin, prompting him to warn of much higher mortality rates when pestilences returned after a long absence than when they recurred more often.[14]

The Count of Lippe-Detmold's court physician, Johann Christian Scherf, considered the containment of smallpox in a context of princes needing inoculation to preserve their children and dynastic succession, and of the bans on the practice being imposed increasingly in cities and towns across Europe. Scherf's proposed approach to inoculation, which was aimed at avoiding such bans, reflects a sympathetic attitude to parents wanting to protect their children before smallpox arrived.[15] In his lengthy evaluation of potential containment strategies, Scherf places a strong focus on the Neapolitan professor Michael Sarcone's measures for isolating smallpox victims and thoroughly cleansing anything they touched.[16] Scherf's own rules aimed at preventing the spread of smallpox from inoculation, which he recommended for incorporation into medical policy, were rare at that time (1783) as pillars of a German policy proposal aimed specifically at the containment of inoculated smallpox.[17]

Dr. Christoph Wilhelm Hufeland (see Figure 8 on p. 88) issued an appeal in *Der Teutsche Merkur* in 1786, quite early in his illustrious career, to focus attention on "diverting the murdering angel from the gates." While offering plaudits for the past success in banishing bubonic plague from Germany, he asserts that the control and quarantine measures proven to be effective against the plague would not halt smallpox because that contagion infected the atmosphere, whereas transmission of the plague required direct contact with a victim. His conclusions about the plague came from his perusal of descriptions of the bubonic plague epidemic in central Russia in 1771–72 that caused at least 100,000 deaths. He makes particular mention of the reports of Count Grigorii Orlov remaining plague-free after riding inside a wagon carrying victims' bodies on the outside, which convinced him that bubonic plague was spread by direct contact, and that the containment of smallpox needed a strategy along the lines of the Hottentots' and the Tartars' exclusion of all afflicted individuals from their villages. Using the analogy of a fire being easily quenched when isolated,

14 Apx 2: Möhsen, part 3 (1775), 138–4. The Prussian king at the time was Friedrich II.

15 Johann C. Scherf, *Archiv der medizinischen Polizey und die gemeinnützigen Arzneikunde*, vol. 3 (Leipzig: Weygand, 1785), 234–5.

16 Scherf, 1:283–92.

17 Scherf, 2:237–41. Scherf's ideas may have been influenced by local regulations issued in Chester six years before John Haygarth discussed those regulations in his book (1784): Haygarth, *Inquiry*, 169–73.

Hufeland proposes that smallpox patients should be housed in premises located away from residential areas.[18]

Hufeland admits that extreme disappointment at the vehement opposition to inoculation arising from the occasional death from the procedure prompted his move toward isolation measures as a primary approach to combating smallpox. For an effective, well-designed containment strategy he recommends Dr. Johann Friedrich Cappel's translation (1785) of the protocol designed by Dr. John Haygarth and his colleagues that succeeded in dampening a virulent smallpox epidemic threatening Chester in the previous year.[19] The core of Haygarth's strategy was the Chester Smallpox Society, which was founded and funded from benevolent donations with the aim of curbing the impact of smallpox in the town through inoculation, isolating all infected individuals, and offering rewards for adherence to a set of 'Rules of Prevention' designed to prevent the spread of the disease. Though inoculation ended up playing only a minor role because of its unpopularity, with the Society failing to reach its anticipated tally of 416 inoculated individuals during 1778–82, the combined strategy nonetheless succeeded in keeping smallpox at bay. Yet the chairman Thomas Falconer considerably understated the Society's achievement, with his pronouncement that "the contagion is now so perfectly extinguished in this city." A better measure of the true magnitude of the Society's success was Falconer's sombre reminder that "the natural small-pox did very lately and probably does at present rage with destructive violence in Liverpool, Manchester, and other towns," which were not far away.[20]

The achievement of Haygarth and his colleagues in halting smallpox turned into a beacon of hope and inspiration for the German intellectual elite. Professor Juncker was so impressed that he repeated Haygarth's inspiring words – "When the publick voice unites and gives vigour to the laws, every eye and tongue would aid and assist their accomplishments" – to underscore his own confidence that the German public would support isolation measures for smallpox.[21] Yet Haygarth's proposed civil regulations aimed at eradicating

18 Hufeland, "Vertilgung," 167 (quote), 174–5, 179–8; John T. Alexander, *Bubonic Plague in Early Modern Russia* (Oxford: Oxford University Press, 2003), 257–8. Möhsen noted in 1774 the Hottentots' habit of isolating smallpox victims to prevent the disease from spreading: Apx 2: Möhsen, part 3 (1775), 135–6.

19 Hufeland, 179–81; John Haygarth, *Untersuchung wie die Blattern zuvorzukommen sey,* trans. Johann F.L. Cappel (Berlin and Stettin: Nicolai, 1785). For earlier discussion of Hufeland and his career, see pp. 87–8 and 155–6 above.

20 Haygarth, *Inquiry*, 165–208, 192, 222 (quotes).

21 Johann C.W. Juncker, *Archiv der Aerzte und Seelsorger wider die Pockennoth,* vol. 2 (Leipzig: Weygand, 1797), 216, n. 3.

smallpox from Great Britain (1793) failed to attract much attention in Germany owing to the belatedness of the translated version, which appeared in 1799 amid the flood of commentary on Edward Jenner's promising new cowpox vaccination approach to solving the smallpox problem.[22] Many German doctors as well as laymen were so inspired by the successful effort to halt the spread of smallpox in Chester in 1785 that they proposed their own strategies aimed toward not only containing the disease but eradicating it altogether. Among the first clergymen to suggest such an approach (1787) was Johann Gottlieb Meißner, the superintendent of churches in the Steinau district of Silesia. While admitting his admiration for inoculation's ability to reduce the severity of smallpox, Meißner conceded that a new strategy based on containment had the advantage of leading toward the potential eradication of the disease. His proposed set of rules for combating the spread of the contagion included not only a payment for adherence to the isolation regulations but an additional bonus if the patient survived, reflecting his awareness that the widespread fatalistic attitudes to smallpox led to the neglect of afflicted children.[23] He also proposed the exclusion of anyone who had not previously had the illness from the group of mourners accompanying the smallpox-dead to their graves, though such a regulation was just as likely to be disobeyed as the Prussian prohibition on open-coffin displays of smallpox victims that was already being regularly flouted.[24]

Pastor Schwager from Joellenbeck gave Haygarth an emphatic vote of confidence by publishing the Chester Smallpox Society's strategy as an attachment to his own sermon celebrating the successful inoculation of the Prussian king's children (1789). In doing so, he highlighted not only his ongoing confidence in inoculation but also his resounding approval of the containment approach.[25] His counterpart from Lüneburg (Hanover), Christoph Friedrich Lindemann, adopted a more assertive stance in issuing a public appeal for action to eradicate smallpox. While offering effusive praise for the Italian professor Michael Sarcone's recommended containment measures, Pastor Lindemann criticises other doctors, particularly the "misleading erudition" of the Breslau doctor Johann Gottfried Hahn, for adhering to the innate smallpox theory that contradicted the very notion of containment. He also accuses the authorities of

22 John Haygarth, *Entwurf, die zufälligen Blattern zu verbannen und eine allgemeine Impfung einzuführen,* trans. Johann B. Bonzel (Gotha: Perthes, 1799).

23 Johann G. Meißner, "Vorschlag, die Blattern zu vertilgen," *Neue BMN* 4 (1787): 358–61; Juncker, *Archiv*, 3:90, 127; 4:166; 5:109; 7:221–2.

24 Meißner, 360; Juncker, 1:281–2; 3:134–5; 4:79; Moritz Pistor, "Geschichte der preussischen Medizinalverwaltung," *DVG* 40 (1908): 243, 780–1.

25 Apx 2: Schwager, *Zur Beherzigung* (1790).

relying on the outdated notion of innate smallpox, as an excuse for inaction in addressing the urgent need for the implementation of containment and quarantine measures, beseeching "you princes and kings; help us eradicate this appalling pestilence from the earth, or at least issue wise laws to keep it at bay like the plague." In an appeal to like-minded Germans to take decisive action, Lindemann urges them to write articles designed to penetrate the public consciousness, which would educate people about the true nature of smallpox, and to send them to the people's journals and fashion magazines. As an example, he highlights Salzmann's delivery of such advice in his fictional love-story *Carl von Carlsberg*, and provides the page reference.[26]

Christian Gotthilf Salzmann was an Erfurt pastor who took up teaching and established an elite school in 1784 on his rural estate near Gotha. He became known for his books promoting his particular brand of moral education, and for his colloquial journal *Der Bote aus Thüringen* that he produced at his own publishing enterprise on his Schnepfenthal estate. He used those publications as well as his lengthy romantic novel *Carl von Carlsberg* (1783–87) as vehicles for public education.[27] He raises the matter of smallpox eradication in that novel in a letter from the fictional heroine Henriette to her beloved Carl recounting her coach trip home after visiting him, in which she was accompanied by her father and cousin, a church deacon. Henriette describes their lunch during a change of horses, noting their sudden loss of appetite when the tavern-keeper serves their food while holding his child who clearly had smallpox, and the ensuing sympathetic discussion of the man's plight in having to earn a living while fulfilling his parental duty to his sick child. She makes particular mention of a fellow-passenger's interjection that smallpox could actually be eradicated through a state-sponsored campaign, and her chaperones' prompt response querying how that could be possible considering that the disease was an integral and necessary part of human nature. Their well-informed new companion's attention-grabbing exclamation: "smallpox is just as necessary to our constitution as bubonic plague" initiates a lesson about the true nature of smallpox, and a recommendation of Dr. Hufeland's article (1786) in *Der Teutsche Merkur* for further explanation of the mechanism of smallpox transmission. The knowledgeable passenger points out that Hufeland advises the isolation of smallpox patients in houses situated away from residential

26 Christoph F.H. Lindemann, "Ueber die Ausrottung der Kinderblattern," *HM* 27 (1789): 565–8, 569 (quotes) –70; Johann G. Hahn, *Variolarum ratio exposita* (Breslau: Korn, 1751).

27 Georg C. Hamberger and Johann G. Meusel, *Das gelehrte Teutschland,* vol. 17 (Lemgo: Meyer, 1798), 17–20; Margot Hochheim, *Der Pädagoge Salzmann* (Berlin: Springer, 1939), 53.

areas, to prevent the spread of the contagion, and that the pursuit of smallpox eradication was just one of the ambitious goals inspired by two remarkable achievements: the elimination of the plague and the introduction of lightning rods, which jointly fostered the belief that anything was possible.[28]

Salzmann made another effort to promote smallpox eradication strategies in his introduction to an extract from Professor Francesco Maria Scuderi's book (in Latin) on the topic (1794), which was translated and published by his son-in-law Christian Ludwig Lenz, a teacher at his school. Lenz's addition of his own smallpox eradication strategy to his translation of the Sicilian professor's ideas aimed toward the same objective, following Salzmann's introduction, resulted in three quite different smallpox eradication plans in the one volume.[29] Reviewers for three highly-respected journals were decidedly unimpressed by not only Salzmann's and Lenz's respective plans but also by the parts of Scuderi's plan that Lenz chose to translate. They judged Salzmann's plan, which was centred on 'smallpox houses' in every town and village and elements from Haygarth's 'Rules,' as not only inferior to the English doctor's strategy but also far too costly. Lenz's plan they regarded as unworkable because the proposed cordons to keep smallpox out of a particular area would trap people who feared catching the disease if they travelled further afield. One reviewer for Professor Johann Jacob Hartenkeil's highly-regarded *Medicinish-chirurgische Zeitung* criticised not only the proffered plans but also the tendency for laymen to issue advice on medical matters, which was epitomised by the addition of two laymen's strategies for smallpox eradication to a volume centred on the ideas aired by a Sicilian professor of medicine.[30] Many more proposals from laymen were yet to come.

Lieutenant Friedrich Ludwig von Pufendorf from the Brunswick-Lüneburg regiment added yet another smallpox eradication plan to the growing collection, albeit a much more detailed proposal than most of the others of the time. In his introduction, Pufendorf praises "the courageous Englishman Haygarth" whose rules for isolating patients and maintaining scrupulous cleanliness he adopted for his own plan.[31] He also expresses regrets that the spread of

28 Christian G. Salzmann, "Twelfth Letter, Henrietta to Carl," *Carl von Carlsberg, oder über das menschliche Elend,* vol. 6 (Leipzig: Crusius, 1788), 150–7, 158 (quote and reference to Hufeland, "Vertilgung," 180–1). For discussion of Hufeland's article, see pp. 195–6 above.

29 Francesco M. Scuderi, *Vorschläge zur Ausrottung der Kinderblattern und anderen ansteckenden Seuchen,* trans. Christian L. Lenz (Schnepfenthal: Erziehungsinstitut, 1794).

30 Reviews of *Vorschläge,* by Scuderi, *ALZ* 1 (1795): 367–8; *GA,* no. 29 (1795): 282–4; *MCZ* 3 (1794): 218–20.

31 Friedrich L. von Pufendorf, *Ausführbare Vorschläge zur gänzlichen Vertilgung der Blattern. Regenten, Staatsmännern, und Menschenfrunden zu reiflicher Erwägung und Beherzigung*

inoculation was thwarted by superstition, fatalism, and other common prejudices, explaining that he omitted inoculation from his plan only because its contagiousness was incompatible with the objective of smallpox eradication.[32] Pufendorf centres his approach largely on smallpox hospitals outside each town to contain the disease contagion, and the distribution of a detailed advice pamphlet that includes a sign to be posted on the door of every house with a smallpox case. He admits to assuming that the less-educated part of society would follow the example of the more enlightened groups if the latter were to obey the rules, explaining that the scarcity of local civic leaders in rural areas, to set an example, necessitated his special rules for peasants.[33] One reviewer hailed Pufendorf's recommendations as very important, though unlikely to be heeded at that time of terrible war; another saw little fundamental difference between Pufendorf's plan and the respective strategies proposed by Scuderi, Salzmann, and Lenz, regarding them all as exceptionally costly and reflecting too much "theoretical humanitarianism." The second reviewer stated that, in his view, smallpox eradication was not feasible and inoculation remained the best approach to the disease.[34]

Professor Johann Samuel Halle mused about the theoretical simplicity of eradicating smallpox by inoculating all non-immune individuals at once. Yet the Berlin historian admitted regretfully that inoculation was too unpopular in Germany to be made compulsory, and could therefore have no part in policies aimed toward the eradication of smallpox. Halle's own proposed strategy (1793) to achieve that objective had much to do with historical measures employed against bubonic plague: border-police, quarantine-gates, public health authorities, and regulations requiring disease notification. Halle also suggested that a writer of popular fiction such as Salzmann or Becker, "whose tone … is the most understandable and convincing for the common man and most certain to press on his heart," should produce a brochure that not only describes in detail the regulations for smallpox containment but also highlights the vital importance of such rules.[35] Perhaps Halle was already aware of Salzmann's delivery of advice about smallpox containment in his novel *Carl von Carlsberg*.

---

empfohlen (Brunswick: Schulbuchhandlung, 1792), third page of (unnumbered) introduction.

32 Pufendorf, 55–67.

33 Pufendorf, 88–94, 99–102. Thirteen of the 128 pages (pp. 72–84) consist of quotes from Haygarth, trans. Cappel, *Untersuchung* (1785).

34 Review of *Vorschlage*, by Pufendorf, *Deutsche Zeitung über moralische Schilderungen der Menschen, Sitten und Staaten unsrer Zeit*, no. 5 (1793): 73–6; joint reviews of *Vorschläge* by Pufendorf, and *Vorschläge* by Scuderi: *MCZ* 3 (1794): 210 (quote), 218, 222.

35 Johann S. Halle, *Fortgesetzte Magie, oder die Zauberkräfte der Natur* (Berlin: Pauli, 1793), 523–5, 526 (quote) –31. The Becker to whom Halle referred was Rudolph Zacharias Becker:

Awareness that inoculation was causing the spread of smallpox prompted increasing calls for bans on the practice outside places where outbreaks of the disease were occurring, after the *Paris Parlement* led the way in 1763.[36] Six years later, the Hamburg *Stadtphysikus* Johann Friedrich Bolten and apothecary Johann Gerhard Andreä voiced concerns about the spread of smallpox from inoculation in their own city.[37] Yet German municipal authorities resisted calls for the kinds of limits being imposed on the practice in other jurisdictions in Europe. Commenting on the matter in 1782, Dr. Albrecht Wilhelm Roth from Bremen argued that bans on inoculation would cause difficulties for doctors attempting to comply with clients' requests for inoculation at a time that may be unsuitable in terms of the disease spread.[38] His like-minded counterpart in Hamburg, the elite Johann Albrecht Reimarus, publicly opposed any limits on inoculation when the matter was raised again in 1793, highlighting the need to protect children before smallpox arrived when the risks from natural infection were low.[39] By 1796 at least four German jurisdictions had imposed bans on inoculation in smallpox-free areas, as the calls for such limitations grew louder with the realisation that the practice was incompatible with the new objective of smallpox eradication.[40] Other municipal and territorial authorities considered the matter.[41] Cautious parents in towns where no bans were in place had little choice other than to take their own avoidance measures if they wanted to protect children from the inoculated contagion, and had the means to do so. Friedrich Schiller and his wife were among the parents who took such precautions, as Schiller indicates in a letter to Goethe in September 1794: "my wife is in Rudolstadt for three weeks with the child, to avoid the smallpox with which Mr. von Humboldt had his little ones inoculated." In another letter three years

Reinhart Siegert, "Aufklärung und Volkslektüre exemplarish dargestellt an Rudolph Zacharias Becker und seinem 'Not- und Hülfsbüchlein,'" in *Archiv für Geschichte des Buchwesens* 19, eds. Berthold Hack, Reinhard Wittman, and Marietta Kleiss (Frankfurt am Main: Buchhändler-Vereinigung, 1978), 1202–14.

36 *Real-Zeitung*, no. 52 (Erlangen), July 2, 1763, 402–3.

37 Apx 2: Andreä and Bolten (1769), 294–6.

38 Apx 2: Roth (1782), 650–53.

39 Johann A.H Reimarus, "Ueber die Ausrottung der Blattern," *Sammlung auserlesener Abhandlungen zum Gebrauch praktischer Aerzte* 16 (1793): 517–19.

40 A regulation issued in 1784 limited inoculation in the Bishopric of Münster: Scherf, *Archiv*, 6:112–17. In 1796 such regulations weres issued in the Rhineland free city, Mühlhausen, the tiny northern principality, Eutin, and the Duchy of Mecklenburg-Schwerin: "Chronik der Reichsstädte," *NZT*, no. 20 (1796), 440–2; Juncker, *Archiv*, 2:229, n. 10; 4:31.

41 Review of *Ueber den nützen der Pocken-Inoculation in Vergleich des Schadens der natürlichen Pocken* (Düsseldorf, 1795), by Bernard J. Reyland, *MCZ* 2 (1795): 463–4; Karl F.W.A. Vater, *Preussisch-Schlesische Civil Medicinal- and Sanitäts-Verfassung*, part 2 (Breslau: Korn, 1800), 556–7.

later when his own child and Mr. Humboldt's other children were about to be inoculated, Schiller tells Goethe of his warning to his brother and sister-in-law not to come for a visit with their child, who was not ready for inoculation.[42] Goethe seems to have overlooked the inoculation of his own son August, born in 1789, who died from smallpox in 1830.[43]

Dr. Johann Valentin Müller from Frankfurt observed as early as 1788 that inoculation had become unfashionable and that stringent isolation measures, which he regarded as impractical, were being promoted instead.[44] A hard-hitting article in 1795 questioning the sudden calls for limiting inoculation underscores the extent to which the practice had been discredited in Germany by the mid-1790s. The anonymous author asks why, when every mother and pastor was quite recently being encouraged to inoculate, was "the beneficial discovery that was generally praised to the skies just a few years ago being condemned in all ways?"[45] The Münden (Hanover) church superintendent Karl David Vasmer posed a similar question:

> where does it come from that inoculation, which is seemingly so worthwhile for mankind and so beneficial to its subjects, has vanished? ... that a family only seldom decides on it without long consideration, and always with a certain fear of it?[46]

Vasmer suggests, in answer to his own question, that inoculation had become unfashionable in large towns because of public opposition to a general adoption of the practice.[47]

Inoculation was reinvigorated to some extent by the extensive virulent smallpox epidemics of 1795–97, when the increasing death toll prompted parents once again to seek protection for their children. Yet the number inoculated came nowhere near the tally in some towns in England, where municipal leaders facilitated the inoculation of everyone in their local community.[48] The largest reported mass inoculation in Germany, arranged by *Kammerherr*

---

42 *Briefwechsel zwischen Schiller und Goethe in den Jahren 1794 bis 1805*, vol. 1, 1794–95 (Stuttgart and Tübingen: Cotta, 1828), 33 (quote); *Briefwechsel*, vol. 3, *vom Jahre 1797* (1829), 39.

43 Peter Boerner, *Goethe*, trans. Nancy Boerner (Haus: London, 2013), 95 (caption), 105.

44 Johann V. Müller, *Medizinisches praktisches Handbuch der Frauenzimmerkrankheiten zum Gebrauch der Aerzte und des schönen Geschlechts* (Frankfurt and Leipzig: Jäger, 1788), 202–3, 206–8.

45 Apx 2: "Nöthige Bemerkungen" (1795), 78, n. (quote), 124–6.

46 Apx 2: Vasmer (1795), 852.

47 Vasmer, 854.

48 John R. Smith, *The Speckled Monster. Smallpox in England, 1670–1970, with particular reference to Essex* (Chelmsford: Essex Record Office, 1987), 52, 60; Peter Razzell, *The Conquest*

von Lepel in 1791, involved 235 peasants and their children on three farming estates in Mecklenburg.[49] Dr. Abraham Zadig recommended a more regular and widespread inoculation of rural populations *en masse*, such as those carried out in the Russian Baltic provinces of Courland and Livonia where the mainly German landowners had the serf children on their estates inoculated every spring, at shearing time.[50] The reported 380 inoculations on Baron Wolf's estate and 680 on other large Livonian farms in 1793 even exceeded the number inoculated annually at the St. Petersburg Smallpox Hospital.[51] The Breslau-born Zadig, who had spent six-years practising in Livonia, seemed puzzled that Silesian landowners had failed to arrive at the same conclusion as their German counterparts in the Russian Baltic states, who crassly equated the value of peasants' lives saved with the monetary value of their wool clip.[52] Yet he recognised that in Prussia "under the benign, glorious sceptre of Friedrich Wilhelm," such insensitive attitudes toward peasants would not be tolerated as they were in Livonia where the serfs endured a state akin to slavery.[53]

With those various issues in mind and Haygarth as his inspiration, Zadig proposed a smallpox eradication strategy of his own design (1797), focused mainly on north-east Germany. Yet it was clear from the outset that preventing smallpox across a vast rural area with a dispersed population raised a different set of challenges than the ones overcome by Haygarth and his colleagues in an urban environment.[54] Zadig's plan relied heavily on the benevolence of the landowning nobility to fund the proposed regional inoculation societies that would not only arrange and conduct the rural mass inoculations at the heart of his strategy, but would also carry out other smallpox-related functions.[55] One of Zadig's more innovative ideas was a thanksgiving festival to be held

---

of Smallpox: the Impact of Inoculation on Smallpox Mortality in Eighteenth-century Britain (London: Caliban, 2003), 101–2.

49 Apx 2: "Nachricht" (1791), 515–6. The ongoing serfdom in Mecklenburg in the 1790s may have influenced the peasants' consent for inoculation.

50 Abraham Zadig, *Plan, nach welchem die Einimpfung der Pocken in eine ganze Provinz allgemein eingeführt, und die längstgewünscht Ausrottung derselben erreicht werden kann* (Breslau: Korn, 1797), 48–9.

51 William C. Friebe, *Physische, ökonomische und statistische Bemerkungen von Lief-und Ehstland, oder von den beiden Staathalterschaften Riga und Reval* (Riga: Hartnoch, 1794), 220–2; Apx 2: Elsner (1787), 38. Courland was a duchy in the region of modern western Latvia.

52 Zadig, *Plan*, 49.

53 Zadig, 49–50. In the Bromberg region of rural East Prussia, where no group inoculations were reported, 33.6 per cent of all deaths in 1796 were recorded as smallpox: Juncker, *Archiv*, 3:45.

54 Zadig, 47–55.

55 Zadig, 63–7, 78–88.

at each contributing large estate if the inoculations went well, to encourage participation in future mass inoculations. His proposed presentation of floral tributes from the local "Inoculation Society" to parents who permitted the inoculation of their children was intended to applaud their contribution while shaming those excluded from the festivities for failing to give their permission. Similarly, the triumphal procession of recently-inoculated children was meant not only as a form of acknowledgement for parental involvement but also as encouragement to resistant parents to participate in future mass inoculations. Zadig envisaged the children draped in flowers and ribbons seated on a long wagon drawn by four horses and accompanied by fiddlers and trumpeters, as they passed through the villages on their way to the estate-owner's manor. On arrival, they would be officially received in front of their waiting parents who would remain for refreshments while the parade continued wending its way around the villages. Zadig's insistence that anyone opposing inoculation should be excluded from the festival, even if he were the mayor, would reinforce the 'message' that maximum participation was imperative.[56]

While conceding that the enterprise would be costly for the estate-owners, Zadig's observation of the reduced incidence of smallpox following the mass inoculations in rural Livonia convinced him of the rewards in lives saved.[57] One reviewer was quite complimentary about the plan, though another disagreed with Zadig's assumption that the estate-owners and urban upper-class would offer the generous contributions required. That reviewer also alluded to the sheer number of proposed smallpox eradication plans causing public confusion about the proffered advice.[58]

2 Two Campaigns Aiming to Eradicate Smallpox

The smallpox epidemics of the mid-1790s, and the recognition that containment of the contagion could potentially eradicate the disease provided the inspiration for two quite different smallpox eradication campaigns that both attracted ardent followers. One was led by Bernhard Christoph Faust, the Bückeburg *Landphysikus* and *Leibarzt* to the widowed Countess Juliane Wilhelmine of Schaumburg-Lippe. The leader of the other campaign was the Halle professor, Johann Christian Wilhelm Juncker. Faust's approach revolved around the establishment of a 'smallpox house' in every town to accommodate patients

56 Zadig, 72–3.
57 Zadig, 74.
58 Reviews of *Plan*, by Zadig, *Neue ADB* 36 (1798): 152–3; *MCZ* 1 (1799): 437.

for the duration of their illness, and a set of rules for infected households to follow, similar to Haygarth's 'Rules.' Faust omitted inoculation from his strategy after estimating that one hundred times more *Blatternhäuser* would be needed if it were part of his plan.[59] Yet he was by no means opposed to the practice, having carried out at least two hundred inoculations before vowing in 1797 not to undertake any more of the procedures outside a *Blatternhaus.*[60] He also continued to include a description of inoculation in the editions of his popular "Health Catechism" published after he made that vow, though he placed his major focus on the new containment approach and on instructing parents about the correct treatment for children with smallpox. Samuel Christoph Wagener, a Prussian military pastor, credited Faust with saving children's lives through his good advice, and praised the schoolmaster in Haina (Hesse-Darmstadt) who reminded his pupils to alert their parents to the smallpox treatment recommendations in Faust's *Gesundheits-Katechismus* when the disease struck the town in 1798.[61]

Faust and his supporters devised several innovative strategies to promote their plan for eradicating smallpox. Faust's own approach was to submit to multiple journals, under his own name, the same hard-hitting article with the same title, explaining the need for 'smallpox houses.'[62] Faust's well-known acolyte, Christoph Gotthilf Salzmann, adopted a similar approach in a more colloquial style, repeating Faust's 'messages' in an article titled "The Start of Smallpox Eradication in Germany and Europe," which was authenticated with Faust's signature. Salzmann first published the article in 1797 in *Der Bote aus Thüringen*, his own *Volksjournal* that aimed to deliver important truths in simple narratives, and it also appeared in at least three other journals.[63] In order

---

59 Bernhard C. Faust, *An den Kongreß zu Rastadt über die Ausrottung der Blattern* (Bückeburg, 1798), 4; Faust, "Versuch," 88–9.

60 Bernhard C. Faust, *An den Herrn Eduard Jenner, über einige Versuche zur weiteren Untersuchung der Wirkungen und zum Beweise der Unschädlichkeit der Kuhpocken-Materie* (Hanover: Hahn, 1802), 38; Juncker, *Archiv*, 2:229.

61 Bernhard C. Faust, *Gesundheits-Katechismus zum Gebrauche in den Schulen und beym häuslichen Unterricht* (Leipzig: Kummer, 1800), 113–6. Faust's catechism was so popular in Germany that it went to nine editions (1794–1802). Samuel C. Wagener, "Der Schulmeister vom Haina," *PAD* 1 (1799): 155–8.

62 Bernhard C. Faust, *Versuch über die Pflicht der Menschen, jeden Blatternkranken der Gesunden abzusondern; und dadurch zugleich in Städten und Ländern und in Europa die Ausrottung der Blatternpest zu bewirken* (Bückeburg: Grimme, 1794; Leipzig: Kummer, 1794). For Faust's articles with the same title as his book, see: *PJ* 4 (1794): 40–95; *Neue MM* 4 (1795): 89–97; *Neue MM* 5 (1796): 345–50, 369–73.

63 Salzmann's journal was published in 1795–99 and intermittently in subsequent years, by his *Erziehungsinstitut* in Schnepfenthal: Hochheim, *Salzmann*, 53. For multiple

to highlight to the 'average reader' of "The Messenger from Thüringen" Faust's 'message' about the urgency of containing the smallpox contagion, Salzmann used the clever device of confusing Dr. Faust's identity with that of the legendary *Dr. Faustus* who achieved notoriety for communing with the devil:

MESSENGER	Today, dear folks, for once I will read to you not about Columbus but about another remarkable man, Doctor Faust.
TAVERN-KEEPER	What is this! How do you come to Dr. Faust?
MESSENGER	It is not the Dr. Faust that the people say summoned the devil. This Faust, a very clever and courageous man, can be seen alive in Bückeburg where he is the physician to the prince's wife. Listen to this…[64]

The 'messenger from Thüringen' then proceeds to describe Faust's smallpox eradication plan in detail.[65] An anonymous later article, again set in a Thüringen inn and again invoking *Dr. Faustus* as a lead-in to Dr. Faust's smallpox eradication plan, was probably also written by Salzmann. That article, purportedly by an elite traveller forced to stay at a basic inn after his carriage broke an axle, describes a fictional discussion initiated by the sight of the innkeeper's smallpox-afflicted daughter lying in front of the fire being offered hot coffee by her mother. The well-informed traveller's question about the wisdom of hot coffee for a feverish child led to a general discussion of smallpox with five other guests. In trying to convince his new acquaintances of the paramount importance of containing the smallpox disease contagion, the traveller found that he first needed to dispel the common myths they raised about smallpox being innate and therefore inevitable. When he moved on to explain the need for the 'smallpox houses' that Dr. Faust believed were so crucial for the eradication of smallpox, the other guests predictably fixated on the legendary *Dr. Faustus*. Once again, the fictional character who 'communed with the Devil' was exploited to draw public attention to Faust's smallpox eradication strategy.[66] The effectiveness of the mode of delivery of Faust's messages, through important truths in simple narratives and through health advice to children,

---

anonymous articles promoting Faust's ideas and undersigned by Faust, see "Anfang der Blatternausrottung in Deutschland und Europa," *Der Bote aus Thüringen*, no. 14 (1797), 209–16; *Berlinisches Archiv der Zeit und ihres Geschmack* 1 (1797): 452–60; *Neues HM* 7 (1797): 1070–80; *Münchner Intelligenzblatt*, no. 33 (1797): 517–20.

64 "Anfang," *Bote*, 209.

65 "Anfang," 209–16; "Doctor Faust," *Neueste Legenden*, vol. 2 (Vienna, 1793), 379–81.

66 "Ueber die Pockeninoculation und die Pockenvertilgung. Ein Gespräch im Wirtshaus zu B…," *DMS* 2 (1798): 184–92.

is evident from a commentator's remark (1798) that the many readers of the "Messenger from Thuringen" and of Faust's "Catechism of Health" linked Faust's name to the concept of smallpox eradication.[67]

Faust, in his own publications, was inclined to adopt a sensationalist approach as a way of attracting attention to his messages about the imperatives of eradicating smallpox. He repeatedly describes in graphic and horrifying detail the excruciating suffering endured by vast numbers of victims of severe smallpox, and highlights attention-grabbing statistics: nineteen million Germans in one generation (33.3 years) would endure 190 million days of fear and pain, and one-fifth would die after the appalling suffering he describes.[68] Having shocked readers in that way, Faust would express his hope and confidence that the smallpox menace could be eradicated by the implementation of his plan. Recognising that the deep-seated belief in innate smallpox contradicted his urgent calls for the isolation and containment of the disease, the first step of his strategy was to inform the people about the true nature of smallpox by explaining in all of the popular journals that the disease "arises only through contagion, and that duty necessitates the removal of all smallpox cases from the community of the healthy into a *Blatternhaus*, in order to achieve the eradication of smallpox." Faust goes on to recommend the establishment of a *Blatternhaus* in every district, with one house per 10,000 of the population in the more densely settled areas.[69]

Pastor Gottlieb Nathaniel Fischer from Halberstadt (Prussia) set about trying to implement Faust's plan in his own town after the high local smallpox mortality in 1796 convinced him of the need for such action. He alerted the public to the urgent need for the isolation of all individuals with smallpox symptoms, to prevent the disease from spreading, in a local newspaper article in which he clearly explains the reasons behind the general consensus among doctors that smallpox was transmitted only through contagion. He follows with a notification that the fund for a local *Blatternhaus* in which to isolate smallpox cases had received a donation of four *Louis d'or* from Minister Dohm to match his own contribution of that amount, as well a donation of one *Friedrichs d'or* from Dr. Faust along with an apology that the publication of his catechism had strained his finances.[70]

67 Johann C. Dolz, *Praktische Anleitung zu schriftlichen Aufsätzen über gegenstände des gemeinen Lebens, besonders für Bürgerschulen* (Leipzig: Barth, 1798), 271.

68 Faust, "Versuch," *PJ* 4 (1794): 49–50, 55–56, 69; *Neue MM* 4 (1795), 350; *Neue MM* 5 (1796): 373; Juncker, *Archiv*, 2:226–7.

69 Faust, *PJ* 4 (1794): 74 (quote) –6.

70 Gottlieb N. Fischer, "Die Pocken können, und also sollen und müssen ausgerottet werden. Aufruf an seine Mitburger," *Halberstädtischen neuen gemeinnützigen Blättern,* no. 46 (1797): 8; One *Louis d'or* = 5 Thaler and 10 Groschen: Juncker, 6:180. One *Friedrichs'd'or*

Faust's plan attracted not only enthusiastic supporters but also many critics, particularly in the medical fraternity. A committee of doctors in Hamburg concluded that smallpox could not be contained in the way Faust proposed in a free city reliant on trade, such as their own. Their local colleague Johann Albrecht Reimarus was similarly sceptical, pointing out that even if Faust's recommended precautions managed to contain smallpox for a time, an eventual lapse would allow the disease to return and it would wreak greater havoc for having been kept away.[71] Other critics pointed to the impossibility of achieving the large number of *Blatternhäuser* that Faust envisaged.[72]

The other smallpox eradication campaign of the 1790s, led by Professor Juncker, also attracted ardent followers keen to do whatever was necessary to further the cause.[73] A primary difference between Faust's and Juncker's approach was inoculation, which Juncker encouraged as long as the inoculator was a doctor who used suitable containment precautions.[74] The schoolteacher Lenz became a devoted supporter of Juncker while his father-in-law Salzmann was busily promoting Faust's ideas, after both men had seemingly abandoned their own respective smallpox eradication strategies.[75] Many other respondents to Juncker's call for volunteers were doctors and pastors who agreed to submit reports regarding the status of smallpox and of prevention strategies in their locality. Judging by the public attention to his campaign and the impressive list of volunteers from across Germany and the borderlands, Juncker's optimistic view that smallpox could indeed be eradicated by the means he proposed was widely shared.[76]

A key element of Juncker's plan was the isolation of everyone infected with smallpox, and the attachment of a large, square sheet of cramped text, the *Pockentafel* (Figure 17), to their door to alert visitors to the presence of the infection. The sheet of advice lists nine detailed points, including warnings

(Prussian) was worth 5 Thaler: Jürgen E. Krusen, *Allgemeiner Hamburgischer Contorist*, vol. 2 (Hamburg: Krusen Erben, 1782–83), 6.

71 F.J.L. Meyer, "Blatternausrottung, in der halbjährigen öffentlichen Versammlung der Gesellschaft, von 9 May 1795, berichten über 1793–94," *VSH* 4 (1797): 142; Reimarus, "Ausrottung," 517–19.

72 Reviews of *Versuch*, by Faust, *Neue ADB* 25 (1796): 533; *MCZ* 2 (1795): 454.

73 Juncker, *Vorschläge. Dritter Versuch*, 1–22; Juncker, *Archiv*, 1:1–7. For Juncker's concerns about surgeons' inoculations, see p. 100 above; for Juncker's appeal for erudite opinions on the morality of inoculation, see p. 117 above.

74 Juncker, *Vorschläge*, 37–48.

75 Christian L. Lenz, *Bemerkungen auf Reisen in Dänemark, Schweden und Frankreich*, part 2 (Gotha: Ettinger, 1801), 488–91; Christian L. Lenz, "Vertheidigung und Berichtigung," *RA* 2 (1799): 2025–7.

76 Johann C.W. Juncker, "Nachricht, die Pockennoth betreffend," *BMS* 28 (1796): 88–93.

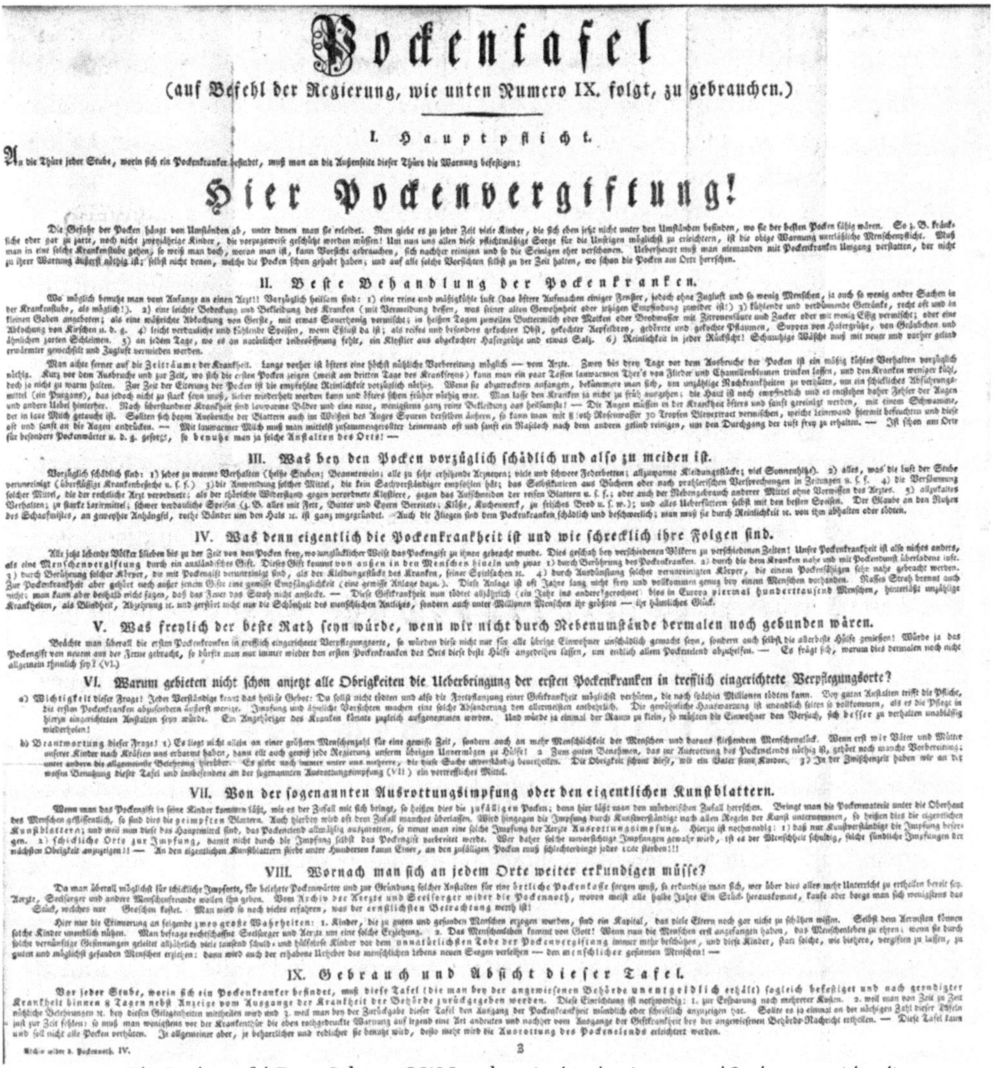

Pockentafel

(auf Befehl der Regierung, wie unten Numero IX. folgt, zu gebrauchen.)

I. Hauptpflicht.

Hier Pockenvergiftung!

II. Beste Behandlung der Pockenkranken.

III. Was bey den Pocken vorzüglich schädlich und also zu meiden ist.

IV. Was denn eigentlich die Pockenkrankheit ist und wie schrecklich ihre Folgen sind.

V. Was freylich der beste Rath seyn würde, wenn wir nicht durch Nebenumstände dermalen noch gebunden wären.

VI. Warum gebieten nicht schon anjetzt alle Obrigkeiten die Ueberbringung der ersten Pockenkranken in trefflich eingerichtete Verpflegungsorte?

VII. Von der sogenannten Ausrottungsimpfung oder den eigentlichen Kunstblattern.

VIII. Wornach man sich an jedem Orte weiter erkundigen müsse?

IX. Gebrauch und Absicht dieser Tafel.

FIGURE 17 *The Pockentafel.* From Johann C.W. Juncker, *Archiv der Aerzte und Seelsorger wider die Pockkenoth*, vol. 4 (Leipzig, 1798)

about the presence and potential severity of smallpox, appropriate treatments, dangers of spreading the illness, precautions to avoid the contagion, advice about prophylaxis including inoculation, directions to sources of additional information, and advice about the purpose and use of the 'smallpox board.' Juncker also promoted what he called 'eradication inoculations,' which were undertaken by doctors adhering to appropriate containment precautions.[77] A

77 Juncker, *Archiv*, 4:293–4 (the *Pockentafel*); 6:1–2; 7:7–37, 132–4.

so-called campaign 'archive' published two or three times per year was another feature of Juncker's strategy. Each volume contained pertinent 'news' such as the progress in spreading the *Pockentafel* and other isolation measures, matters related to inoculation, strategies for educating the lower classes about smallpox, the campaign's financial status, lists of new subscribers, letters to various leaders, replies received, relevant publications, and a summary of reviews of previous volumes of the 'archive.' Other issues to do with smallpox were included as well, particularly the reports Juncker had requested from the widely-dispersed cohort of doctors, clergyman, and officials who assiduously gathered details of local smallpox cases, treatments, patient care, inoculations, disease transmission, and other smallpox-related matters.[78]

By 1799 Juncker's campaign stretched from Hamburg in the north to Tirol in the south and from Lithuania and Bohemia in the east to Kleve in the west. Its spread across German-speaking regions not only generated publicity about Juncker's objective but also aroused a sense of German unity and patriotism at a time of war and the threat of a full-scale French invasion.[79] Anticipation of an accord at the Peace Conference in the Rhine border town of Rastatt, which commenced in December 1797, inspired a sense of optimism that the imminent new century would usher in an age of not only justice, peace, and prosperity but also a future free from smallpox. The utopian notion that a united effort was all that was needed to overcome the challenge of smallpox eradication was inspired by not only the commentators' copious reminders of past success in banishing bubonic plague, but seemingly also by the audacious overthrow of the ruling elite in France a decade earlier that had given rise to a movement for social reform in Germany.[80] That sense of optimism is epitomised in an emotional appeal in 1797 to the 'guardian spirit of the end of the century,' in verse, to ensure that smallpox was eradicated before the imminent resignation of that 'spirit:'

Wenn die Pest in tödesschwangern Lüften	When the plague blew over hills and dales
Ueber Flur und Hugel weht,	In the air infused with its deadly breath,

78 The first volume of 'Juncker's archive' was published in September 1796, exactly three years before the seventh and final volume; volumes two and three appeared in 1797, and volumes four to six in 1798: Juncker, *Archiv* (Leipzig: Weygand, 1796–99).

79 Juncker, *Archiv*, 3:27–34, 173; 4:82–3, 190–4; 7:252–3, 259; Peter Watson, *The German Genius* (London: Simon and Schuster, 2010), 261–2.

80 Wagener, "Schulmeister," 158; Parhysius, "Ueber die mancherley Mißgriffe derer, welche aus Reformationssucht überall stürmend zu Werke gehen," *PAD* 1 (1799): 290–3.

Mit gesenktem Haupt die Heerde steht	The masses stood with hanging heads
And verschmachtet auf den Tristen,	And languished in their sadness.
Sorgt der Volkesväter weiser Rath,	The leaders cared. With wise advice
Menschlicher Erbarmung voll, die Seuchen	And deep compassion they chased the plague
Aus der Horden und der Flur zu scheuchen:	From the hordes of people and the fields:
Aber wenn der Menschheit junge Saat	Yet – when mankind's younger brood
Unter der Erynne Geisselstreichen	Is claimed while you self-flagellate,
Hekatombenweis zum Orkus sinkt	To sink in masses down to Orkus
Und die geilen Todtenäcker düngt; –	And fertilize obscene graveyards; –
Ha! wer kümmert sich um solche Leichen? –	Ha! Who cares about such dead? –
Die ihr Menschenwohl in Händen trägt,	You who hold the common good,
Fürsten, und ihr Väter, Mütter, Brüder	You princes, fathers, mothers, brothers
Der Erwürgten, legt das Haupt nicht nieder,	Of the strangled ones, don't lay your head
Bis ihr diese Höllenbrut verjagt! ... [81]	'Til you've hunted down this hellish thing! ...
Träfen Männer ihre Schlangenbisse,	If this snake's bite affected men,
Wäre gegen euch ihr Dolch gerückt,	If it aimed its dagger straight at you,
O – das Unthier wäre längst erstickt,	Oh – that monster would have long been choked,
Wie in jener Zeit der Finsternisse,	As in those times of darkness when
Ihre Schwester Pest der Bannstrahl traf.[82]	Its sister, plague, was cast asunder.

Leading up to those lines accusing society and its leaders of lacking compassion for smallpox victims because most were mere children, the anonymous poet expresses the fervent hope that the imminent nineteenth century would be a more humane period:

Nimm sie mit, entschlummerndes Jahrhundert!	Take them with you, dying century!

81 *Aufruf an den Genius des scheidenden Jahrhunderts zur Ausrottung der Blattern* (Thorn: Bollmer, 1797), 19.

82 *Aufruf*, 29.

Jede Plage, die die Menschheit drückt ...	Every plague that afflicts mankind ...
Sklaverey und Krieg und Blattern mit![83]	Take slavery, war, and take smallpox!

The mood of the time was also captured in a satirical theatrical parody (1799) depicting a new society where the ruler and his subjects are like a family, complaints of oppression or despotism have ended, and peace prevails. In that happy nation, courageous, loyal Germans unite behind their wise, just, virtuous, magnanimous princes whom they support with warmth and enthusiasm while honouring and loving them as fathers.[84] Samuel Christian Wagener's admission that his new journal *Patriotisches Archiv für Deutschland* was inspired by a "desire to revive the dying sense of unity and true patriotism" was another reflection of the nationalistic mood nurtured by the lengthy Rastatt peace talks.[85]

Juncker seized on the opportunity offered by the gathering of Europe's leaders for the Peace Conference to appeal to them directly for a united effort to eradicate smallpox. In the hope that a peace resolution would leave the princes free to tackle the smallpox problem, he sent a submission to the conference highlighting the importance of smallpox containment, to which he attached a copy of his *Pockentafel* (see Figure 17 on p. 209).[86] His urging of like-minded campaigners to send to Europe's leaders at Rastatt their own pleas for action to eradicate smallpox elicited a number of other submissions as well. Faust sent a convincing appeal for the establishment of 'smallpox houses' in towns across the landscape, while the Gotha official, Johann Christoph Reinecke, beseeched the leaders (1799), in verse, to address the smallpox problem "on behalf of all mankind from the Alps as far as the Andes:"[87]

83 *Aufruf*, 14.

84 *Erscheinungen und Träume am Ende des 18. Jahrhunderts. Ein grosses Trauerspiel in 'Isslandscher und Kotzebuescher Manier'* (Germanien, 1799), 59–66, 74–80.

85 Samuel C. Wagener, "Ein vorläufiger Gedanke," *PAD* 1 (1799): second page (unnumbered).

86 Johann C.W. Juncker, *Mémoire addressée au Congrès de Rastadt concernant la petite vérole – affiche concernant la petite vérole à employer conformement aux ordres du gouvernement/ Pockentafel, auf Befehl der Regierung zu gebrauchen* (Halle, 1798).

87 Bernhard C. Faust, *An den Congrès de Rastadt sur l'extirpation de la petite vérole/ An den Congreß zu Rastadt über die Ausrottung der Blattern* (Bückeberg, 1798); Juncker, *Archiv*, 6:142–9, 157–79; Johann C.M. Reinecke, "Epistel an den Congreß zu Rastadt," *PAD* 1 (1799): 159.

Millionen flehen Euch am Frieden –	Millions entreat you that freedom be sent –
Sey er ihnen bald und ganz beschieden! …	May it be soon and leave them content! …
Gebt der Kindheit ihren Frieden wieder!	Give back to childhood the freedom it craves!
Rettet sie von jener grausen Hyder,	Save it from that cruel hydra-like snake
Die aus Afrika's Gefilden drang,	That pushed its way from Africa's plains,
Und in wilder Wuth um ihre Glieder	And in its wild rage, twines round the limbs
Hundertfach verworrne Knoten schlang …	Hundreds of knots in confused arrays …
Euch den Ruf der Menschheit dann zurück:	The cry of mankind comes back to you:
"Gebt der Kindheit ihren Frieden wieder!"[88]	"Return the freedom to childhood!"

The delegates at Rastatt probably never saw any of the submissions urging action to eradicate smallpox, before the conference disbanded in 1799 owing to a resumption of the war. In one commentator's words: "the misery of smallpox was neither controlled nor helped, thus the issue must likely be entrusted, with God's will, to another congress."[89] Critics of the very idea of appealing to the peace congress for action on smallpox raised the pertinent question of why the forty princes waging war for seven years would be likely co-operate to eradicate smallpox when they showed no urgency to save lives by ending their own conflict.[90]

3 Disputes over Prospects for Eradication

Juncker's campaign aroused much debate over whether the eradication of smallpox using the adopted strategy was a realistic goal or a utopian dream

88 Reinecke, 158, 160. The poem was also published in Juncker, *Archiv*, 7:271–3.

89 *Der Engel Gabriel und die Gebrüder Schlegel nebst einem Durchflug Gabriels von Jena über Halle und Wittenberg nach Berlin* (1799), 125.

90 "Fifty Articles of Literary and Philosophical Intelligence," *The Monthly Magazine* 7 (1799): 150–1; Review of *Archiv*, vols. 3–6, by Juncker, *MCZ* 5 (1798): 372–3.

raising vain hopes.[91] Reviewers of Juncker's publications detailing his approach criticised his overly optimistic assessment of not only the future political and social environment but also of the public morality, which were all fundamental to the achievement of his goal.[92] Professor Friedrich Benjamin Osiander highlighted Juncker's failure to recognise that his strategy would not succeed in eradicating smallpox, and reiterated earlier warnings that keeping the disease at bay for a time would cause the population to become more vulnerable, and would thus worsen the impact when it inevitably returned.[93] Other high-ranking sceptics accused Juncker of presenting a misleading image of a united group of like-minded doctors dedicated to eradicating smallpox, when his recruits were merely gathering information of questionable value for the reports he requested.[94] Juncker's professorial colleague at Halle, Kurt Sprengel, joined his Göttingen counterpart Osiander in objecting to Juncker's request for each final-year medical student to donate one *Louis d'Or* to his campaign fund, the *Pockencasse*. Other high-ranking doctors criticised the very act of collecting funds for a campaign that, in their view, was unable to achieve its objectives using the proposed strategy.[95] Juncker was so angry at the disparaging comments levelled at his *Pockencasse,* particularly by Professors Christian Gottfried Gruner from Jena and Johann Jacob Hartenkeil from Salzburg, that he issued both men with a lawsuit.[96] Yet the subscriptions kept coming. The social pressure on doctors to join the subscribers is evident from the fund's expansion from 368 Thaler in October 1797, to more than 1,400 in December, and to 1,665 Thaler in September 1798.[97]

Even though the reviewers' assessments of the various volumes of 'Juncker's archive' were usually well argued and the criticisms quite justified, each negative

---

91 "Gesundheitskunde,"*RA* 2 (1797): 2661–4; "Berichtigungen und Streitigkeiten," *RA* 2 (1798): 1890–1; "Abgedrungene Erklärung," 135–43.

92 "Erklärung," 140–1; Review of *Gemeinnützige Vorschläge. Dritter Versuch,* by Juncker, *MCZ* 4 (1796): 214–7; Review of *Archiv*, vols. 3–6, by Juncker, *MCZ* 4 (1798): 372–3.

93 Osiander, "Urtheil," 1269.

94 Review of *Vorschläge. Dritter Versuch,* by Juncker, *MCZ* 4 (1796): 190–2; Vater, *Verfassung*, 2:552; Osiander, "Urtheil," 1274–5; Review of *Archiv*, vols. 3–6, by Juncker, *MCZ* 4 (1798): 372.

95 Osiander, 1274–5; Review of *Archiv*, vols. 3–6, 387–8; Georg W. Sponitzer, "Bemerkungen über das leidenschaftliche höchst unedle Benehmen des Prof. Juncker gegen die Dissenters seiner Meinungen," *RA* 1 (1799): 775–8.

96 Christian G. Gruner, *Ein Paar Worte zur Belehrung, Beherzigung und Besserung an den Herrn Ex-Professor Fichte* (Jena, 1799), 27–8; Johann C.W. Juncker, "Nachricht für Aerzte von den neuesten und beyspiellosen Ungerechtigkeiten in der Hartenkeil'schen (Salzburger) Zeitung, in Betreff der Pockenangelegenheit," *RA* 1 (1799): 285; Juncker, *Archiv*, 6:240–61.

97 Juncker, *Archiv*, 3:202; 4:280; 6:180.

review escalated Juncker's feuds with his peers.[98] Some journal editors even avoided reviewing newly-published volumes because of Juncker's unedifying public hostility to any criticism of his campaign, and even to constructive suggestions. Dr. Georg Wilhelm Sponitzer from Küstrin (Prussia) tried to convince those editors to reconsider, arguing that the public needed their journals' unbiased reviews of Juncker's strategy.[99] Sponitzer's choice of the widely-distributed daily *Reichs-Anzeiger* for airing his objections to Juncker's approach widened the disputes beyond the medical fraternity into the broader public sphere. An anonymous contributor sensibly called for a calmer debate about the achievability of smallpox eradication, but his appeal was to no avail.[100] Juncker continued to escalate the animosity, with accusations that critics of his 'archive' lacked compassion for smallpox victims, and that their "unwarranted" criticisms disparaged his good intentions.[101] Professor Hartenkeil, the editor of the *Medicinisch-chirurgische Zeitung*, defended his reviewers accused of such indifference, reminding Juncker that they had indeed acknowledged his benevolent intentions but were obliged to point out the insurmountable obstacles that would prevent his campaign from achieving its ultimate goal.[102] Juncker's critics were further offended by the insulting insinuations in the last eight lines of an extract from a lengthy anonymous poem that Juncker published in his 'archive:'

Kommt ihr alle, die ihr um verlorne	Come, all of you who lament your
Brüder, Schwestern, Freunde, Kinder, klagt,	Brothers, sisters, friends, or children's passing,
Oder jetzt noch für ihr Leben zagt;	Or still chase around to save their lives;
Auf! verschwört euch gegen die geschworne	Get up and swear against the foe
Feindin einer Menschheit nackt und bloß …	Of a humankind left stripped and bare …

98 Review of *Archiv*, vols. 1–2, by Juncker, MCZ 3 (1797): 142–60, 293–9; Review of *Archiv*, vols. 3–6, MCZ 4 (1798): 401–5; Review of *Archiv*, vol. 3, *Medicinisches Journal* 2, no. 4 (1797): 39–47; Juncker, *Archiv*, 1:30–1, 275–6; 2:142–62, 293–9; 5:252–62; 6:240–61.

99 "Abgedrungene Erklärung," 135–8; Georg W. Sponitzer, "Freymüthige Erklärung an den Herrn Professor Juncker und andere Gegner der artigen Bemerkungen zu den jetzigen Verhandlungen über die Blattern im XI Stück des J. d. Erfindung," RA 1 (1798): 1549–55.

100 "Berichtigungen und Streitigkeiten," RA 2 (1798): 1890–1.

101 Johann C.W. Juncker, "Antwort an den hrn. Dr. Sponitzer auf die an mich gerichtete Erklärung im RA d. J. Nr. 134," RA 2 (1798): 1711–3.

102 Johann J. Hartenkeil, "Nachricht für Nicht-Aerzte, die von der beyspiellosen Geschwätzigkeit und Zankzucht des Prof. Junckers in Halle sich überzeugen wollen, da es die Aertze schon längstens sind," RA 1 (1799): 613–5. At least nine articles focussing on the dispute were published in *Reichs-Anzeiger* during ten months of 1798–99.

Reicht die Hand zu diesem edlen Bunde!	Reach out your hand to this noble band!
Sammlet euch von nah und fern …	Gather yourselves from near and far …
Ihr nur, feile Söldlinge der Hölle,	Just you, weak hirelings of the Hell
Die ihr, zitternd für den schnöden Sold,	That makes you yearn for vile rewards,
Jene Hyder nicht verbannen wollt, –	You don't want that hydra stopped, –
Weg von dieses Bundestempels Schwelle!	Go from this Order's temple porch! –
Keinen Fluch! – Wer Mensch ist, richtet nicht.	You'll not be cursed! – the worthy do not judge.
Doch durch Hohngelächter und durch Lügen	Yet a humankind cheated of being healed,
Eine Menschheit um ihr Heil betrügen	Through scornful mocking and through lies,
Trägt in sich schon Fluch und sein Gericht.[103]	Carries its own curses and its judgements.

That appeal for volunteers to join the honourable band of humanitarian campaigners seeking to eradicate smallpox, and the suggestions that deliberate non-participants were outsiders audaciously mocking the noble campaign encapsulate the divisions that Juncker's approach was causing. Osiander deplored the *Kreuzfahrtsprediger* (crusade preacher) mentality that the campaign had adopted, and Sponitzer was outraged by the insinuations that deliberate non-subscribers to Juncker's fund were mercenary types seeking to profit from the misery of smallpox. Although the anonymous poet, rather than Juncker, cast those aspersions, Sponitzer accused Juncker of the insult, expressing his fury at being "excluded from participating in the society of doctors, and excommunicated under Juncker's anathema" because he criticised the collection of funds for a campaign with an impossible goal.[104] Regular readers of the *Reichs-Anzeiger* could hardly have missed Sponitzer's angry tirade that occupied nine of the sixteen pages in a March 1799 issue, nor Juncker's irate response.[105] Readers taking sides on the question of whether Juncker's strategy

103 Juncker, *Archiv*, 2:140–1; *Aufruf*, 30–2. The quoted lines conclude the anonymous poem cited on pp. 210–1 above.

104 Osiander, "Urtheil," 1273–5; Sponitzer, "Bemerkungen," 775 (quote) –79.

105 Sponitzer, 770–9; Johann C.W. Juncker, "Einige Bemerkungen über die Ansatz des Dr. Sponitzer in *RA* nr. 67," *RA* 1 (1799): 1090–2. The dispute was assessed in "Abgedrungene Erklärung," 139–43.

could actually attain its goals largely showed support for the campaign.[106] One (anonymous) contributor cited the theologian Johann Gottfried Herder, to reinforce a personal view that the worthy objective of smallpox eradication transcended disputation:

"Dieß ist einer von uns: dieß ist ein Fremder" – So sprechen	"This is one of us: this is an outsider" –
Niedere Seelen. Die Welt ist nur ein einziges Haus.	As those with lower minds say. The world is just a single house.
Wer die Sache des Menschengeschlechts als seine betrachtet,	He who regards mankind's cause as his own
Nimmt an der Götter Geschäft, nimmt am Verhängnisse Theil.[107]	Engages in matters divine and takes part in its destiny.

Juncker's critics would have been well-aware that compliance with 'mankind's cause' was a guiding principle of leaders of the French Revolution, and that citizens were sent to the guillotine for 'transgressions' of that principle.[108] It may have been somewhat disquieting to be regarded, just a few years after those beheadings, as an 'opponent' of the 'cause' that had come to characterise Juncker's smallpox eradication campaign, which represented in some minds the mood of hope for reconstruction and regeneration in Germany in the approaching new century.[109]

An anonymous satirist's jest in 1799 that Juncker and Faust, along with their respective ardent supporters Lenz and Fischer, were "the people with the strongest lungs in Germany" for their involvement in "The Outcry about the Smallpox Problem" underscores the public awareness of both leaders and their respective campaigns.[110] Another observation, that most smallpox eradication plans were largely forgotten amid the attention being captured by Juncker's

106 "Erfreuliche Nachrichten in Betreff des Pockenelends!," RA 2 (1799): 1897; Christian H. Janis, "Nachtrag zu meiner kleinen Schrift: Was müssen wir bey den jetzigen Bemuhungen deutscher Aerzte, die gänzliche Ausrottung der Blattern vorzubereiten, zur Mitwürkung thun?," RA 2 (1799): 1713–7; Christian L. Lenz, "Vertheidigung und Berichtigung," RA 2 (1799): 2025–7; "Sollte nicht gegen Orte, worin die Blattern-Epidemie herrscht, die Sperrung engeführt werden?," RA 1 (1800): 104.

107 "Ausrottungs-Impfung der Blattern," RA 1 (1800): 382.

108 Christoph Girtanner, *Historische Nachrichten und politische Betrachtungen über die Französische Revolution* (Berlin: Unger, 1792), 32; Jonathan I. Israel, *Radical Enlightenment* (Oxford: Oxford University Press, 2002), 78–80, 717.

109 Samuel C. Wagener, "Staatsdiener! Schriftsteller! Leser jedes Standes!," PAD 1 (1799), 1–15; Watson, *Genius*, 261–2.

110 *Gabriel*, 124 (quote); review of *Vorschläge*, by Scuderi, MCZ 3 (1794): 210.

campaign, was a reminder that smallpox eradication had been topical for quite some time. How much ink had been expended on the topic, and for how long is indicated by a commentator's remark in 1797:

> So much has been said and written about the eradication of smallpox by considerate German men, both doctors and laymen, for many years, and this important topic is so hotly discussed, especially now, with so much written for and against the feasibility of the project, that a small library of writings could be collected.[111]

While the dispute about Juncker's approach was in full swing, the news of Edward Jenner's latest experiments inoculating cowpox as a smallpox prophylactic changed the whole outlook for smallpox eradication. Faust's and Hufeland's respective reviews of Jenner's late-1798 report of his first experiment indicating that cowpox prevented smallpox had initially alerted German doctors to the emergence of a potential new weapon against the deadly disease.[112] More attention was focused on the innovative prophylactic during the second half of 1799 following the publication of Jenner's latest promising report and the results of two cowpox vaccination trials carried out in London, one by Dr. George Pearson and the other by Dr.William Woodville.[113] The Weimar *Stadt-* and *Landphysikus* Paul Johann Helmershausen clearly explained the effects and intent of inoculating cowpox into humans, in a bland article in the *Reichs-Anzeiger* in July 1799, which Helmershausen based on "a publication from London." Yet he gave no credit to Jenner for the discovery of the prophylactic that he himself concluded was a means to eradicate smallpox, nor to

111 Reviews of *Von dem Ursprung und der Ursache der ansteckenden Krankheiten, insbesondere der Blattern, und deren leicht zu bewerkstelligenden Ausrottung*, by Francesco M. Scuderi, and *Vorschläge*, by Scuderi, *Neue ADB* 2, Anhang (1797): 123.

112 Edward Jenner, *An Inquiry into the Causes and Effects of the Variolae Vaccinae, a Disease Discovered in the Western Counties of England, and Known by the Name of the Cow Pox* (London: Sampson Low, 1798); Christoph W. Hufeland, "Neuer Vorschlag zur Verhütung der Blattern durch Inoculation der Kuhpocken," *JAW* 6 (1798): 907–9; Bernhard C. Faust, "Von den *variolis vaccinis*, die den Menschen vor den Pocken schützen sollen; nach Edward Jenner," Juncker, *Archiv*, 6:278–80.

113 Review of *Further Observations on the Variolae Vaccinae, or Cow Pox*, by Edward Jenner, *MCZ* 4 (1799): 141–2; Review of *Reports of a Series of Inoculations for the Variolae Vaccinae, or Cow-pox, with Remarks and Observations on this Disease, considered as a Substitute for the Small-pox*, by William Woodville, *MCZ* 4 (1799): 129–39; Review of *An Inquiry Concerning the History of the Cow-pox, Principally with a View to Supersede and Extinguish the Small-Pox*, by George Pearson, *MCZ* 4 (1799): 139–41.

Dr. Pearson who was presenting himself as the leading authority on cowpox vaccination.[114] In February of the following year, the Hanover royal court physicians Christian Friedrich Strohmeyer and Georg Friedrich Ballhorn reported the promising results of their own cowpox vaccine trial on eleven children, leaving no doubts about the respective roles of Jenner in discovering the vaccine and bringing it into use, and of Pearson and Woodville as the leaders of the London trials of the vaccine.[115] In the same month, in the same Hanover journal, Dr. Bönig published an enthusiastic account of progress in England, pointing out that more than 5,000 vaccinations had been carried out since Jenner first inoculated cowpox material to test its effectiveness in preventing smallpox. Bönig explained that Jenner's experiments were inspired by the observation that Gloucestershire milkmaids seemed resistant to smallpox after developing a pustule on the hand and a mild fever when they had milked cows showing signs of cowpox.[116] Faust, too, reported optimistically on the prospect of a new weapon against the "appalling murdering angel," in a *Reichs-Anzeiger* article in August 1800 in which he recounted a report from the "Institution for the Inoculation of the Vaccine Pock" in London.[117] Juncker responded to the publications by Jenner, Woodville, and Pearson by requesting some cowpox material from Dr. Pearson who was distributing the material.[118] He announced enthusiastically in November 1800 that he had successfully inoculated a group of children with cowpox, including his own daughter, and that he envisaged a new approach to smallpox eradication that involved a combination of cowpox inoculation and isolation measures.[119] Although Juncker's sudden death just five weeks later brought his dreams and his campaign to a sudden end, at least he lived to see the beginning of the end of smallpox.[120]

114 Paul J.F. Helmershausen, "Auszug eines Schreibens aus London in Betreff der Kuh-Pocken," *RA* 2 (1799): 1793–5.

115 Georg F. Ballhorn and Christian F. Strohmeyer, "Uebersicht der in Hannover mit der Kuhpockenimpfung angestellten Versuche," *Neues HM* 10 (1800): 221–2.

116 Bönig, "Etwas zur Empfehlung der Kuhpockenimpfung," *Neues HM* 10 (1800): 874–5.

117 Bernhard C. Faust, "Resultate der Kuhpockenimpfung in Großbrittanien während des Jahrs 1799," *RA* 2 (1800): 2401–8, 2409 (quote) –11.

118 Johann C.W. Juncker, "Celeberrimo Doctori G. Pearson," *Medical and Physical Journal* 4 (1800): 141–5; for an English translation, see MS 6914, Wellcome Library London, Archives and Manuscripts.

119 Johann C.W. Juncker, "Nachricht für die respectiven Regierungen," *RA* 2 (1800): 3481–4.

120 The final eradication of smallpox in 1978 is described in: Donald A. Henderson, *Smallpox: the Death of a Disease* (New York: Prometheus, 2009); Frank Fenner et al., *Smallpox and its Eradication* (Geneva: World Health Organization, 1988).

Germany moved rapidly to vaccination with *Kuhpocken,* though the name of the infectious material being used was quickly changed to allay fears associated with inoculating animal material. The new name *Schutzpocken*, perhaps best translated as 'protective pox' or 'guardian pox,' was apparently in use as early as 1801.[121] The spread of vaccination with *Schutzpocken* was expedited by the decades of discussion and practice of inoculation that had familiarised the public in many regions with inoculating infectious matter into the skin to prevent severe smallpox. Inoculation had also equipped a considerable number of medical men and even some country pastors with hands-on experience, providing a widespread body of expertise that enabled vaccinations to commence quickly, confidently, and on a relatively large scale once the cowpox lymph was available.[122] The impact of vaccination was felt as early as 1802 when the Weimar poet, von Hinzberg, had this to say in his "Hymn to Dr. Jenner:"

Durch Dich ernährt der Sonne goldner Seegen	Millions are blessed by the golden sun's warmth
Einst millionen in der Lauf der Zeit,	Through you, during the passage of time,
Die längst im Schooß der dunkeln Erde lägen,	Who would long have lain in the lap of dark earth
Als zarte Kinder schon dem Tod geweiht.	As small children doomed before their time.
Und unentstellt an jügendlichen Wangen,	And without disfigurement of their young cheeks,
An Gliedern und an Sinnen ungeschwächt,	Or weakness in their limbs and minds,
Wird einst im Morgenroth des Lebens prangen	New generations in the dawn of life will be
Durch deine Kunst ein schöneres Geschlecht.[123]	Lovelier, owing to your clever find.

Before the arrival of cowpox vaccination, curbing smallpox across the vast German landscape with its myriad governments and regulations proved to be an

121 Sebastian J.L. Döring, *Kurzer Unterricht für die lieben Bürger und Landleute der fürstlich Oranien-Nassauische Lände über die Schutzpocken* (Herborn, 1801).

122 Faust, *An den Herrn Eduard Jenner,* 34–7; Rolf Gehrmann, *Bevölkerungsgeschichte Norddeutschlands zwischen Aufklärung und Vormärz* (Berlin: Spitz, 2000), 297; Claudia Huerkamp, "The History of Smallpox Vaccination in Germany: a First Step in the Medicalization of the General Public," *JCH* 20 (1985): 623.

123 Von Hinzberg, "An den Urheber der Kuhpockenimpfung, Doktor Jenner," *Der neue teutsche Merkur* 1 (1802): 5–6.

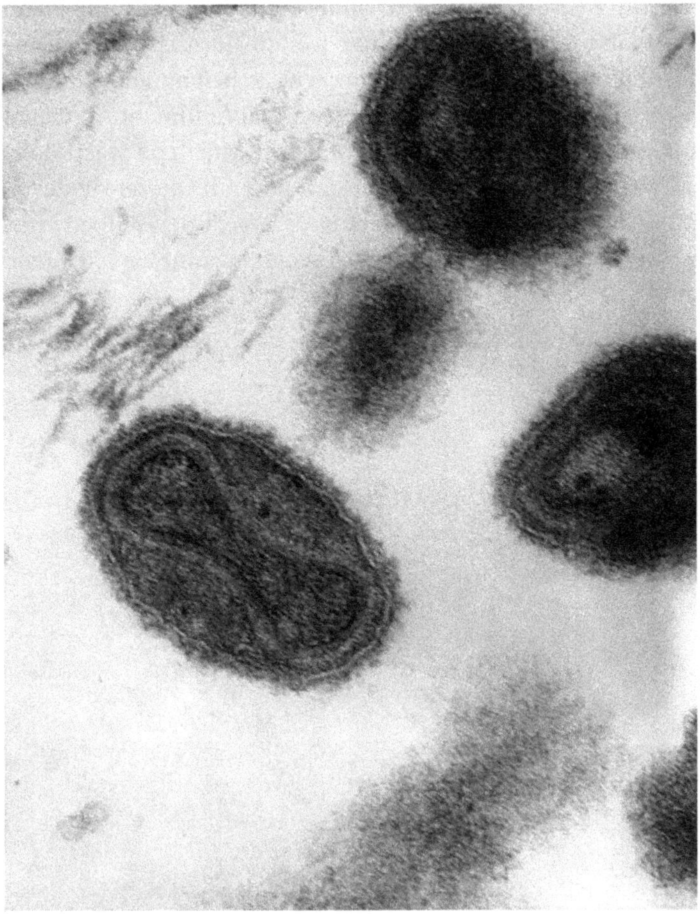

FIGURE 18 Transmission electron micrograph of smallpox virus particles magnified × 370,000
CREATED BY DR. FRED MURPHY AND SYLVIA WHITFIELD. COURTESY OF U.S. CENTRES FOR DISEASE CONTROL PUBLIC IMAGE LIBRARY

insurmountable challenge when the only options were inoculation and containment measures. In the 1790s, groups of proud, self-proclaimed 'humanitarians' accepted the challenge, at least in theory, by formulating strategies that they envisioned would actually eradicate smallpox, even without any new tools at hand. Their inspiration for attaining that seemingly impossible goal came not only from the impending new century but also from a unity of purpose helped along by a rising sense of patriotism forged by the war with France and the threat of military invasion. Even before Edward Jenner revealed his new tool for defeating smallpox, that 'noble band' of humanitarian campaigners was optimistically foreshadowing 'victory' in the 'battle' of a despairing humankind against the *Hydra* poisoning so many children. It was indeed an accident of history that cowpox vaccination arrived in Germany at the time the utopian idealism of eradicating smallpox was at its height, and that Jenner's momentous discovery was the key to the eventual fulfilment in 1978 of that seemingly impossible goal.[124] Thirty years before smallpox was finally extinguished, the cause of the disease was visualised with the newly-developed electron microscope (Figure 18). The relatively large, brick-shaped virus was named *Variola major* to distinguish it from a second strain, *Variola minor,* which caused a mild disease.[125]

124 Ian Glynn and Jennifer Glynn, *The Life and Death of Smallpox* (London: Profile, 2004), 184–9, 228.

125 Fenner et. al., *Smallpox,* 96–7, 110–1.

Conclusion

The eighteenth-century smallpox mortality and disability rates alongside graphic poetic accounts of loved-ones dying in excruciating agony underscore the death and damage wrought by the 'murdering angel' at that time. Most families had the misfortune to witness the demise of children from smallpox, and sometimes adults, whom doctors were helpless to save with their medicines, which were quite inadequate for the task. The prevalence and horror of smallpox illustrated so vividly in emotive verse underscores the efforts of German doctors to understand the disease, to improve the treatments, to encourage inoculation, and eventually to push for isolation measures aimed at curbing the spread of the contagion. Joining the doctors in their efforts to ameliorate the impact of smallpox was a broad cohort of Germans assiduous in their belief that inoculation could halt the suffering and deaths.

Princes across Germany led the way in having their children inoculated, and court physicians spread inoculation beyond the court to the local elite. Princes' wives were often the driving force behind the inoculation of their own children, as revealed in their correspondence with well-known inoculation advocates. Less well-publicised was the support for inoculation among the nobility, particularly the rural landlords who arranged for extensive inoculations on their estates. Some landlords' wives and other female relatives volunteered to help the peasant mothers care for the inoculated children, along with the local pastor and sometimes his wife. The reports of such 'inoculation events' present an uncommon view of co-operation between the landed nobility and other sections of rural society during the 1790s.

Apart from the princes' and noblemen's initiatives, the effort to promote inoculation was driven largely by the university-educated cohort of German society, who were the main contributors to the inoculation discourse. An emerging intelligentsia influential in education and government service promoted the humanitarian, social, and economic benefits of inoculation in various ways, both overt and subtle. In their roles as government officials responsible for the appointment of doctors to publicly-funded positions, such men were well-placed to select candidates with inoculation expertise. Similarly, the inoculation supporters who established new kinds of generally-targeted journals tended to choose like-minded editors and reviewers, ensuring that a pro-inoculation viewpoint was kept before the public gaze. Nor were like-minded translators likely to endanger their proudly progressive credentials by translating anti-inoculation views expressed by someone else.

 | DOI:10.1163/9789004465374_010

The literary sources reveal that poets and writers encouraged inoculation in subtle ways too. Fictional young women with glowing complexions found love and happiness after being inoculated to save their beauty from the ravages of smallpox, and maternal 'inoculation heroines' embraced inoculation to protect their children. By portraying women making decisions in favour of inoculation, the literary elite not only promoted inoculation but also used it as a vehicle to encourage society to free women from the paternalistic shackles it imposed on them. Such interweaving of inoculation into a vision of aspirational social change for women reveals a collective way of thinking among some graduates of universities sponsored by enlightened princes. Links between enlightened absolutism, German territorial universities, and the promotion of inoculation in the broader society, and more specifically among women through the encouragement provided in poetry and works of literature, suggest that the enlightened princes' greatest contribution to the spread of inoculation, albeit inadvertent, was their support for the universities that adopted their own social outlook.

Professors at university medical schools across Germany, particularly the two largest schools, played a significant role in encouraging the expansion of inoculation during the 1750s-70s when the practice was neither simple nor widespread. Yet some doctors who specialised in inoculation experienced considerable stress when called upon to inoculate noble and aristocratic children, judging by their actions in arranging to share the responsibility with another practitioner. Surgeons too engaged in inoculation, independently as well as in various co-operative arrangements with doctors. By reporting successful inoculations carried out by local surgeons as well as by doctors, and by arguing in their sermons and in articles that inoculation was morally and ethically sound and was permitted by the Christian religion, pastors too encouraged parents to have their children inoculated. The country pastors sometimes backed up their words by inoculating their own children, particularly in areas where medical men were scarce, occasionally admitting that they offered to do the same for their parishioners. Country pastors were also instrumental in convincing groups of peasants to agree to have their children inoculated by a doctor brought in at the landlord's cost.

A broad range of sources collectively reveals an intricate communication web forged throughout society in relation to the effort to combat smallpox, particularly through the encouragement and practice of inoculation. Many kinds of interactions were involved in addition to the direct link between the inoculators and those they inoculated, and parents in many cases acting as intermediaries. Grandparents, husbands, and wives discussed whether or not to inoculate the children. Medical boards deliberated about inoculation, passing their ideas to the prince who discussed inoculation with his officials and physicians at his court. Professors taught students about inoculation, medical students conversed about inoculation, and doctors discussed inoculation with their colleagues, friends, and sometimes with local surgeons. Pastors talked with their parishioners about inoculation, including rural landlords who discussed inoculation with their tenants and in some cases summoned a doctor to inoculate the children. Noblewomen and pastors' wives helped to care for inoculated peasant children, on occasion, and pastors kept the doctor informed of the children's health. Enlightened pedagogues directed literature about inoculation and smallpox treatments to schoolchildren, and teachers encouraged their pupils to communicate the treatment advice to their mothers, sometimes directing them to copy the recommendations. Women were informed by doctors as well as by poets and writers that inoculation could save their beauty and their children from smallpox, and the occasional female writer, a rarity at the time, introduced themes of smallpox and inoculation into her work. Considering the vast number of articles, books, and literary works about inoculation, many people who may not have been discussing the matter in person were writing or reading about it, underscoring the pervasiveness of the topic in German society during the second half of the eighteenth century. Such a broad picture of the interactions integral to the efforts to ameliorate smallpox at that time can be painted only through the use of a wide variety of sources.

Despite the concerted efforts to encourage it, inoculation remained generally unpopular. The limited 'trickle-down' effect of princely inoculations, which rarely penetrated below the elite level, was largely due to doubts and fears about inoculation that were rooted to some extent in traditional notions that well-educated Germans had largely cast aside. Yet, by the mid-1780s, changing ideas about the nature of smallpox prompted even some of the staunchest supporters of inoculation to admit the need for a new approach in addressing the smallpox problem. The longstanding notion that smallpox was innate had by then been discarded in the face of overwhelming evidence that the disease was a contagious fever, inspiring comparisons with the feared bubonic plague that had been banished by means of quarantine and containment measures. German minds made a considerable contribution to the idea that smallpox could potentially be eradicated in the same way, though it was a well-publicised new smallpox prevention strategy from the English town of Chester that prompted the flood of German plans and proposals for smallpox eradication during the last fifteen years of the eighteenth century.

The smallpox epidemics and political climate of the 1790s jointly gave rise to the notion that smallpox could be eradicated by a united effort, even though no new medicines or other weapons had yet been devised. Crucial to that sense of unity were the coalition wars ensuing from the French Revolution, which gave rise to a sense of nationalism among Germans fearing a foreign takeover if their princes and allies were defeated. Another element prompting the sense of utopian optimism was the approaching new century, which aroused hope for a coming age of peace, prosperity, and unity of purpose that would enable the achievement of common goals. Smallpox eradication was one of those goals. As Juncker's 'archive' and other contemporary publications indicate, a pan-German network of enthusiastic 'believers' was working toward the eradication of smallpox while the realists were proclaiming that the achievement of that objective using the proposed strategy was a utopian dream. Serendipitously, the arrival of Jenner's cowpox vaccination at the turn of the nineteenth century not only gave credence to the previously unfounded optimism that the 'murdering angel' could indeed be defeated, but also led eventually to the World Health Organisation's welcome announcement in 1980 that smallpox had been eradicated from the global population.

APPENDIX 1

German University Dissertations about Inoculation: 1720–1798

1720 Vater, Abraham. *Methodus nova transplantandi variolas per insitionem. Das Blatter-Beltzen.* Respondents: Johann H. Ulrici and Carl H. Stoll. Wittenberg, 1720.

1721 Fischer, Johann A. *Praeses: curiosa variolarum transplantatio earumque emtio venditio; das sogennante Blatterbeltzen und der Blatterhandel.* Erfurt, 1721.

1722 Detharding, Georg C. *Dissertatio, historia inoculationis variolarum.* Respondent: J.G. Kindler. Rostock, 1722.

1725 Morasch, Johann A. *Proempticon academicum de inoculatione variolarum.* Respondent: Bartholomew Golling. Ingolstadt, 1725.

1725 Mülich, Johann F. *Dissertatio de variolarum insitione modesta epicrisis.* Altdorf, 1725.

1725 Waldschmid, Wilhelm H. *Dissertatio de singularibus quibusdam variolarum et nova earundem insitionis.* Respondent: Christian Waldschmidt. Kiel, 1725.

1729 Nebel, Wilhelm B. *De insitione variolarum.* Heidelberg, 1729.

1729 Schumacher, Werner F. *Dissertatio de nova methodo praeservationis variolarum.* Duisburg, 1729.

1735 Lembke, Johann. *Dissertatio de cautelis quibusdam practicis circa curationem variolarum observandis, cum quaestione: Num quis variolarum inoculationem salva le committere, ac medicus jure eandem suadere et commendare possit.* Greiphswald, 1735.

1737 Bauer, Johann F. *Dissertatio, problema medicum inaugurale sistens inoculationem variolarum in utramque partem disputatam.* Respondent: Caspar Krisch. Leipzig, 1737.

1745 Hilscher, Simon P. *Historia variarum methodorum defendendi homines a variolis iisdemque medendi.* Jena, 1745.

1757 Röderer, Johann G. *Dissertatio utrum naturalibus praestent variolae artificiale.* Respondent: Heinrich A. Nissen. Göttingen, 1757.

1757 Schott, Christoph F. *Dissertatio juris naturalis de eo, quod licitum est circa insitionem variolarum.* Respondents: Chistoph F. Rössler, Wilhelm E. Strasheim, and Ludwig F. Biberstein. Tübingen, 1757.[1]

1 Schott's dissertation was from the theology faculty.

1760 Kessler, Friedrich L. *Dissertatio inauguralis de nonullis ad variolarum insitionem pertinentibus*. Halle, 1760.

1762 Krause, Karl C. *Dissertatio inauguralis de variolarum extirpatione, insitioni substituenda*. Respondent: Friedrich G. Beer. Leipzig, 1762.

1762 Oettinger, Friedrich C. *Problema practicum an anchorum insitio, imitando variolarum insitionem pro curandis pueritae morbis rebellibus tuto tentari possit*. Respondent: Samuel T. Gmelin. Tübingen, 1762.

1763 Murray, Johann A. *Dissertatio fata variolarum insitionis in Suecia*. Göttingen, 1763.

1765 Wrisberg, Heinrich A. *Dissertatio de insitione variolarum nonulla momenta recenset et simul ad sermonem academicum de physologia errores quosdam expurgante*. Göttingen, 1765.

1765 Schröder, Philipp G. *Dissertatio exhibens ephemeriden variolarum corpori proprio insitarum*. Respondent: Heinrich H. von Borstell. Göttingen, 1765.

1766 Büchner, Andreas E. *Dissertatio de nonullis ad morbillorum insitionem spectantibus*. Respondent: Johann A.B. Böhme. Halle, 1766.

1766 Schröder, Philipp G. *Dissertatio praemissae sunt variolarum duobus adultis insitarum historiae nonullis observationibus illustratae*. Respondents: Moritz F. Houth, Johann P. Rüling, and Friedrich L. May. Göttingen, 1766.

1766 Schröder, Philipp G. *Praemissima est variolarum adulto insitarum historia variis observationibus illustrata*. Respondent Johann C. Grimman. Göttingen, 1766.

1768 Diez, Carl P. *Dissertatio de nova methodo inserendi variolas Anglicans*. Respondent: E. Gmelin. Tübingen, 1768.

1768 Kannegiesser, Gottlob H. *Dissertatio de instione variolarum*. Respondent: C.A. Carstens. Kiel, 1768.

1770 Lenhardt, Joseph. *Dissertatio de commodis ex variolarum insitione*. Jena, 1770.

1776 Baumer, Johann W. *Monita quaedam de variolis, earumque curatione ac insitione*. Respondent: H. Tabor. Gießen, 1776.

1780 Hartmann, Peter. *Dissertatio de contagio naturali ab insitivis variolis circumspecte arcendo*. Respondent: Samuel G. Leissner. Frankfurt (Oder), 1780.

1782 Panzerbieter, Johann F.C. *Dissertatio inauguralis de variolarum insitione, extra epidemiam instituenda*. Jena, 1782.

1784 Reiter, Joseph. *Dissertatio inauguralis de insitio variolarum*. Ingolstadt, 1784.

1785 Overkamp, H. de. *Dissertatio de variolis earumque inoculation*. Heidelberg, 1785.

1786 Herckenruth, G.A.J. *Dissertatio de variolarum inoculation*. Duisburg, 1786.

1788 Vogelsang, Christoph. *Dissertatio, medica momenta quaedam de efficacia insitionis variolarum in curandis nonullis morbis chronicis exhibens*. Göttingen, 1788.

1791 Zirtzow, Friedrich. *Dissertatio inauguralis de variolis natura et insitione productis*. Breslau, 1791.

1792 Balz, Jakob F. *Dissertatio de praestantia methoda, variolas ope vesicatorii inserendi.* Tübingen, 1792.

1792 Schmidt, L.A. *Dissertatio de inutilitate praeparationis communis ad insitionem variolarum.* Göttingen, 1792.

1794 Lindau, Leberecht. *Dissertatio inauguralis exhibens omnis insitioni variolarum obici fere solita esse falta.* Frankfurt (Oder), 1794.

1795 Hager, K.W.H. *Dissertatio de vera praeparationis ubi variolarum insitionem indole.* Göttingen, 1795.

1797 Alexander, Sigmund. *Observationem quaedam circa variolarum insitionem.* Duisburg, 1797.

1798 Otto, Bernhard C. *Dissertatio de variolarum lue insitionis beneficio proscribenda.* Respondent: Johann C. Bretge. Frankfurt (Oder), 1798.

1798 Schäffer, Friedrich G. *Dissertatio inauguralis de variolarum insitione.* Jena, 1798.

1798 Titius, Salomo C. *De inoculatione variolarum epidemico contagio varioloso longe praeferenda.* Respondent: C.A. Flemming. Wittenberg, 1798.

APPENDIX 2

Original German Publications about Inoculation: 1714–1800

Abbreviations

Journals

AA *Auserlesene Abhandlungen, praktischen und chirurgischen Inhalts, aus den philosophischen Transaktionen und Sammlungen.* Lübeck and Leipzig

AAC *Acta Academiae Caesarae Naturae Curiosorum, Ephemerides.* Nuremberg.

ABC *Annalen der Braunschweig-Lüneburgischen Churlande.* Hanover.

ABL *Auserlesene Biblothek der neuesten deutschen Litteratur.* Lemgo.

ADB *Allgemeine deutsche Bibliothek.* Berlin and Stettin.

AEL *Acta Eruditorum Lipsiae.* Leipzig.

AGN *Allgemeine gelehrte Nachrichten.* Hamburg.

ALZ *Allgemeine Literatur-Zeitung.* Jena and Leipzig.

AMB *Acta medicorum Berolinensium.* Berlin.

AMN *Allgemeines Magazin der Natur, Kunst und Wissenschaft.* Leipzig.

AWS *Die königliche schwedische Akademie der Wissenschaften, Abhandlungen aus der Naturlehre, Haushaltungskunst und Mechanik.* Leipzig.

BA *Braunschweigisches Anzeigen.* Brunswick.

BB *Beiträge zur Beruhigung und Aufklärung über diejenigen Dinge, die dem Menschen unangenehm sind oder sein können.* Leipzig.

BM *Bremisches Magazin.* Hanover (to 1757), Bremen and Leipzig.

BMN *Bunzlauische Monatsschrift zum Nutzen und Vergnügen.* Bunzlau.

BMS *Berlinische Monatsschrift.* Berlin.

BNM *Berlinisches Magazin.* Berlin.

BRM *Braunschweigisches Magazin.* Brunswick.

BSA *Berlinische Sammlungen zur Beförderung der Arzneywissenschaft, der Naturgeschichte, der Haushaltungskunst, Kameralwissenschaft und der dahin einschlagende Litteratur.* Berlin.

BWN *Anton Friedrich Büsching's Wöchentliche Nachrichten von neuen Landcharten, geographischen, statistischen und historischen Büchern und Sachen.* Berlin.

BWR *Berlinische wöchentliche Relationen.* Berlin.

CB *Chronic von Berlin, oder Berlinische Merkwürdigkeiten.* Berlin.

CC *Collectanea chirurgica.* Hildesheim.

CLN *Commentaria Litteraria Norimburgensis.* Nuremberg.

CN *Critische Nachrichten*. Greifswald.

CRM *Commentarii de Rebus in Scientia Naturali et Medicina Gestis*. Leipzig.

DA *Der unterhaltende Arzt; über Gesundheitspflege, Schönheit, Medizinalwesen, Religion und Sitten*. Copenhagen and Leipzig.

DJ *Dänisches Journal*. Leipzig.

DBB *Die Brittische Bibliothek*. Leipzig.

DM *Deutsches Museum*. Leipzig.

DMS *Deutsche Montasschrift*. Leipzig.

DNA *Der nordische Aufseher*. Copenhagen and Leipzig.

EA *Erlangische gelehrte Anmerckungen und Nachrichten*. Erlangen.

EM *Ephemeriden der Menschheit oder Bibliothek der Sittenlehre, der Politik, und der Gesetzgebung*. Leipzig.

FAE *Fränkische Acta Erudita et Curiosa*. Nuremberg.

FF *Für die Frau, eine sittliche Wochenschrift*. Leipzig.

FNW *Fortgesetzte Nachrichten von dem Zustände der Wissenschaften und die Künste in dänischen Reichen und Ländern*. Copenhagen and Leipzig.

FS *Fränkische Sammlung von Anmerkungen aus der Naturlehre, Arzneygelahrheit, Oekonomie und den damit verwandten Wissenschaften*. Nuremberg.

GA *Göttingische Anzeigen von gelehrten Sachen*. Göttingen.

GB *Gelehrte Beyträge zu den Braunschweigishen Anzeigen*. Brunswick.

HAM *Hamburgisches Magazin, oder gesammelte Schriften aus der Naturforschung und den angenehmen Wissenschaften überhaupt*. Leipzig.

HB *Hannoverische Beyträge zum Nutzen und Vergnügen*. Hanover.

HJ *Hamburgisches Journal*. Hamburg

HM *Hannoverisches Magazin*. Hanover.

HUC *Gelehrte Nachrichten, Hamburgischen unpartheyischen Correspondenten*. Hamburg.

HUN *Hamburgische freye Urtheile und Nachrichten zum Aufnehmen der Wissenschafte und Historie überhaupt*. Hamburg.

HW *Helmstädter gelehrte Wochenblatt*. Helmstedt.

JE *Journal der Erfindungen, Theorien und Widersprüche in der Natur und Arzneiwissenschaft*. Gotha.

JLM *Journal des Luxus und der Moden*. Weimar.

JMC *Journal de médecine, chrirurgie, pharmacie, etc*. Paris.

LM *Lausizitsches Magazin oder Sammlung verschiedener Abhandlungen*. Görlitz.

LZ *Leipzige Zeitung von gelehrten Sachen*. Leipzig.

MA *Mannigfaltigkeiten*. Berlin.

MF *Gemeinnütziges Magazin für die Freunde der nützlichen und schönen Wissenschaften und Künste*. Hamburg.

MM *Monatsschrift von und für Mecklenburg*. Schwerin.

NS	*Nützliche Sammlungen.* Hanover.
NZ	*Nürnbergische gelehrte Zeitung.* Nuremberg.
NVB	*Neue Verfassungen und Bemerkungen aus der Arzneykunst und übrigen Gelehrsamkeiten.* Altenburg.
PA	*Physikalisch-ökonomische Auszüge aus den neuesten und besten Schriften.* Stuttgart.
PJG	*Philosophisches Journal einer Gesellschaft teutscher Gelehrten.* Jena and Leipzig.
PP	*Physikalische und ökonomische Patrioten.* Hamburg.
RN	*Rostocker gelehrte Nachrichten.* Rostock.
RNS	*Das Reich der Natur und der Sitten.* Halle.
SAW	*Sammlung Auserlesene Wahrnehmungen aus der Arzneywissenschaft, der Wundarzneykunst und des Apothekerkunst.* Frankfurt am Main and Leipzig.
SHB	*Schleswig-Holsteinische Blätter für Polizei und Kultur.* Altona.
SHP	*Schleswig-Holsteinische Provinzialberichte.* Altona.
SNM	*Sammlung von Natur und Medicin-, auch Kunst- und Literatur-Geschichten.* Leipzig and Bautzen.
SP	*Schlesische Provinzialblätter.* Breslau.
STB	*Supplement zu den Tübingischen Berichten von gelehrten Sachen.* Tübingen.
TM	*Der teutsche Merkur.* Weimar.
VAM	*Vermischte Anmerckungen über einige auserlesene Materien zu Beförderung der nützlichen Wissenschaften.* Leipzig.
VUR	*Vollständiges und accurates Universal-Register aller wichtigen und merckwürdigen Materien veröffentlicht in der Sammlung von Natur- und Medicin-Geschichte.* Erfurt.
WHA	*Wöchentliche hallesche Anzeigen.* Halle.
WUN	*Wöchentliche Unterhaltungen zum Nutzen und Vergnügen.* Nuremberg.
WVN	*Wahrnehmungen zum Vortheil der Naturkunde und des gesellschaftlichen Lebens.* Leipzig.

Abbreviations Showing the Origin and Nature of the Listings

A	Austria	I	Italy
Am	America	L	Livonia
B	Britain	N	Netherlands
D	Denmark	S	Switzerland
F	France	Sp	Spain
G	Germany	Sw	Sweden
H	Hungary	T	Turkey
R	review		
+	multiple journals publishing the same work, in some cases in a later year		

Publications[1]

1714 T R Review of *Historia variolarum, quae per insitionem excitantur*, by Emmanuel Timoni (Constantinople, 1713). *AEL* (August 1714): 382–84.

1717 T Klaunig, Gottfried and Emmanuel Timoni. "Historia variolarum quae per insitionem excitantur." *AAC* 5 (1717): 3–13.

1717 I R Review of *Nova et Tuta Variolas Excitandi per Transplantationem Methodus, Nuper Inventa et in Unum Tracta*, by Jacob Pylarini (Venice, 1715). *AAC* 5–6 (1717): 13–20.

1719 G "Nachricht von der neuen Inventio der Inoculationis Variolarum" (August, 1717). *SNM* (1719): 4.

1721 G Vater, Abraham. *Das Blatter-Beltzen oder die Art und Weise, die Blattern durch künstliche Einpfropffung zu erwecken: welche vor 50 Jahren her in Orient gebräuchlich gewesen und von daraus vor einigen Jahren durch der dasigen Medicorum an die Königl. Societät in London abgestatteten Bericht in Europa bekandt worden; nebst der völligen Nachricht zu procediren.* Wittenberg, 1721.

1722 B à Castro, Jacob. *Dissertatio in novam tutam ac utilem methodum inoculationis.* Hamburg, 1722. R: *AEL* (1723): 220–23.

1722 G Boretius, Matthias E. *Observatio de inoculatione variolarum, in carcere Londinensi (Vulgo Newgate) auctoritate publica in sex personis capite damnatis feliciter instituta.* Königsberg, 1722.

1722 B R Review of *Peste dissertatio, cui accessit descriptio inoculationis variolarum*, by Walter Harris (London, 1721). *AEL* (February, 1722): 87–90.

1722 B Steigerthal, Johann G. "Observationem per inoculationem." *CC* 2 (1722).

1723 G Boretius, Matthias E. "Special-Nachricht von der neuen Inventio der 'Inoculationis variolarum' oder das Blatter-Peltzens, wie solche in London execiret worden" (August, 1721). *SNM* (1723): 204–12.

1723 G "Quid de variolarum adeo per Europam celebrata insitione medico-practice sit sentiendem." *AMB* Decad 2, 11 (1723): 5–41.

1723 H Reimann, Johann A. "Historia der in Eperjes an. 1721 grassirten Blatter-Seuche, nebst kurtzem Reflexionibus von deren Ursprung im Curatione per Vomitum und durchs Peltzen oder Inoculation" (August–September, 1721). *SNM* (1723): 136–45 and 246–55.

---

1 This list does not include dissertations from German universities, which are listed in Appendix 1, nor articles in newspapers or clerical journals, nor articles in medical journals published after 1750.

1723 N R Review of *Dissertationes in novam, tutam ac utilem methodum inoculationis sive transplantionis variolarum*, by Jacob à Castro, Walter Harris, and Anton le Duc (Leiden, 1722). *AEL* (May, 1723): 220–23.

1723 B R Review of *Lettre au Dr. Freind, montrant le danger et l'incertitude d'inserer la petite vérole*, by William Wagstaffe (London, 1722). *LZ*, nos. 87, 98 (1723): 854, 959.

1723 G Vater, Abraham. *Ausführliche Nachricht von der Beschaffenheit und Success des Blatter-beltzens in neu-Engelland, beschrieben von Herrn Benjamin Colmann, Predigern zu Boston.* Wittenberg, 1723.

1723 G Wreden, Johann E. "Report of inoculations in Hanover." *CC* 2 (1723).

1724 G "Problema de variolarum inoculatione." *AMB*, Decad. 2, III (1724): 30–32.

1724 B R Review of *An account of the success of inoculating the small-pox, in a letter to Dr. William Whitaker*, by Thomas Nettleton (London, 1722). *SNM* (1724).

1724 G Wreden, Johann E. *Vernünftige Gedanken von der Inoculation der Kinderblattern, vier Abhandlungen.* Hanover, 1724.

1725 B Maitland, Charles. *Bewährte Einpfropfung der Blattern; zu Widerlegung der von dem Doctor Wagstaff und Herrn Massey wider diese Cur verfertigten Schrifft und Predigt herausgegeben.* Trans. Weber. Bremen, 1725.

1726 G "Fernere Nachricht vom Blatter-Belzen" (October, 1723). *SNM* (1726): 254–55.

1726 G "Methode, die Blattern zu inoculiren, deren man sich bishero in Anspach bedient hat." *FAE* 1 (1726): 130–36.

1726 G R Review of *Dissertatio qua curioso variolarum per insitionem nostri temporis prophylaxis sistitur; von Einpfropfung der Kinderblattern*, by Johann A. Fischer (Erfurt, 1726). *SNM* (September, 1726): 384–85.

1726 G Wolff, Christian S. "Von ungefähr geschehener Inoculation der Blattern" (August, 1724). *SNM* (1726): 207–8.

1727 G Behrens, Conrad B. "De insitione variolarum." *AAC* 1, Obs. 75 (1727): 133–40.

1727 G "Epicrisis in conspectum mortuorum Berolinensium per annum 1724." *AMB*, Decad. 2, VII (1727): 28–31.

1727 G Seip, Johann P. "Von Einpfropffung der Blattern zu Pyrmont im Sommer 1725" (August, 1725). *SNM* (1727): 235–41.

1727 G "Vom Blatter-Belzen" (April, 1726). *SNM* (1727): 516.

1730 G Löber, Emmanuel C. *Gründliche Anweisung zu einer glücklichen Blatter Cur nebst einen Anhang der Schriften die vor diese Seuche und deren inoculation handelt.* Jena, 1730.

1730 G "Problema de variolarum inoculatione." *AMB*, Decad. 2, X (1730): 53.

1736 G "Chirurgische Operationes: Variolarum inoculationem." *VUR*, part 15 (1736): 298–99.

1737 G "Anonymi observationes de variolarum inoculatione." *CLN* 16, no. 4 (1737): 323–25.

1741 G Vater, Abraham. *Das Blatter-Beltzen oder die Art und Weise die Blattern durch künstliche Einpfropffung zu erwecken, welche vor 50 Jahren her in Orient gebräuchlich gewesen und von daraus durch der dasigen Medicorum an die Königl. Societät in London abgestatteten Bericht in Europa bekandt worden.* Wittenberg, 1741.

1744 B R Review of *An Essay on Inoculation occasioned by the Small-Pox being brought into South-Carolina in the Year 1738*, by James Kilpatrick (London, 1738). *Neuer Zeitungen von gelehrten Sachen, Leipzig.* Part 1 (1744): 701–02.

1745 G Neumann, Caspar. *Die Einpfropfung der Pocken, oder Art und Weise, wie man derjenigen, welche noch nie die Pocken gehabt, solche durch Kunst zu Wege zu bringen und gleichsam zu inoculiren pfleget, worbey noch eine kleine Nachricht wegen des Gefängniß Newgate hinzugefüget.* Berlin, 1745.

1750 B R Review of *Practice and Theory of Inoculation with an Account of its Success*, by Thomas Frewen (London, 1749). *GA*, no. 59 (1750): 466–67.

1751 B R Review of *The Case of Receiving the Smallpox by Inoculation, Impartially Considered, Especially in a Religious view*, by David Soame (London, 1751). *GA*, no. 64 (1751): 596.

1752 B R + Review of *A Sermon Preached Before his Grace Charles Duke of Marlborough, the President, Vice-president and Governors of the Hospital for Small-pox and Inoculation*, by the Bishop of Worcester (London, 1752). *HUC*, no. 43 (1752): 2–3. *GA*, no. 53 (1753): 485–86.

1753 B Maddox, Isaac, the Bishop of Worcester. "Gründe für das Inoculiren der Blattern." *HAM* 12 (1753): 346–52.

1753 Am "Nachricht von der im Jahre 1752 in America vorgenommenen Inoculation der Blattern." *HUC*, no. 13 (1753): 3.

1754 S R Review of "Extract of a Letter to Dr. Maty from Geneva, Concerning the Introduction and Success of inoculation in that City," *Philosophical Transactions* 47 (1751–52). *CRM* 3, part 1 (1754): 54–55.

1754 S R + Review of *L'inoculation justifiée, ou dissertation pratique et apologétique sur cette méthode* (Lausanne, 1754), by Samuel-Auguste D. Tissot. *GA*, no. 120 (1754): 1032–37. *CRM* 5 (1756): 261–66.

1754 S R + Review of "Mémoire historique sur l'inoculation de la petite vérole, pratiquée à Genève, depuis le mois d'Oct. 1750, jusqu'au mois de Nov. 1752 inclusivement," by Daniel Guiot. *Mémoires de l'Académie Royale de chirurgie* 2 (1753). *CRM* 3, part 4 (1754): 617–18.

1754 F R + Review of *Mémoire sur l'inoculation de la petite vérole, lû à l'assemblée publique de l'Académie Royale de Sciènces, le Mercredi 24 Avril, 1754*, by Charles-Marie de la Condamine (The Hague, 1754). *GA* 5 (1754): 386–88. *CRM* 4, part 1 (1755): 159–60. *GA*, no. 124 (1755): 1152–54. *CRM* 9, part 3 (1761): 397.

1754 B R + Review of *The Analysis of Inoculation,* by James Kirkpatrick (London, 1754). *HUC*, nos. 26, 35 (1754): 1–2, 1–2. *CRM* 4, part 1 (1755): 125–53. *GA*, no. 91 (1755): 843–49. *GA*, no. 106 (1755): 991–92.

1753 F R Review of *Traité de la petite vérole,* by Jean-Antoine Butini (Paris, 1752). *CRM* 2, part 1 (1753): 58–61.

1755 G Büscher, J.G. "Zweifel gegen das Einpfropfen der Pocken." *NS* 1 (1755): 747–52.

1755 F + De la Condamine, Charles-Marie. "Abhandlung von der Einpfropfung der Kinderblattern." *NS* 1 (1755): 529–82. *BA*, nos. 94, 95, 97 (1755): 1181–91, 1945–53, 1985–96.

1755 G Justi, Johann H.G. von. "Erfahrung vom Einpfropfung der Pocken." *WVN* 8 (1755): 166–73.

1755 G Neuenhahn, Carl L. "Anmerckung von der Versetzung der Pocken." *VAM* 3 (1755): 1003–62.

1755 B Porter, Jacques. "Neue Nachrichten von dem Gebrauch der Inoculation in Georgien." *AGN,* no. 37 (1755).

1755 B R Review of *An Account of the Preparation and Management necessary to Inoculation* (London, 1754), by James Burges. *CRM* 4, part 1 (1755): 153–58.

1755 F R Review of "Extrait du rapport de M. Hosty, pendant son sejour à Londres, au sujet de l'inoculation," by Ambrose Hosty, *Mercure de France* (1755). *GA,* no. 124 (1755): 1154.

1756 G "Bestätigende Abhandlung vom Einpfropfung der Blattern." *NS* 2 (1756): 1067–80.

1756 B Burges, James A. *Nachricht von der Vorbereitung und Behandlung welche der Einpfropfung der Blattern nothwendig sind.* Bremen, 1756.

1756 N Chais, Charles. *Vertheidigung der Methode, die Blattern durch die Einpfropfung zu geben.* Brunswick, 1756.

1756 F + De la Condamine, Charles-Marie. "Abhandlung von der Einpfropfung der Pocken." *HAM* 17 (1756): 14–75. *NS*, nos. 34–37 (1757).

1756 B Kirkpatrick, James. *Erläuterung der Einpfropfung.* Trans. P.J. Heineken. Leipzig, 1756.

1756 G Matthiä, Georg. "Antwort auf den Zweifel des Herrn D. Büschers gegen das Einpfropfen der Pocken, in den *Nützl. Sammlungen* 1755, 47. Stück, S. 747, und folgende, worauf wieder in denselbigen *Sammlungen* 1756, 68. Stück, S. 1067, eine Antwort verlangt worden." *NS* 2 (1756): 1225–36.

1756 B Mead, Richard. "Kurze Abhandlung von dem Einpfropfen der Blattern." *NS*, 2 (1756): 1257–70.

1756 G "Nachricht, wie man in China die Blattern inoculiret." *NS,* no. 91 (1756): 1441–48.

1756 B Ranby, John. "Aussatz von der Einpfropfung der Kinderblattern, von Hans Sloane." *AMN* 8 (1756): 360–66.

1756 N R Review of *Noodig Bericht over de intentinge der Kinderpockjes in 's Hage*, by Thomas Schwenke (The Hague, 1756). *AGN* (1756).

1756 F R + Review of *Pièces concernant l'inoculation de la petite vérole, et propres à en prouver la securité et l'utilité*, by Morisot Deslandes, Pierre Joseph, and Jean Etienne (Paris, 1756). *AGN*, no. 49 (1756). *GA*, no. 4 (1757): 36–39.

1756 F R Review of *Tractatio chirurgico-medica proponens quaestionem: An variolas in nostris regionibus inoculare sit consulendem?*, by Joseph R.M. Joachim (Strasburg, 1755). *CRM* 5, part 1 (1756): 266–67.

1756 Sw Schultz, David. "Bericht von der Pocken Einpfropfung." *Neueste Geschichte der Gelerhrsamkeit in Schweden* 1 (1756): 407–36.

1756 G Schulze, Friedrich A. *Abhandlungen von dem Ursprung und der Inoculirung der Kinderpocken*. Lüneburg, 1756. R: *RN* 12 (1757): 478–80. *ADB* 13 (1770): 257.

1756 Am Thomson, Adam. "Abhandlung von der Vorbereitung des Körpers zu den Pocken, und der Art und Weise, wie das Anstecken derselben geschieht." *HAM* 16 (1756): 115–59.

1756 S Tissot, Samuel-Auguste D. *Praktische Vertheidigung des Einpfropfens der Pocken*. Trans. Friedrich S. Morgenstern. Halle, 1756.

1756 A Tralles, Balthasar L. *Vexatissimum de insitione variolarum argumentum, vel admittenda, vel repudianda*. Breslau, 1756.

1756 G "Von der Inoculation der Kinderblattern." *FF* 1 (1756): 97–112.

1757 I "Auszug eines Schreibens aus Sienne, die Inoculation der Blattern betreffend." *PP* 4 (1757): 191f.

1757 Sw Bergius, P.J. "Ansteckung der Pocken welche eine Einimpfung ahnlich ist." *SAW* 18 (1757): 38–43.

1757 G Constantini, Friedrich G. "Der besondere Vorzug der künstlichen Blattern vor den natürlichen." *NS* 3 (1757): 673–724.

1757 G Delius, Heinrich F. "Gedanken vom Einpfropfen der Blattern." *FS* 8 (1757): 17–19.

1757 F "Dissertatio, an virus variolarum intra corpus inoculatione debeat intrudi." *SAW* 2 (1757): 75–93.

1757 F "Entwurf, Wie man sich in Ansehung des Einpfropfens der Blattern verhalten solle; an H***Paris." *SAW* 2 (1757): 312–35.

1757 F "Frage von der Einpfropfung der Blattern samt derselben Beantwortung." *SAW* 2 (1757): 75–99.

1757 F Hosty, Ambrose. "Bericht von der Einpfropfung der Blattern." *BA*, no. 88 (1757): 1409–15.

1757 G *Gutachten über das Einbelzen der Kinderblattern*. Augsburg and Munich, 1757. R: *RGN*, no. 42 (1758): 476–78.

1757 G Haller, Albrecht von and Johann G. Röderer. "Auszug aus der Hrn. Präsident von Hallers Aussatz von verschiedenen Beobachtungen und Anmerckungen über das Einpfropfen der Blattern, welche er den 5. November 1757 in den Versammlung der königlich Gesellschaft der Wissenschaft zu Göttingen abgelesen hat." *HUN*, no. 92 (1757): 732–34. R: *GA*, no. 137 (1757): 1297–1301.

1757 G "Nachricht von der in Greiz von Hrn. Dr. Sturm vorgenommenen Einpfropfung der Blattern." *LZ*, no. 7 (1757): 60ff.

1757 G "Nachricht von einer Art der Einpfropfung." *FF*, no. 46 (1757): 363–66.

1757 B + Porter, John. "Beantwortung der Frage, wie es mit der Einpfropfung der Blattern im Morgenlande stehe." *HAM* 18 (1757): 150f. *BM* 2 (1758): 65–67.

1757 B R + Review of *Dissertation sur l'inoculation, pour servir de réponse à celle de M. de la Condamine, sur le même sujet,* by Andrew Cantwell (Paris, 1755). *GA*, no. 26 (1757): 263f. *GA*, no. 39 (1758): 375–76. *GA*, no. 147 (1759): 1284–86. *HUN*, no. 36 (1759): 281–85.

1757 F R Review of *L'inoculation de la petite vérole, deferée à l'église et aux magistrats* (Paris, 1756). *HUN*, no. 25 (1757): 193–96.

1757 T Timoni, Emmanuel. "Auszug eines Schreibens..., worinnen von der daselbst gewöhnlichen Einpfropfung der Kinderblattern Nachricht ertheilet wird." Trans. C.F. Schulze. *HAM* 18 (1757): 99–107.

1757 F "Von der Einpfropfung der Blattern bei der Chinesern." *AMN* 9 (1757): 181–90.

1758 B + Bracken, Henry. "Versuch über die Einpfropfung der Kinderblattern." *BM* 3 (1758): 165–80. *DBB* 4 (1759): 424–35. *Neues MF* 1 (1760): 442–49.

1758 F "Brief des H*** des ARD zu Paris an Hrn. Missa, von dem Einpfropfen der Blattern; Paris den 6. Aug, 1755." *SAW* 3 (1758): 257–60.

1758 B + Gilchrist, Ebenezer. "Antwort auf einen Einwurf wider das Einpfropfen der Blattern." *NVB* 2 (1758): 448–56. *BM* 2 (1758): 94–101.

1758 F + Hosty, Ambrose. "Nachricht von einer zu Paris vorgenommenen Einpfropfung, ohne darauf erfolgte Pocken." Trans. Johann G. Krünitz. *HAM* 21 (1758): 425–39. *BA*, nos. 88, 89, 90 (1758): 1409–15, 1425–29, 1441–44.

1758 D "Nachricht von der in den dänischen Reichen und Landen seit 1754 eingeführten Einpfropfung der Pocken." *FNW* 33 (1758): 282–84.

1758 G Rahlwes. "Vom Einpfropfen der Kinderblattern." *BA*, nos. 28, 29 (1758): 433–41, 449–58.

1758 F Raulin. "Brief über das Einpfropfen der Blattern, an den Hrn. Dario, den Vater, Paris." *SAW* 3 (1758): 240–57.

1758 B R Review of *Ad abjectionem contra inoculationem variolarum factam, responsionem*, by Ebenezer Gilchrist (Edinburgh, 1757). *CRM* 7, part 1 (1758): 98–99.

1758 I R + Review of *In variolarum inoculationem dissertatio epistolaris*, by Count Francesco Roncalli-Parolino. *CRM* 7, part 1 (1758): 536–38. *GA*, no. 127 (1759): 112. *LZ*, no. 29 (1759): 257–59. *HUC* (November 23, 1759), and no. 26 (1760). *Nova AEL* (January, 1759): 29–32.

1758 A R + Review of *Quaestiones saepius motae super methodo inoculandi variolas, ad quas directa eruditorum responsa hucusque desiderantur; indirecta minus satisfacere videntur: orbi medico denuo proposita*, by Anton de Haen (Vienna, 1757). *GA*, no. 99 (1758): 249–51. *STB*, no. 10 (1758): 142. *HUN*, no. 35 (1759): 273f. *LZ*, no. 20 (1761): 177–79.

1758 G Schott, Christoph F. "Dissertatio juris naturalis de eo quod licitum est circa insitionem variolarum." Tübingen, 1757. *HUN*, nos. 12–13 (1758): 95f.

1758 Sw Schultz, David. "Abhandlung von der Einpfropfung der Pocken." *Neueste Gechichte der Gelehrsamkeit in Schweden* 3 (1758): 407–34; 4 (1759): 525–57.

1759 D Cramer, Johann A. "Schutzschrift für die Inoculation der Blattern, oder Beweis, daß die Inoculation der Blattern nach der Religion und Moral erlaubt sey." *DNA* 2 (1759): 498f.

1759 G Delius, Heinrich F. "Gedanken von Einpfropfen der Blattern (vertheidigt)." *FS*, no. 26 (1759): 100–102.

1759 F Hosty, Ambrose. "Auszug aus dem Bericht des Hrn. Hosty, den er während seinem Aufenthalt in London von dem Einpfropfen der Blattern aufgesetzt hat." *SAW* 3 (1759): 321–34, 382–91.

1759 B R Review of "Account of inoculation, given by Sir Hans Sloane to Mr. Ranby for publication in 1736, read to the Royal Society in 1756." *BM* 3 (1759): 260–61.

1759 B R Review of *Letter to a Friend on the Subject of Inoculation*, by S. Cox (London, 1757). *GA*, no. 3 (1759): 975f.

1759 S R Review of *Lettre à M. de Haen, en réponse à ses questions sur l'inoculation*, by Samuel-Auguste D. Tissot (Lausanne, 1758). *GA*, no. 98 (1759): 846–48.

1759 B R Review of *Remarks on a serious address concerning the means of avoiding the dangers of inoculation*, by Thomas Cooper (London, 1758). *GA*, no. 149 (1759): 1303.

1759 F R + Review of *Seconde memoire sur l'inoculation de la petite vérole*, by Charles-Marie de la Condamine (Geneva, 1759). *GA*, no. 93 (1759): 805–807. *CRM* 4 (1759): 59.

1759 Sw Schultz, David. "Abhandlung von der Einpfropfung der Pocken." Trans. Johann A. Murray. *AWS* 18 (1759): 190–2.

1759 G Voigt, Johann C. *Send-Schreiben an den Dr. Mathias Georg Pfann, den Grund-Stoff der Blattern und derselben Einpfropfung betreffend.* Culmbach, 1759.

1759 G Voigt, Johann C. "Auszug aus seinem Schreiben an Herrn Prof. Pfann in Erlangen über den Grundstoff der Blattern und derselben einpfropfen." EA, no. 19 (1759): 153–59.

1760 G Büscher, J.G. "Erwiederung auf die S. 1280 in dem 81. Stück der *Nützl. Saml.*, vom Jahre 1756 ergangene Antwort des Herrn Professors Matthiä, gegen dessen wider die Einpfropfung der Blattern im 47. St. gedachter Samlungen, vom Jahre 1755 gemachten Einwürfe." HB 2 (1760): 1417–48.

1760 D Cramer, Johann A. "Ist die Inoculation die Blatter nach der Religion und der Moral erlaubt?" HB 2 (1760): 321–42.

1760 G Delius, Heinrich F. "Erläuterung der Göttingische Beurtheilung." FS 5 (1760): 99–102.

1760 F Deslandes, Morisot and M.N. de Courveault. "Auszug aus dem Streitschrift, 1755, in dem Morisot Deslandes behauptet: schickt sich das Einpfropfen der Blattern für die Einwohner von Paris." SAW 4 (1760): 180–88.

1760 G Herbart, J.M. *Ueber die Einimpfung der Pocken.* Oldenburg, 1760.

1760 D "Lettre de M. Mallet à Copenhagen, à M. Condamine." *Neues* MF 8 (1760): 124f.

1760 F R Review of "Addressé à Msgr. le Prince Royal de Dannemarc, au sujet de l'heureux succès de son inoculation," by Paul H. Mallet. *Neues* MF 2 (1760): 124f.

1760 Sw R Review of *Beraettelse om koppor sympando, öfverlämnad till högloslige Kongl. Sundhets. Comm*, by David Schultz (Stockholm, 1756). GA, no. 5 (1760): 37–40.

1760 S R + Review of *De morbo nigro, scirrhis viscerum, cephalaea, inoculatione irritabilitate, cum cadaverum sectionibus*, by Samuel-Auguste D. Tissot (Lausanne, 1760). GA, no. 130 (1760): 115–17. LZ, no. 14 (1761): 121–23.

1760 I R Review of *Nuova scoperta a felicemente suscitare il vajuolo per artificiose concatto*, by Francesco Berzi (Padua, 1758). GA, no. 132 (1760): 1135f.

1760 A R + Review of *Réfutation de l'inoculation. La première réponse concernant une dissertation lûe dans la Société de l'Académie Royale de Sciènces de Paris, par M. de la Condamine; la seconde réponse, une lettre de M. Tissot, à l'auteur de la présente réfutation*, by Anton de Haen (Vienna, 1759). GA, no. 9 (1760): 79–80. CRM 9 (1761): 436–39. LZ, no. 21 (1761): 185. ADB 5 (1767): 264–66.

1761 G Matthiä, Georg. "Untersuchung der Frage: Ob durch die inoculirten Blattern der Leib nicht so gut gereiniget werden als durch die natürlichen?" HB 3 (1761): 1177–222, 1225–36.

1761 I Roncalli-Parolino, Count Francesco. "In variolarum inoculationem dissertation epistolaris, nobili et sapienti viro." *Nova* AAC 4 (1761): 133–72.

1761 A R + Review of *De methodo medendi variolas hactenus cognita saepe insufficiente magno pro inoculatione argumento, dissertatio epistolaris ad Joh. Casp. Sulzerum*, by Balthasar L. Tralles (Bratislava, 1761). *HW*, no. 35 (1761): 278–80. *LZ*, no. 16 (1762): 124f. *CRM* 10, part 3 (1762): 508–13. *GA*, no. 23 (1763): 181–82. *ADB* 5 (1767): 260.

1762 G + Büchner, Andreas E. " Abhandlung von dem Einpfropfen der Blattern." *Neues HAM* 12 (1762): 105–8; *RNS* 12 (1762): 175–76, 208; *WHA* 20 (1762): 306f; *WHA* 38 (1766): 649.

1762 D Cramer, Johann A. "Schutzschrift für die Inoculation der Blattern, oder Beweis, daß die Inoculation der Blattern nach der Religion und Moral erlaubt sey." *DNA* 2 (1762): 667f.

1762 F De la Condamine, Charles-Marie. "Verhandlung von der Einpfropfung der Kinderblattern, welche 1754, den 24. April, der königlichen Akademie der Wissenschaft zu Paris vorgelesen worden." *BM* 5 (1762): 356–410.

1762 B R Review of *Analysis of Inoculation Comprising the History, Theory, and Practice of it*, by James Kirkpatrick (London, 1762). *GA*, no. 43 (1763): 345–50.

1762 F R Review of *Lettres à M. Bernoulli*, by Charles-Marie de la Condamine (Paris, 1760). *GA*, no. 54 (1762): 486–87.

1762 Sw Schultz, David. "Abhandlung von der Einpfropfung der Pocken." Trans. Johann A. Murray. *HAM* 26 (1762): 1–83, 115–87.

1763 I R Review of *Della inoculazione del vajuolo*, by S. Manetti (Florence, 1761). *GA*, no. 65 (1763): 527–28.

1763 I R Review of "Dell' Innestare il Vajuolo Discorso," by Francesco Caluri et al., in *Gli Atti del Academia delle Scienze de Siena, anno 1760* (1761), 1–193. *GA*, no. 49 (1763): 400, 511–12.

1763 I R Review of *Diario dell'innesta del vajuolo satto, ne due figli del Dr. Tadini, nel mese di Maggio 1761*, by F. Tadini (Milan, 1762). *GA* 1 (1763): 88.

1763 F R + Review of *Réflexions sur l'inoculation de la petite vérole, et sur les moyens qu'on pourroit employer pour délivrer l'Europe de cette maladie*, by J.B.A. Rast (Lyon, 1763). *Altenburgische gelehrte Mercur*, no. 38 (1763): 321f. *GA*, no. 8 (1764): 63f.

1763 B R Review of *The Analysis of Inoculation*, by James Kirkpatrick (London, 1762). *GA* 1 (1763): 345–50.

1764 B "Bedenken über die Einpfropfung der Blattern." *HJ* 10 (1764): 880–84.

1764 A R + Review of *Ad perillustris Balthasar Ludwig Tralles, epistolam apologeticam responso, cuius pars prior circa variolarum inoculationem versatur*, by Anton de Haen (Vienna, 1764). *GA*, no. 149 (1764): 1201–04. *ADB* 5 (1767): 264–66.

1764 D R Review of "Le conseil de la raison, ou lettre de Mr... de l'Académie de Danemark a M.E.M., de l'Académie Royale de Paris, sur l'inoculation de la petite vérole." *GA*, no. 40 (1764): 320.

1764 F R + Review of *Lettre de M. Gatti à M. Roux,* by Angelo Gatti (Paris, 1763). GA, no. 40 (1764): 319f. CRM 13, part 2 (1766): 210. PA 8 (1766): 441–45.

1764 F R Review of *Observations sur la nature, les causes et les effets des epidémies varioliques, et réfutation de quelques ecrits contre l'inoculation de la petite vérole,* by J.P. David (Paris, 1764). GA, no. 139 (1764): 1125f.

1764 N R Review of *Recherches sur la nature de l'inoculation de la petite vérole,* by M.J.C. Robert (The Hague, 1763). GA, no. 35 (1764): 279f.

1764 F R + Review of *Réflexions sur les préjuges, qui s'opposent aux progrès, et à la perfection de l'inoculation,* by Angelo Gatti (Paris, 1764). GA, no. 108 (1764): 876–78. PA 8 (1766): 441–45.

1764 I R Review of *Relazioni d'innesti del vajuolo sarti in Firenze dell'autonno del anno 1756,* by G.T. Tozetti (Florence, 1757). GA, no. 37 (1764): 296.

1764 F R Review of "Réponse à une des principales difficultés ou objections qu'on oppose maintenant aux partisans de l'inoculation de la petite vérole," by de Chantelii. GA, no. 40 (1764): 318–19.

1765 N Chais, Charles. *Versuch, einer Vertheidigung der Einpfropfung der Blattern.* Gotha, 1765.

1765 G de Redern, Count Sigismund E. "Réponse à la dissertation de M. Le Comte Roncalli, sur l'inoculation de la petite vérole." In *Histoire de L'Academie Royale des Sciences et belles Lettres, Année 1758,* 71–88. Berlin, 1765.

1765 G Hensler, Philipp G. *Briefe über das Blatterbelzen.*Vols. 1–2. Altona, 1765–66. R: ADB 5 (1767): 183.

1765 G Tralles, Balthasar L. *De methodo medendi variolas hactenus cognita saepe insufficiente magno pro inoculatione argumento.* Breslau, 1765. R: GA, no. 23 (1763): 181–2.

1765 F R Review of "Abhandlung von der Einpfropfung der Kinderblattern," by K. Strack. JMC 23 (1765). GA, no. 118 (1765): 948.

1765 B R Review of *An Account of the Inoculation of the Small-pox in Scotland,* by Alexander Monro (Edinburgh, 1765). GA, no. 141 (1765): 1132f.

1765 F R Review of "G. de l'Epine's réfutation de A. Roux, les avantages et les désavantages de l'inoculation." JMC 22 (1765). GA, no. 148 (1765): 1185.

1765 I R Review of *Primi selioli successi dell'inoculazion del vajuolo nella Rezia di qua dell Alpi,* by V.A. Levizzari (Lugano, 1764). GA, no. 141 (1765): 1136.

1765 F R Review of *Recherches für quelques points d'histoire de la Médicine, qui peuvent avoir rapport à l'arrêt de la grande chambre du Parlement de Paris, concernant l'inoculation,* by Théophile de Bordeu (Liège and Paris, 1764). GA, no. 50 (1765): 379–81.

1766 G "Empfindungen und Gedanken eines zärtlichen Vaters, der ein Kind, welchem er die Blattern geben lassen, in der Gefahr des Todes sahe." HM 4 (1766): 1281–88.

1766 G	Hensler, Philipp G. "Geschichte der Einpfropfung der Kinderblattern." BMS 3 (1766): 480–85.
1766 F	Hosty, Ambrose. "Bericht von den Anmerckungen und Betrachtungen, die er bey seiner vor einiger Zeit nach London gethanen Reise über die in England so übliche Einpfropfung der Kinderblattern gemacht hat." BWR 3 (1766): 890f.
1766 G	Linekogel, Simon F. "Rückfällige Pocken." HM 4 (1766): 447–48.
1766 G	"Medicinische Merkwürdigkeiten." BMN 2 (1766): 146–48.
1766 B	Monro, Alexander. *Nachricht von der Einimpfung der Kinderblattern in Schottland.* Trans. Johann E. Wichmann. Altenburg, 1766. R: LZ, no. 21 (1766): 165–67. ADB 5 (1767): 219.
1766 A R	Review of *Das bestrittene Vorurtheil in zwey Abhandlungen, die Einpfropfung der Kinderpocken betreffend* (Vienna, 1764). ADB 1 (1766): 257.
1766 Sp R	Review of *Dissertación de la Inoculatión, y de la inoculada, Doña María Pérez, Pastor Rodríguez de Vera, hija única de Don Francisco Pérez Pastor,* by Antonio Capdevila (Valencia, 1765). GA, no. 105 (1766): 838–9.
1766 F R	+ Review of *Lettre de M. Belletête, sur les inoculations faites à Nîmes,* by Razoux (Nîmes, 1764). GA, no. 72 (1766): 573. CRM 13, part 2 (1766): 215.
1766 F R	Review of *Mémoire sur l'inoculation de la petite vérole, addressée à Messieurs les Commissaires, chargés par la Faculté de Médecine d'examiner les avantages et les désavantages de cette pratique,* by A. Roux (Amsterdam and Paris, 1765). CRM 13, part 2 (1766): 224f.
1766 F R	Review of "Nouveaux éclairissemens sur l'inoculation de la petite vérole, pour servir de réponse à un écrit de M. Rast," by F.J. de Chastelleux. CRM 13, part 1 (1766): 56–58.
1766 Sw	Review of "Om sarloter som mäst härja ibland rikets, allmoge, presented to the Royal Society, Stockholm in July, 1764," by A. Baeck. GA, no. 41 (1766): 327f.
1766 F R	Review of *Premier rapport en faveure de l'inoculation, lû dans l'assemblée de la Faculté de Medicine de Paris en l'année 1764, et imprimé par son ordre,* by A. Petit (Paris, 1766). GA, no. 121 (1766): 966–68.
1766 F R	Review of *Réfutation, d'Anthony Relhan, des Réflexions sur l'inoculation de la petite vérole,* by J.B.A. Rast (Lyon, 1763). GA, no. 5 (1766): 37f.
1766 F R	Review of *Tentamen juvenile de variolarum extirpatione quaerenda primum, illique subnectenda variolarum insitione,* by Johannes B. Richard (Montpelier, 1764). CRM 13, part 1 (1766): 59.
1766 B R	Review of *The practice of Inoculation Impartially Considered, its Advantages Proved, and the Objections Against it Confuted,* by J. Andrew (Exeter, 1765). GA, no. 56 (1766): 446–48.

1766 F "Schreiben, des Hrn. Grafen von Toutnon, von 16 Jan. 1766, und Anmerckungen von des Hrn. Hachete, Leibchirurgi des Grafen von Albon, Prinzen von Yvetot, vorgenommene Heilung der natürlichen bösartigen Blattern durch die Einpfropfung." BMN 3 (1766): 471–80.

1766 G Triller, Daniel W. *Geprüfte Pockeninoculation, ein Physicalish-Moralisch Gedicht mit nöthigen Anmerckungen und Zusätzen.* Frankfurt and Leipzig, 1766. R: GA, no. 98 (1766): 783. ADB 8 (1768): 288–90.

1766 G Wichmann, Johann E. "Neuigkeiten, die Einpfropfung der Blattern betreffend, an einen Arzt auf dem Lande." HM 4 (1766): 433–36.

1767 B Baker, George. *Untersuchung was von der jetzt in verschiedenen Provinzen von England üblichen Methode die Kinderblattern einzupfropfen zu halten sey.* Leipzig, 1767.

1767 G Bolten, Johann F. "Anmerkungen über das 39ste Stück dieses Magazins, die Einimpfung der Blattern betreffend." *Neues* HAM 5 (1767): 1601–16.

1767 G Bütesisch, J.U. "An das Publikum, die Einimpfung der Blattern betreffend." GB 7 (1767): 309–12.

1767 G Evers, E.J.A. "Auszug eines Schreibens an den Herrn Dr. Reimarus in Hamburg vom Blatterbelzen." HM 5 (1767): 529–44.

1767 Am Gale, B. "Historische Nachricht von der Einimpfung der Blattern, wie dieselbe in den brittischen Provinzen in Amerika, besonders in Neuengland ausgeübet worden." *Neues* HAM 3 (1767): 265–81.

1767 G Gery. "Schreiben an Hrn. Petit in Paris über die Einpfropfung der Blattern." HM 5 (1767): 459–62.

1767 G Kleine, J.O. "Von der Einpfropfung der Blattern." HM 5 (1767): 609–22.

1767 G Löber, Christian J. *Sendschreiben von wiedergekommenen Pocken nach geschehener Einimpfung.* Erfurt, 1767.

1767 B R Review of *Inquiry into the Merits of a Method of Inoculating the Smallpox*, by George Baker (London, 1766). ADB 7 (1767): 276.

1767 A R Review of *Vexatissimum nostra aetate de insitione variolarum, vel admittendo vel repudianda, argumentum, occasione quastionum ab illustrissimo viro Antonia de Haen et al, sibi propositarum, abjecto omni partium studio curatius evolutum*, by Balthasar L. Tralles (Bratislava, 1765). ADB 5 (1767): 260–64.

1767 D Rotböll, Christian F. "Abhandlung von den Blattern." DJ 1 (1767): 71–85.

1767 G Wichmann, Johann E. "Fortsetzung, Neuigkeiten, die Einpfropfung der Blattern betreffend, an einen Provinzialarzt." HM 5 (1767): 817–40.

1768 F + D'Alembert, Jean le Rond. "Ueber die Anwendung der Berechnung wahrscheinlicher Fälle auf die Einpfropfung der Blattern." HM 6 (1768): 818–31; 834–43; 849–64; 865–74. R: GB, no. 4 (1768): 25–32.

1768 G Brückmann, Urban F.B. "Ob es dem gemeinen Besten zuträglicher sey, die Blattern zu den Zeiten einzuimpfen, wenn der natürlichen Blattern bereits im Schwange gehen, oder zu solchen Zeiten, wenn an den natürlichen Blattern ferne oder wenige Kränke vorhanden sind." GB 8 (1768): 425–36.

1768 B Dimsdale, Thomas. *Unterricht von der gegenwärtigen Methode, die Kinderblattern einzupfropfen: nebst einigen Versuchen, die natürlichen Blattern auf eine ähnliche Art zu behandeln.* Trans. Carl F. Tiemann. Leipzig, 1768. R: ADB 10 (1769): 220f.

1768 G "Des berühmten Herrn d'Alembert Gedanken über die Blattern-Inoculation." GB 8 (1768): 25–32.

1768 G Eberhard, Johann P. "Von denen Kindblattern, deren Kur und Ausrottung." *WHA* 37, 39 (1768): 626–29, 661–69.

1768 N Gaub, Hieronymus D. "Einpfropfung der Pocken, verrichtet und bis zur völligen Wiederherstellung behandelt." *Neues HAM* 4 (1768): 260–301.

1768 G Krünitz, Johann G. *Verzeichniß der vornehmesten Schriften von den Kinderpocken und deren Einpfropfung.* Lepizig, 1768.

1768 G Morgenbesser, Johann G. *Betrachtung über die Art der Zubereitung von der Einpfropfung der Kinderblattern.* Breslau, 1768.

1768 G "Nachricht von den fernern glücklichen Fortgange der Blattern-Inokulation in Braunschweig." GB 8 (1768): 345–60.

1768 G "Nachricht von der hieselbst wieder vorgenommenen öffentlichen Blatterninokulation, in der neuen Lazarete vor dem Wendenthore." GB 8 (1768): 705–28.

1768 G "Nochmalige Beantwortung der in dem 77. Stück der gelehrten Beyträge geschehenen Anfrage, ob die Einpfropfung der Blattern solchen, welche ein Fontanelle tragen, zuträglich sey?" GB 8 (1768): 679–88.

1768 G Plitt, Johann J. "Kann die Blattern Einpfropfung mit gutem Gewissen vorgenommen sein?" *Theologische Untersuchungen* 2, no. 4. (1768).

1768 G Pott, Johann F. "Nachricht von einer hieselbst abermals glücklich verrichteten Einpfropfung der Blattern." GB 8 (1768): 289–92.

1768 G Rahlwes, G.C. "Fortsetzung der bey der Blattern-Einimpfung hieselbst gemachten Beobachtungen," GB 8 (1768): 449–54.

1768 Sw Rosenstein, Nils R. von. *Abhandlung über die Einpfropfung der Blattern.* Trans. Johann A. Murray. Göttingen, 1768.

1768 S and Sw Tissot, Samuel-Auguste and Nils R. von Rosenstein. *Abhandlungen über die Einpfropfung der Blattern zum gemeinnützigen Gebrauch.* Translated by Ernst G. Baldinger and Johann A. Murray. Langensalza, 1768. 2nd ed. Leipzig, 1778. R: ADB 11 (1770): 227.

1768 G Topp, Johann F.J. "Von einigen Privat-Inokulationen." GB 8 (1768): 725–28.

1768 G "Weitere Nachricht von einer glücklich allhier unternommenen Blatter-Inokulation." *GB* 8 (1768): 57–64.

1768 G Wolf, Johann H.K. *Die Pflicht durch die Einpfropfung der Künstlichen, den natürlichen Blattern zu entgehen.* Grünstadt, 1768.

1769 G Andreä, Johann G.R. and Johann F. Bolten. "Von zweymaligen natürlichen Blattern: und gewisse Gedanken von einer nöthig scheinenden Einschränkung des Inoculations-gebrauchs." *Neues HAM*, no. 28 (1769): 291–98.

1769 G Bolten, Johann F. "Anmerkungen über vorhergehendes Stück (J.O Kleine), die Einimpfung der Blattern betreffend." *Neues HAM*, no. 28 (1769): 311–25.

1769 G Danneil, Johann F. *Vergleichung der natürlichen und eingepfropften Blattern.* Quedlinburg, 1769. R: *ADB* 13 (1770): 256.

1769 B Dimsdale, Thomas. *Auszug von den heutigen Inoculations-geschichte in Engeland.* Trans. Johann N.A. Leuthner. Munich, 1769.

1769 G "Etwas von der Inoculation der Pocken." *EI*, no. 44 (1769): 346–48.

1769 B Hewit, Andrew. *Apologie de la nouvelle méthode d'inoculer la petite vérole.* Bremen, 1769.

1769 B Holwell, John Z. "Nachricht von der Einimpfung der Blattern, wie sie die Braminen in Bengalen verrichten." *BSA* 1 (1769): 266–9.

1769 G Kleine, J.O. "Von der Einpfropfung der Blattern." *Neues HAM*, no. 28 (1769): 299–310.

1769 G Körber, Peter F. "Beiträge zur neuen Geschichte der Blattern-Einimpfung." *PA* 7 (1769): 60–130.

1769 G Löber, Gotthilf F. *Predigt von der ächten Gewissenhaftigkeit älterlicher Sorgen für die Gesundheit der Kinder: besonders in Absicht auf die Blattereinpfropfung, am Sonntag Reminiscere 1769, über das Evangelium in der Brüderkirche zu Altenburg.* Altenburg, 1769.

1769 G Mann, Christoph D. *Beglückwünschende Nachricht von Einpfropfung der Kinderblattern in Oberschwaben.* Ulm, 1769.

1769 G Murray, Johann A. "Beiträge zur neuern Geschichte der Blattern-Einimpfung." *PA* 10 (1769): 60–118.

1769 Sw Schultz, David. *Unterricht von der Einpfropfung der Pocken.* Trans. Johann A. Murray. Göttingen, 1769.

1769 A R + Review of *Observationes practicae circa inoculationem variolarum in neonatis institutam; continuatio prima et altera experimentorum de inoculatione*, by Maximilian Locher (Vienna, 1768). *ADB* 10 (1769): 217. *GA*, no. 36 (1769): 351–52.

1769 B Watson, William and Thomas Glass *Versuche und Abhandlungen von der neuesten und besten Art die Kinderblattern glücklich einzupfropfen.* Trans. Christian H. Schütte. Halle, 1769. R: *ADB* 13 (1770): 258.

1770 G Bock, Friedrich S. *Von der vorzüglichen Geschichtlichkeit Herrn Motherby bey Einpfropfung der Pocken* (Königsberg, 1770). R: *TM*, no. 12 (1775): 283–92.

1770 G Brecht, Karl L. *Specimen heureticae medicae ad pleuritidem applicatae; nebst angehängten Schreiben, die Einimpfung der künstlichen Blattern betreffend.* Hamburg, 1770.

1770 N Chais, Charles. "Kurze Nachricht von der Art, auf der Küste der Barbarey, und in Bengalen in Ostindien, die Blattern einzupfropfen." Trans. Johann E. Wichmann. *HM* 8 (1770): 357–62.

1770 G Dunze, A. "Practische Bemerkungen über die Einpfropfung der Blattern." *HM* 8 (1770): 545–52.

1770 G Mosheim, Johann L. von. "Gründe von der Moralität der Einpfropfung der Kinderblattern." In vol. 9 of *Sitten-Lehre der heiligen Schrift*, ed. J.P. Miller, 176–85. Göttingen, 1770.

1770 B Spring, Johann P. *Akademische Rede von einem der Inoculation entgegen gesetzten neuen Rettungsmittel.* Munich, 1770.

1770 G Weinland, Erhard F. *Die Vortheile welche der Staat durch die Einführung des Blatterbelzens erlangt.* Zelle, 1770. R: *ADB* 13 (1770): 256f. *GA* (1770): 903–04.

1770 G "Zu der Geschichte der Blatterbelzens in Schwaben." In *Sammlung von Beobachtungen aus der Arzneygelartheit und Naturkunde.* Ed. Johann A.P. Gesner, 185–236. Nördlingen, 1770.

1771 G Ackermann, Johann F. *Commentatio epistolaris de insitione variolarum.* Kiel, 1771.

1771 G Croll. "Beantwortung einiger Vorurtheile gegen die Einpfropfung der Blattern." *GB* 11 (1771): 689–704.

1771 L Eisen, Johann G. "Ein neuer Versuch, die wohlthätige Blatterimpfkunst bis unter den gemeinen Volk auszubreiten." *GB* 11 (1771): 65–72.

1771 G "Gedanken von der Einimpfung gewißer Krankheiten überhaupt." *BS* 3 (1771): 581–94.

1771 G Hirschel, Leon E. "Gedanken über die Einimpfung der Pocken." *MA* 2 (1771): 654–61.

1771 G Rosenbach, P.D. "Von einer bösartigen Blattern-Epidemie, und zu selbiger Zeit geschehenen Inokulationen." *HM* 9 (1771): 1301–10.

1771 A Störck, Anton von. *Abhandlung von der Einpfropfung der Kinderblattern.* Nuremberg, 1771.

1771 G Tiemann, Carl F. "Nachricht von einer auf dem Fürstlichen Amte Warberg vorgenommenen glücklichen Blattereinimpfung." *GB* 11 (1771): 333–40.

1771 G Thümmel, Moritz A. von. *Die Inoculation der Liebe. Eine Erzählung.* Leipzig, 1771. R: *GA*, no. 61 (1771): 523–4. *ADB*, no. 2 (1771): 352–58.

1771 S Tissot, Samuel-Auguste D. *Vertheidigte Einpfropfung der Blattern, wider den Graf Roncalli* (Leipzig, 1771).

1772 N Camper, Petrus. *Anmerckungen über die Einimpfung der Blattern; durch Beobachtungen erläutert.* Trans. J.C.W. Redlich. Leipzig, 1772. R: *ABL* 3 (1773): 597–601.

1772 G + Gravenhorst, C.J. and J.H. Gravenhorst. "Nachricht von der Einimpfung der Blattern an vier Kindern." *HM* 10 (1772): 305–26. *GB*, nos. 29–31, 33 (1772): 128–48, 157–160.

1772 G Hannes, Christian R. *De insitione variolarum in urbe patria Vesaliensi tentata.* Wesel and Leipzig, 1772. R: *ADB* 24 (1774): 367.

1772 G Leporin, Johann P. "Erfahrungen von Einpfropfung der Blattern." *HM* 10 (1772): 1273–80.

1772 G Gatti, Angelo and Carl G. Wagler. *Neue Betrachtungen über das Verfahren bey der Inoculation der Blattern.* Hamburg, 1772. R: *ADB* 22 (1774): 498–504.

1773 G Ackermann, Johann F. *Programmata analecta ad variolarum insitionem.* Kiel, 1773.

1773 G Murray, Johann A. "Ob nach einem, ohne vorgängige bedenkliche Zufälle, erfolgten Ausbruch der Pocken nach der Einpfropfung weiter keine Gefahr zu befürchten sey?" *HM* 11 (1773): 713–20.

1773 A R Review of *Abhandlung von der Einpfropfung der Kinds-Blattern*, by Anton von Störck (Vienna, 1771). *ABL* 3 (1773): 591–92.

1773 S R + Review of *Sendschreiben an Herrn Anton von Störck, über die Einpfropfung der Kinderblattern*, by Salomon Schinz (Zürich, 1773). *ABL* 3 (1773): 595–96. *ADB* 24 (1774): 62.

1773 G Schröter, Luwig P. *Kurzer Unterricht von der gegenwärtigen, nachgekünselten Methode die Blattern einzupfropfen.* Bremen, 1773. R: *ADB* 24 (1774): 390.

1773 G Weis, Christian G. *Versuch eines Beweises, daß die Gefährlichkeit der Kinder-Pocken in einer beschwerlichen Veränderung des Pocken-Gifts in wahren und guten Eiter bestehe.* Duisburg, 1773.

1773 G Wichmann, Johann E. "Von der Wahl des Alters bey der Einpfropfung der Blattern." *HM* 11 (1773): 481–94.

1774 G "Auszug eines Briefes an den Herausgeber von der Einpfropfung der Pocken." *TM* 8 (1774): 218–21.

1774 G Bolten, Johann F. *Sammlung merkwürdiger Erfahrungen, die den Werth und großen Nutzen der Pocken-Inoculation näher bestimmen können.* Part 1. Lübeck, 1774.

1774 G Brinckmann, Johann P. *Brief über die Wirkung des Blattereiters bey der Inoculation.* Düsseldorf, 1774.

1774 N Camper, Petrus. *De emolumentis et optima methodo insitionis variolarum.* Bremen, 1774.

1774 N + Chais, Charles. *Versuch einer Vertheidigung der Einpfropfung der Blattern.* Trans. H. Beneze. Hersfeld, 1774. Gotha, 1775.

1774 B "Die Geschichte der Einimpfung der Blattern, Auszüge aus den Briefen von Drs. E. Timoni und J. Pylarini." AA 1 (1774): 323–31.

1774 G Opitz, Rudolph C.F. *Geschichte der in Minden angefangenen und mit dem glücklichsten Erfolge eingeführten Einpfropfung der Kinderblattern.* Minden, 1774. R: ADB 25 (1775): 209.

1774 L R Review of *Fortsetzung von der erleichterten und den Müttern selbst übertragenen Blatternimpfung*, by Johann G. Eisen (Riga, 1774). ADB 24 (1774): 390–91.

1774 F R Review of *Histoire de l'inoculation de la peite verole*, by Charles-Marie de la Condamine (Amsterdam, 1773). GA, no. 3, appendix (1774): 21–24.

1774 F R Review of *Poème en quatre chants*, by M.L.R (Amsterdam, 1773). GA, no. 84 (1774): 719–80.

1774 L "Von der Blatterimpfung in Lifland." *Russische Bibliothek* 2 (1774): 475–6.

1775 F Gardane, Joseph-Jacques. *Entdeckdes Geheimniß derer Suttons, oder die der ganzen Welt bekannt gemachte Einimpfung der Pocken.* Trans. Rudolph C.F. Opitz. Berlin, 1775. R: GA, no. 31 (1775): 269–72. *Neue* MA 3 (1775): 128.

1775 G Möhsen, Johann K.W. *Sammlung merkwürdiger Erfahrungen die den Werth und großen Nutzen der Pocken-Inoculation näher bestimmen können.* Parts 2–3. Berlin, 1775. R: BWN 3 (1775): 335–36, 345–48. ADB 28 (1776): 462. GA, no. 5 (1777): 75–76.

1775 B Neumann, H., Thomas Nettleton, James Jurin, and B. Davis. "Von der Einpfropfung der Pocken." AA 2 (1775): 237–50.

1775 G "Nöthige Erinnerung in Betreff eines Falls wo die Eingeimpften Blattern wiedergekommen seyn sollen." TM, no. 6 (1775): 4–5.

1775 G Wieland, Christoph M. et al. "Antwort auf das Ansuchen eines gelehrten Arztes im *Teutschen Merkur*, betreffend den Fall der wiedergekommenen natürlichen Pocken nach vorhergegangener Einimpfung." TM 2 (1775): 279–92.

1776 G Baylies, William. *Nachrichten über die Pockeninoculation zu Berlin, worinnen der Fall, den jungen Herrn von Blumenthal geprüft wird.* Trans. Johann G. Krünitz. Dresden, 1776. R: ADB 30 (1777): 507.

1776 G Bytanus, Guelpher. "Gedanken bey Lesung des Aufsatzes im 42ten Stück dieses Magazins vom gegenwärtigen Jahre, über die Zuläßigkeit der Blattern-Inoculation." HM 14 (1776): 1087–88.

1776 G Hausen, G.L. "Nachricht von einer, an vier Kindern verrichteten Inoculation der Blattern." HM 14 (1776): 129–42.

1776 F Villiers, Jacques-François de. *Eine geheime Handschrift der Suttons, und raisonnierende Erläuterung der Mittel, welche sie sich bey der Einimpfung der*

Blattern bedienen. Trans. Johann G. Fritze. Frankfurt and Leipzig, 1776. R: *Neue Critische Nachrichten* 2 (1776): 318–9. GA, no. 150 (1776): 1295–96. ADB 32 (1777): 431.

1776 G Ziegler, Christian J.A. *Wahrnehmungen bey der Einimpfung der Blattern*. Quedlinburg, 1776. R: ADB 32 (1777): 433.

1777 B Brooke, R. "Letter to James Parsons, concerning Inoculation." AA 4 (1777): 133–37.

1777 G "Etwas von der Einimpfung der Blattern." BMN 4 (1777): 303–07.

1777 G Merkel, Gottlieb D. *Zwei Predigten für die Einpfropfung der Blattern*. Leipzig, 1777. R: *Gothaische gelehrte Zeitung*, no. 31 (1777): 249–50.

1777 B Porter, John. "Letter Containing some New Facts, Tending to Clean up the Accounts Relating to the Practice of Inoculation among the Georgians." AA 4 (1777): 237f.

1777 B Sloane, Hans. "An Account of Inoculation." AA 4 (1777): 310f.

1778 G Hauck, Christian G. *Sendschreiben, Beantwortung der Frage: Was ist von den Impf-Predigern und von Empfehlung der Blatter-Einimpfung auf der Kanzel zu halten? Von zween Freunden der Wahrheit*. Leipzig, 1778. R: ADB 38 (1779): 445–46.

1778 G Klärich, Friedrich W. "Etwas über die Pockenepidemie zu Göttingen 1777, und über die Inoculation der Pocken." HM 16 (1778): 209–22.

1778 B Mudge, John. *Untersuchung warum geimpfte Blattern gelinder und sicherer werden, als die natürliche*. Danzig, 1778. R: GA, no. 118 (1779): 955–59.

1778 S and Sw Tissot, Samuel-Auguste and Nils R. von Rosenstein. *Abhandlungen über die Einpfropfung der Blattern zum gemeinnützigen Gebrauch*. Translated by Ernst G. Baldinger and Johann A. Murray. 2nd ed. Leipzig, 1778.

1779 G Murray, Johann A. *Observationum et animadversionum super variolarum insitione satura*. Göttingen, 1779. R: ABL 18 (1780): 134–42.

1780 G Heinsius, Johann A. *Gründe für und wider die Pockeninoculation gesammelt und verglichen*. Leipzig, 1780. R: NZ, no. 30 (1781): 233–35.

1780 B Jurin, James. "Wie der Verunstaltung des Gesichts durch die natürlichen Pocken vorzubeugen." *Neues* HAM 20 (1780): 92–93.

1780 D R Review of *Etwas zur Empfehlung der Blattereinimpfung* (Flensburg, 1779). ADB 44 (1780): 445.

1780 S R Review of *Über die Einpfropfung der Pocken*, by Jacob Christian Scherb (Zürich, 1779). ADB 43 (1780): 452.

1781 F "Beobachtungen über das Einimpfen der Blattern." *Auszüge aus den besten französischen periodischen Schriften* 3 (1781): 102–15.

1781 G Büsching, Anton F. "Bericht des Wundarztes B. Kratzsch zu Irkutzk in Sibirien, an den Statthalter zu Irkutzk, von der Einimpfung der Pocken, welche er unternommen. Vom Julius 1771." BWN 9 (1781): 337–41.

1781 G Grot, Joachim C. *Petersburgische Kanzelrede von der Rechtmaßigkeit der Blattern-einmpfung aus allgemeinen Gründen.* Leipzig and Riga, 1781.

1781 G H.J.J. "Inokulation." *EM* 2 (1781): 368–9.

1782 B Dimsdale, Thomas. *Schriften über die Einpfropfung der Blattern.* Leipzig, 1782. R: *ADB* 54 (1783): 387–90.

1782 A Leon, Gottlieb von. "An Herrn Maximilian Stoll, als am 18. Brachmonden 1781 das Fest der Blatterneinimpfung gefeyert ward." *DM* 2 (1782): 353–57.

1782 F Maret, Hugo. *Abhandlung von den Mitteln wider die Wuth der Pocken.* Jena, 1782.

1782 G Roth, Albrecht W. "Beantwortung der Frage: 'ob es erlaubt und unbillig sey, an einem Orte, wo die natürliche Blattern nicht sind, Blattern einzuimpfen?'," *Medizinisches Wochenblatt* (1782): 650–53.

1782 G Gatti, Angelo and Carl G. Wagler. *Neue Betrachtungen über das Verfahren bey der Inoculation der Blattern.* 2nd ed. Bremen, 1782.

1783 G "Empfehlung der Blattereinimpfung." *MF* 2 (1783): 19–75.

1783 G Meyer, K. "Etwas über des Herrn Doctor Paris in Berre Vorschlag, über die Inokulation der Kinderblattern." *HM* 21 (1783): 929–44.

1783 G + Möser, Justus. "Also sollte man die Einimpfung der Blattern ganz verbieten. Schreiben einer jungen Matrone." *BMS* 2 (1783): 39–43. *WUN*, no. 41 (1783): 680–84. In *Patriotische Phantasien,* ed. Johanne W.J. Voigt, 64–67. Berlin, 1786. R: *ADB* 57, part 2 (1787): 329–30.

1783 G Paris, J.F. "Ueber die Kinderblattern." *EM* 1 (1783): 257–67.

1783 Am Rush, Benjamin. *Die neueste Methode die Blattern einzuimpfen; eine aus der Universität Philadelphia gehaltene Vorlesung.* Ansbach, 1783. R: *ADB* 78 (1787): 78.

1784 G "Etwas von der Inokulation der Blattern." *Neueste MA* 3 (1784): 17–26.

1784 S R Review of *Inoculations-Catechismus für das Landvolk,* by Johann M. Aepli (Zürich, 1782). *ADB* 58 (1784): 109.

1784 G Schwager, Johann M. *Ist die Inokulation der Pocken Pflicht oder Nicht? Ein Sendschreiben an den gemeinen Mann.* Herford, 1784.

1784 B Timony, Anton. "Abhandlung von der Einpfropfen der Pocken." *AA* 1B (1784): 323.

1785 G *Anpreisung der Inoculation der Blattern nach Gründen der Natur und Religion, von einem wahren Kinderfreunde.* Dresden, 1785. R: *LM* 18 (1785): 322.

1785 G "Pockenimpfung während der Epidemie." In *Almanach für Aerzte und Nichtärzte, auf das Jahr 1785,* edited by Christian G. Gruner, 189–98. Jena, 1785.

1785 Am R Review of *Defense de l'inoculation, et rélation de progrès, qu'elle a fait à Philadelphia,* by Thomas Bond (Strasburg, 1784). *ALZ* 85 (1785): 265.

1785 G Tode, Johann C. "Feiles Blatterimpfen." *DA* 1 (1785): 24–42.

1786 G Klose, Christian G. “An Schlesiens Mütter. Bey Gelegenheit der mörderischen Pocken im Jahre 1785 bis 1786.” *SP* 4 (1786): 393–422.

1786 G Migula, Johann C.R. “Etwas über die Inoculation der Blattern, nach der neuen vortreflichen Methode des Herrn Gatti, nebst einer kurzen Nachricht von einem glücklichen Versuch derselben an 8 Kindern.” *SP* 4 (1786): 206–14.

1786 A R Review of *Ueber die Pocken und deren Einimpfung für Unerfahrene in der Arzneiwissenschaft*, by Johann N. Stunzer (Vienna, 1784). *ADB* 70 (1786): 460.

1786 B Roe, Charles. *Abhandlung von den natürlichen Blattern, nebst Bemerkungen über die Einimpfung derselben.* Lemgo, 1786.

1786 G Schwager, Johann M. “Noch etwas über das Blatterbelzen.” *DM* 1 (1786): 533–52.

1786 G Schwager, Johann M. “Patriotische, aber von den Aerzten gemißbilligte, Pocken-inokulation des Herrn Pastor Schwagers zu Joellenbeck in der Grafschaft Ravensberg.” *DM* 1 (1786): 201–38.

1787 Am Bond, Thomas. *Vertheidigung der Einpfropfung der Pocken und Geschichte ihres glücklichen Erfolgs in Philadelphia.* Trans. Johann C.G. Ackermann. Nuremberg and Altdorf, 1787. R: *ADB* 53, suppl. (1787): 657. *ALZ* 3 (1787): 17–20.

1787 G “Die Geschichte der Einimpfung.” In *Bemerkungen und Erfahrungen über die Bestandtheile und Kräfte der Arzneysubstanzen*, 141–92. Vienna and Leipzig, 1787.

1787 G Elsner, Christoph F. *Ein paar Worte über die Pocken und die Inoculation derselben.* Königsberg, 1787. R: *ALZ* 2 (1788): 349. *ADB* 114 (1793): 77–79.

1787 G Fischer. “Warnung und Vorsichtsregel bei Einimpfung der Blattern.” *HM* 25 (1787): 1473–76.

1787 G “Frage ans Publikum, und insoderheite an die Aerzte.” *SP* 5 (1787): 53–54.

1787 G Gramberg, Gerhard A. “Einiges über die Inokulation der Pocken.” *DM* 1 (1787): 72–77.

1787 G Guericke. “Beitrag zur diesjährigen Blattern-Inokulations-Geschichte in hiesiger Gegend.” *GB*, no. 94 (1787): 383–85.

1787 G Klose, Christian G. “Ein glücklicher Versuch mit der Inokulation in Goldberg an vier Kindern des Herrn Rector Steigers.” *SP* 5 (1787): 457–60.

1787 G Lichtenstein, Heinrich von. “Wider eine Blatterimpfung nachtheiliges Gerücht.” *GB* 27 (1787): 397–402.

1787 G Migula, Johann C.R. “Inokulation der Blattern.” *SP* 6 (1787): 244–47.

1787 G Migula, Johann C.R. “Noch etwas über die Inokulation der Blattern, nebst der Nachricht von einem anderweitigen glücklichen Versuch derselben an 13 Kindern.” *SP* 5 (1787): 409–34.

1787 G “Neueste Blattern-Inokulation zu Zelle.” *ABC* 1 (1787): 158–59.

1787 B R Review of *Inquiry how to Prevent the Small-Pox and Proceedings of a Society for Promoting General Inoculation at Stated Periods*, by John Haygarth (Chester, 1784). GA 2 (1787): 1005–6.

1787 G Steiger. "Inoculation der Blattern." SP 6 (1787): 161–63.

1787 G "Tödlichkeit der Blattern." SP 6 (1787): 91.

1787 G "Ueber Blattern und Inokulation." *Neue* BMN 4 (1787): 14–22.

1787 G Vogel, Samuel G. "Von den Ursachen der Todesfälle bei eingeimpften Pocken." HM 25 (1787): 17–32, 49–62.

1787 G Vogler, J.P. *Geschichte einer Blatterninoculation die mit Gefahr verknüpft war, und einen fatalen Ausgang hatte.* Göttingen, 1787.

1788 G "Bericht." SP 7 (1788): 293–95.

1788 G "Blattern-Epidemie und Inoculation (mit Tabelle)." ABC 2 (1788): 98–101.

1788 G "Blattern-Inoculation an den Werkhaus-Kindern zu Hannover." ABC 2 (1788): 164–67.

1788 G "Blattern-Vorfälle." ABC 2 (1786): 190–92.

1788 G Engelmann, C.F. "Ein Beherzigungswürdiger Vorschlag zur Beförderung der Blatterinoculation." SP 7 (1788): 69–71.

1788 G Fein, C.H. "Also sollte man den Kindern nicht auf der Hand die Blattern einimpfen?" HM 26 (1788): 369–82.

1788 G Künzel, J.K. "Blattern." SP 8 (1788): 74–77.

1788 A R Review of *Medizinischer Versuch, die bisher eingeführte Inokulation oder Einimpfung der Blattern entbehrlich zu machen*, by Joseph L. Kerndt (Vienna, 1787). GA 3 (1788): 1768.

1788 A R + Review of *Versuch über die Einimpfung der Pocken*, by H.J. Raffler (Graz, 1787). GA 3 (1788): 1754–55. ADB 86 (1789): 104–105. ALZ 89 (1789): 191.

1788 G Thebesius, Adam S. "Schreiben an den Herrn Professor Schummel. Warum ich meinen Kindern die Blattern nicht einimpfe." SP 8 (1788): 122–33.

1789 G Brinckmann, Johann P. *Brief über die Wirkung des Blattereiters bei der Inoculation.* 2nd ed. Düsseldorf, 1789. R: ADB 25 (1775): 210–11.

1789 G Ehrhart, Friedrich. *Darstellung der Gründe für und gegen die Blatterneinimpfung fürLeser aus allen Ständen.* Memmingen, 1789. R: ADB 102 (1791): 72. ALZ 92 (1792): 170.

1789 G Hufeland, Christoph W. *Bemerkungen über die natürlichen und geimpften Blattern zu Weimar im Jahre 1788.* Leipzig, 1789. R: ALZ 4 (1789): 305–308. GA, no. 29 (1791): 281–85.

1789 G Hufeland, Christoph W., Hlodowich, and Friedrich J. Bertuch."Empfehlung eines wichtigen und ganz unfelhbaren Schönheits-Mittels." JLM 4 (1789): 76–88.

1789 I R Review of *Diss. de variolarum refellenda inoculatione*, by Pietro Orlandi (Rome, 1788). ALZ 89 (1789): 234.

1789 A R + Review of *Vollständige Geschichte der Einimpfung der Blattern in Wien*, by Anton J. Rechberger (Vienna, 1788). ADB 89 (1789): 68–69. ALZ 89 (1789): 145f.

1790 G Baczko, Ludwig von. “Empfindungen eines durch die Blattern blind gewordenen, bei der Genesung des Kronprinzen, des Prinzen Ludwig und der Prinzessin Augusta von Preußen, königliche Hoheiten, von den Blattern.” BB 2 (1790): 436–38.

1790 G Giese, Johann R. *Untersuchung, warum eingeimpfte Pocken eine gelindere Krankheit verursachen*. Münster, 1790. R: ADB 101 (1791): 402–03.

1790 G “Kurze Geschichte der Pockeninoculation.” CB 7 (1790): 859–72.

1790 G Migula, Johann C.R. “Merkwürdige Inokulation der Blattern.” SP 12 (1790): 42–51.

1790 I R Review of *Della inoculazione del Vajuolo in tempo di Epidemia del Morbo stesso. Discorso physico-practico*, by L. di Basilea (Verona, 1790). ALZ 90 (1790): 114.

1790 G Scheliha, von. “Einimpfung der Blattern zu Perschütz im Trebnitzischen.” SP 11 (1790): 364–68.

1790 G Schwager, Johann M. “Diesmalige Inoculationsgeschichte von Joellenbeck, in der Grafschaft Ravensburg.” *Jahrbuch für die Menschheit* 2 (1790): 1–31.

1790 G Schwager, Johann M. *Zur Beherzigung der Güte Gottes bey entdeckten Heilmitteln und zur Empfehlung des Einimpfens der Kinderpocken. Eine Predigt am 4. Sonntage Advents 1789*. Bremen, 1790. R: GA (1790): 910–11.

1790 G Sintenis, C.F. “Gespräch zwischen ein paar Eheleuten über das Einimpfen der Blattern.” *Neue* BMN 7 (1790): 109–14, 141–47.

1790 G “Waldenburg, den 1. Februar, 1790.” SP 11 (1790): 165–70.

1791 G *Anleitung zu einer schicklichen und angemessenen Behandlung der Pocken bey Gelegenheit der jetzigen Pockenepidemie*. Halle, 1791.

1791 G “Blattern-Einimpfung.” SP 14 (1791): 261–62.

1791 G Harrhausen, J.G.G. *Ueber die Pockeninoculation, ein Gespräch*. Minden, 1791.

1791 G Lueder, August F. “Was ist von der Inokulation oder Einimpfung der Blattern zu halten?” BRM, nos. 6–8 (1791): 81–95, 97–112, 123–8.

1791 G “Nachricht von einer nachahmungswürdigen Blattern-Inoculation.” MM 4 (1791): 515–16.

1791 G Olberg, Franz. *Beiträge zur Litteratur der Blattern und deren Einimpfung: vom Jahre 1768 bis 1790*. Halle, 1791. R: GA, no. 1 (1792): 400.

1791 G “Pocken-Inoculation.” SP 14 (1791): 368–70.

1791 G “Rettung der Blatter-Einimpfung.” SP 14 (1791): 524–30.

1791 G Reyland, Bernard J. *Ueber den Nutzen der Pockeninoculation*. Aachen, 1791.

1791 G Rimann. “Auszug aus den Antwortschreiben des Herrn Chirurgus Rimann in Hirschberg an den Verfasser (anonym) des vorstehenden Briefes ‘Rettung der Blatter Einimpfung.’” SP 14 (1791): 523–32.

1791 B Walker, Robert. *Untersuchung der Pocken, in medicinischer und politischer Rücksicht, nebst einer glücklichen Methode diese Krankheit zu heilen.* Trans. Karl H. Spohr. Leipzig, 1791. R: ADB 108 (1792): 433.

1791 G Winterfeld, M.A. "Fortsetzung des Tagebuchs eines Vaters." *Braunschweigisches Journal*, no.12 (1791): 476–84.

1792 G Bandelow, A.D. *Ueber die Pocken und deren Einimpfung: dem Dessauischen Publikum gewidmet.* Dessau, 1792. R: *Neue* ADB 4 (1793): 468. ALZ 93 (1793): 583–84.

1792 G Finke, Leonard L. *Specimen medicum historiam sistens insitionis variolarum in comitatibus Tecklenburgensii atque Lingensii.* Leipzig, 1792. R: GA 2 (1793): 1912–14. *Neue* ADB 8 (1794): 377–79. ALZ 95 (1795): 207–8.

1792 G Michaelis, John D. *Rechtmäßigkeit der Inoculation der Blattern.* Göttingen, 1792.

1792 G Opitz, Rudolph C.F. *Fortschritte der Blattern-Impfung in dem Fürstenthum Minden.* Minden, 1792. R: ALZ, no. 138 (1793): 362.

1792 G "Ueber einige Vorurtheile und Bedenklichkeiten gegen die Blatterinoculation." *LM*, nos. 7, 9 (1792): 123–124, 133–135.

1792 G Vogler, Friedrich A. "Nachricht von einer Blattern-Einimpfung, welche an acht und fünfzig, in Erkerode vorgenommen ist." BRM 5 (1792): 293–98.

1793 G "Bemerkung über die Einimpfung der Pocken." *JE* 4 (1793): 137–39.

1793 G Hufeland, Christoph W. *Bemerkungen über die natürlichen und geimpften Blattern zu Weimar im Jahr 1788, nebst einem Anhang über die wesentlichen Vorzüge der Inoculation, und einige andere Kinderkrankheiten.* 2nd ed. Leipzig, 1793. R: *Neue* ADB 2 (1793): 521–25. ALZ 93 (1793): 360–68. *PJG* 2 (1795): 170–72.

1794 G Bürde, Samuel G. "Die inoculierte Braut. Eine Erzählung." *SP* 20 (1794): 21–36, 120–35, 234–52, 497–514.

1794 G Harrhausen, J.G.G. *Ueber die Pockeninoculation, ein Gespräch. Zum Unterricht und zur überzeugung von dem Nutzen der künstlichen Blattern; und wie der Gebrauch dieses heilsamen Mittels für den Menschen eine Pflicht sey, ausgesetzt für die lieben Landleute.* Hanover, 1794.

1794 G Piccard, G.F. "Etwas von Blattern." *Neues* HM 4 (1794): 665–76.

1794 G Werbe, J.G. "Die glücklichen Blattern zu Bramel, im Herzogthum Bremen, im Jahre 1794." *Neues* HM 4 (1794): 1321–26.

1795 G Henschel, Elias. *Ueber das Blatterpfropfen. Ein Wort an Nichtärzte und auch an Aerzte, von einem Freund der guten Sache.* Breslau, 1795. R: *Neue* ADB 27 (1796): 370. *GA*, no. 161 (1796): 1604–07. ALZ, no. 155 (1799): 412–15.

1795 G Johnston, von. "Etwas zur Beförderung der Blatter-Inoculation." *SP* 21 (1795): 175–80.

1795 G "Nöthige Bemerkungen zu den jetzigen Verhandlungen über die Blattern, auch für die nicht Eingeweihte." *JE* 3, no. 11 (1795): 74–133.

1795 G Reyland, Bernard J. *Ueber den Nützen der Pocken-Inoculation in Vergleich des Schadens der natürlichen Pocken.* Düsseldorf, 1795. R: *Neue* ADB 24 (1796): 261–62.

1795 B *Unterricht für Eltern über die Behandlung ihrer Kinder in den natürlichen Blattern und während der Eingeimpften, nebst einigen praktischen Fällen zur Bestätigung.* Leipzig, 1795. R: *Neue* ADB 15 (1795): 263.

1795 G Vasmer, Karl D.J. "Prüfung der Gründe gegen die Inoculation der Blattern, und was eigentlich dazu auffordert." *Neues* HM 5 (1795): 849–76.

1796 G Bail, J.S. "Ueber die Blattereinimpfung in religiöser Rücksicht." SP 23 (1796): 219–28.

1796 G "Blattern Einimpfung." SP 24 (1796): 190–92.

1796 G Dietrich. "Ueber Blatter Impfung." SP 24 (1796): 537–50.

1796 G Dietrich. "Ueber Pokkenimpfung." SP 23 (1796): 228–60.

1796 G Girtanner, Christoph. "Einige Gründe für die Impfung der Säuglinge in den ersten 4 Monaten des Lebens." JE, no. 14 (1796): 37–42.

1796 G Nickisch, von. "Empfehlung der Blatter Einimpfung." SP 23 (1796): 578–79.

1796 G "Pokkeneinimpfung unter den Landleuten." SHP 10 (1796): 160–67.

1796 G "Versuch zur Hemmung der Blattern im Eutinschen." SHP 10 (1796): 221.

1796 G Zedlitz u. Neukirch, von. "Pocken Einimpfung bey sieben Geschwistern." SP 23 (1796): 579–82

1797 G "Abhandlung von der Inokulation der Blattern." *Kleines Magazin von ökonomischen Gegenständen und bewährten Hausmitteln* 7 (1797): 92–103.

1797 G Brinckmann, A.C. "Nachricht von einer glücklich vollendeten Blattereinimpfung in der Kalebuyer Gemeine unweit Schleswig." SHP 11 (1797): 125–27.

1797 G Dietrich. "Ueber Blatter Impfung." SP 25 (1797): 112–27.

1797 G + "Ein Wort über die Blattern an die guten Einwohner Eutins." SHP 11 (1797): 142–44. *National-Zeitung der Teutschen*, no. 15 (1797): 331–4.

1797 G Matthiä, E.E. "In welchem Lebensalter und zu welcher Zeit soll man Kindern die Blattern einimpfen?" *Neues* HM 7 (1797): 297–326.

1797 G Zadig, Abraham. *Plan, nach welchem die Einimpfung der Pocken in eine ganze Provinz allgemein eingeführt, und die längstgewünscht Ausrottung derselben erreicht werden kann.* Breslau, 1797. R: *Neue* ADB 36 (1798): 152–53.

1798 G Masius, G.H. "Erklärung, die Pocken-Impfung betreffend." *Neue* MM 7 (1798): 241–43.

1798 G Nickisch, von. "Pokken Einimpfung." SP 28 (1798): 189–90.

1798 G "Pocken Inoculation." SP 28 (1798): 385–87.

1799 G "Die inokulation der Blattern. Eine Erzählung." SP 29 (1799): 499–525.

1799 B Haygarth, John. *Entwurf, die zufälligen Blattern zu verbannen und eine allgemeine Impfung einzuführen; nebst einem Briefwechsel über die Natur des Blatterngifts, mit einem Anhang von G.C. Reich.* Trans. Johann B. Bonzel. Gotha, 1799.

1799 N Oskamp, Dirk L. *Zwey Vorlesungen über die natürlichen und geimpften Kinderblattern.* Trans. Sebastian J.L. Döring. Herborn, 1799. R: ALZ 2 (1800): 380. *Neue* ADB 48 (1801): 337.

1799 G Richter, Johann S. "Ueber die Blatter-Einimpfung." SP 30 (1799): 242–6.

1799 G Vogler, Friedrich A. "Ueber eine dritte Blattern-Einimpfung in Lucklum und Erkerode." BRM 12 (1799): 689–94.

1800 G Coldiz. "Blattereinimpfung im Christianspflegehaus zu Ekkernförde." SHB 1 (1800): 70.

1800 B R Review of *History of the Inoculation of the Small-pox in Great Britain*, by William Woodville. (London, 1796). ALZ 1 (1800): 309–12.

1800 F R + Review of *Instruction sur la pratique de l'inoculation de la petite vérole*, by Mathieu-Antoine Salmade (Paris, 1799). ALZ 1 (1801): 282. *Neue* ADB 65, part 1 (1801): 41–42.

1800 F Salmade, Mathieu-Antoine. *Anleitung zur Einimpfung der Blattern, nebst einer Abhandlung über die natur und Behandlung dieser Krankheit.* Trans. Emmanuel W. Wallich. Frankfurt, 1800.

1800 N Sowden, Benjamin C. *Abhandlung über die Einimpfung der Blattern.* Dortmund, 1800.

1800 G Wissel, F. von. "Ein Beytrag zum Besten der Blatter-Inoculation." SP 32 (1800):150–52.

Bibliography

Primary Sources (Excluding Publications Listed in Appendices)

"Abgedrungene Erklärung über die Pockenangelegenheit, besonders in Rücksicht des Junckerschen Ausrottungsplans." *Journal der Erfindungen, Theorien und Widersprüche in der Natur und Arzneiwissenschaft* 21 (1799): 135–43.

Abschatz, Hans Aßmann von. "Die Blattern oder Kinder-Pocken." In Part 3 of *Hans Aßmann von Abschatz: Poetische Uebersetzungen und Gedichte*, 84–87. Leipzig und Breslau: Bauch, 1708.

Allgemeines Repertorium der Litteratur für die Jahre 1785 bis 1790. Jena: Expedition der ALZ, 1793. *Repertorium 1791 bis 1795*. Weimar: Industrie-Comptoir, 1799. *Repertorium 1796 bis 1800*. Weimar: Landes Industrie-Comptoir, 1807.

Al-Rází, Abú Becr Mohammed Ibn Zacaríyá. *A Treatise on the Small-pox and Measles*. Translated by William A. Greenhill. London, 1868.

"An alle gut gesinnte vernünftige denkende Eltern wegen Einimpfung der Blattern." *Reichs-Anzeiger* 2 (1800): 3145–48.

"An den Gnomen Uriel." In *Lyrische Muse an der Saale*, 182–4. Jena: Schill, 1759.

"Anfang der Blatternausrottung in Deutschland und Europa." *Der Bote aus Thüringen*, no. 14 (1797): 209–16.

"Anfrage, die diesjährige Blattern-Impfung in Darmstadt betreffend." *Reichs Anzeiger* 2 (1800): 2549.

Astronomische-Physicalischer Kalender. Munich, 1762.

Aufgefangener litterarische Briefwechsel der Dodsleyschen Kunstrichter und anderer Gelehrten. Schöppenstadt, 1772.

"Auf eine Pocken-grubichte." In part 6 of *Herrn Hoffmannswaldau und anderer Deutschen auserlesener und ungedruckter Gedichte*, 75. Leipzig: Fritsch, 1709.

Aufruf an den Genius des scheidenden Jahrhunderts zur Ausrottung der Blattern. Thorn: Bollmer, 1797.

"Aus Oesterreich." *Der poetische Zeitungsfabrikant, oder des Münchnerischen Wochenblatts in Versen*. Neunter Jahrgang 1 (1767): item 24.

"Ausrottungs-Impfung der Blattern." *Reichs Anzeiger* 1 (1800): 382.

"Auszug eines Schreibens von Wien, Juli, 1780." *Medizinisches Wochenblatt für Aerzte, Wundärzte, und Apotheker* 2 (1781): 111–2.

Ballhorn, Georg Friedrich and Christian F. Strohmeyer. "Uebersicht der in Hannover mit der Kuhpockenimpfung angestellten Versuche." *Neues hannoverisches Magazin* 10 (1800): 223–36.

"Beantwortung der Frage: Welches sind die gewöhnlichen Ursachen, warum der gemeine Landmann bey vorfallenden Krankheiten seine Zuflucht lieber zum Pfuscher, als zu einem ordentlichen Arzt, nimmt?" *Neue Monatsschrift von und für Mecklenburg* 4 (1795): 133–6.

Becker, R.Z. "Versuch über die Aufklärung des Landmannes." *Der teutsche Merkur* 3 (1785): 109–31.

"Begräbniß Carme." In *M. Francisco Wokenius: Anleitung zur teutschen Poesie,* 22–25. Leipzig, 1715.

Berends, Carl A.W. *Handbuch der praktischen Arzneiwissenschaft.* Vienna: Hapkul, 1830.

Bergius, Johann H.L. and Johann Beckmann. *Sammlung auserlesener Landesgesetze, welche das Policey und Cameralwesen zum Gegenstände haben.* Frankfurt am Main: Andreä, 1792.

Block, G.W. "Sollen die Landprediger auch Aerzte seyn?" *Neues hannoverisches Magazin* 6 (1796): 1559–80.

Block, G.W. and J. Müller. "Beitrag zur Entscheidung der Frage: 'Sollen die Landprediger auch Aerzte seyn?'" *Neues hannoverisches Magazin* 7 (1797): 325–48.

Blum, Joachim C. "An den Komates, 1771." In Joachim C. Blum: *Sämmtliche Gedichte,* 276–88. Karlsruhe: Schmieder, 1781.

Bönig. "Etwas zur Empfehlung der Kuhpockenimpfung." *Neues hannoverisches Magazin* 10 (1800): 869–84.

Bredal, Peter von. *Cantate welche bey der, wegen glücklicher Wiederherstellung Sr. Kaiserl. Hoheit aus den Allerhöchstdenenselben eingeimpften Blattern, von dem herrn Jagd-Junker von Bredal, am 14ten Jenner 1769, in dem grössern Academischen Hörsaal gehaltenen Rede, aufgeführet wurde.* Kiel: Bartsch, 1769.

Briefwechsel zwischen Schiller und Goethe in den Jahren 1794 bis 1805. Vol. 1: 1794–95. Vol. 3: 1797. Stuttgart and Tübingen: Cotta, 1828–29.

Brockes, Barthold H. "Bei dem 1732sten Jahres-Wechsel." In part 5 of *Barthold H. Brockes: Irdisches vergnügen in Gott,* 401–30. Hamburg, Herold, 1740.

Brockes, Barthold H. "Letzte Gedanken über einen kranken und sterbenden Sohn Johann Bernhard Brockes." In vol. 6 of *Weichmann's Poesie der Nieder-Sachsen,* edited by J.P Kohlen, 265–70. Hamburg: Herold, 1738.

Brockes, Barthold H. "Selbstbiographie." *Zeitschrift des Vereines für hamburgische Geschichte* 2 (1847): 167–229.

Brown, John. *Anfangsgründe der Medizin.* Translated by Andreas Roschlaub. Frankfurt am Main: Andreä, 1806

Bürde, Samuel G. "Die Bräutigamsprobe. Eine Erzählung." In *Samuel G. Bürde: Erzählungen,* 57–140. Berlin, 1796.

Burges, James. *An Account of the Preparation and Management necessary to Inoculation.* London: Vaillant, 1754.

Caraccioli, the Marquis. *The Life of Pope Clement XIV* (Ganganelli). 2nd ed. London: Johnson, 1778.

Christan, Thomas. *Beiträge zur Geschichte und Behandlung der natürlichen Pocken.* Vienna: Obelen, 1781.

"Circulare wegen Einführung der Blatter-Inoculation." Vol. 12 of *Sammlung aller Ordnungen, Edicte, Mandate, Rescripte, etc. der Regierung Friedrichs II,* 47–54. Breslau: Korn, 1770.

Cloß, Johann F. *Neue Heilart der Kinderpocken.* Ulm: Bartholomai, 1769.

Coelln, L.F.A. von. "Beytrag zur Charakteristik des Lippeschen, Ritbergischen und Paderbornischen Bauern." *Westphälisches Magazin zur Geographie, Historie und Statistik* 1 (1784): 105–16.

Colman, Benjamin. *A Narrative of the Method and Success of Inoculating the Small-Pox in New England, with a reply to the Objections made against it from Principles of Conscience.* Dublin: Grierson, 1722.

Conradi, Georg C. "Unterricht über die Behandlung der Blattern und Empfehlung der Inoculation, dem Landmanne bestimmt." In *Neuer Volkskalender, oder Beytrage zur nützlichen, lehrreichen, und angenehmen Unterhaltung für allerley Leser, zunächst für den Bürger und Landmann,* 199–220. Hanover: Hahn, 1795.

Contius, Christian G. "Der Spiegel, eine Fabel." In *Christian G. Contius: Gedichte,* 83–86. Dresden: Gerlach, 1782.

De Haen, Anton. *Réfutation de l'inoculation servant de réponse a deux pièces qui ont perçu cette année 1759.* Vienna: Trattner, 1759.

De Haen, Anton and Ernst Platner. *Anton von Haen's kaiserlichen Leibarztes Heilungsmethode, in dem kaiserlichen Krankenhaus zu Wien.* Vol. 5. Leipzig: Weygand, 1782.

De la Condamine, Charles-Marie. *Histoire de l'inoculation de la petite vérole.* Amsterdam: Typographic Society, 1773.

De la Condamine, Charles-Marie. *Journal of a Tour of Italy.* Dublin, 1763.

De la Condamine, Charles-Marie. *Seconde mémoire sur l'inoculation de la petite vérole.* Geneva: Du Villard, 1759.

Dedekind, Johann J.W. "Ueber Königslutters angenehme und gesunde Lage." *Curart der natürlichen Pocken,* no. 2 (1791): 21–39.

Der Engel Gabriel und die Gebrüder Schlegel nebst einem Durchflug Gabriels von Jena über Halle und Wittenberg nach Berlin. 1799.

Detharding, Georg C. *De facie a variolarum insultibus praeservanda.* Rostock: Adler, 1754.

"Die Blattern. Eine Idylle." *Magazin der sächsischen Geschichte* 7 (1790): 300–304.

Die heilige Schrift. Translated by S.G. Dom. Part 3. Berlin and Basel, 1782.

"Die Merkwürdigsten am Kaiserlich-Königlichen Hof 1768." Part 96 of *Fortgesetzte neue Genealogish-historische Nachrichten von den vornehmesten Europäishen Hofen,* 783–800. Leipzig: Heinsius, 1769.

"Die Regierungs-Geschichte der Russischen Kaiserin im Jahre 1768." Part 97 of *Fortgesetzte neue Genealogish-historische Nachrichten von den vornehmesten Europäishen Hofen*, 1–15. Leipzig: Heinsius, 1769.

"Die Wallfahrt zum Monddoktor in Berlin." *Berlinische Monatsschrift* 1 (1783): 368–85.

Dimsdale, Thomas. *Neue Methode für die Einpfropfung der Pocken, auch Anhang.* Zürich: Füssli, 1768.

"Doctor Faust." *Neueste Legenden.* Vol. 2. Vienna, 1793.

Dolz, Johann C. *Praktische Anleitung zu schriftlichen Aussätzen über gegenstände des gemeinen Lebens, besonders für Bürgerschulen.* Leipzig: Barth, 1798.

Dover, George A-E., 1st Baron, ed. *Letters of Horace Walpole, Earl of Orford, to Sir Horace Mann, His Britannic Majesty's resident at the court of Florence.* Philadelphia: Lea and Blanchard, 1844.

Drais, Karl W.L.F. von. *Geschichte der Regierung und Bildung von Baden unter Carl Friedrich.* Karlsruhe: Müller, 1818.

Eisen, Johann G. *Der erleichterten und den Müttern selbst übertragenen Blatternimpfung.* Riga: Hartnoch, 1774.

Eller, Johann T. *Observationes de cognoscendis et curandis morbis, praesertim acutis.* Königsberg and Leipzig: Woltersdorff, 1762.

Engelhard, Philippine. "Eine wahrscheinliche Historia. Erster Gesang, 1779." In vol. 2 of *Philippine Engelhard: Gedichte*, 116–32. Göttingen, Dieterich, 1782.

"Erfreuliche Nachrichten in Betreff des Pockenelends!" *Reichs Anzeiger* 1 (1799): 1897.

Erhard, Friedrich. "Anfrage, die medicinischen und ökonomischen Predigten betreffend." *Neue Miscellaneen historischen, politischen, moralischen, auch sonst verschiedenen Inhalts* 20 (1785): 189–95.

Ersch, Johann S. *Litteratur der Medicin seit der Mitte des achtzehnten Jahrhunderts.* Amsterdam and Leipzig: Kunst- und Industrie-Comptoir, 1812.

Erscheinungen und Träume am Ende des 18. Jahrhunderts. Ein grosses Trauerspiel in 'Issländischer und Kotzebuescher Manier.' Germanien, 1799.

Eser, Friedrich. Aus Meinem Leben (1798–1873), edited by P. Beck. Ravensburg: Alber, 1907.

"Etwas zur Berichtigung der Anfrage, die diesjährige Blattern-Impfung in Darmstadt betreffend." *Reichs Anzeiger* 2 (1800): 2857–58.

"Etwas zur Characteristik des Landmanns in der westphälischen Grafschaft Mark." *Neues westphälisches Magazin zur Geographie, Historie und Statistik* 3 (1792): 185–202.

Faust, Bernhard C. *An den Congrès de Rastadt sur l'Extirpation de la petite vérole / An den Congreß zu Rastadt über die Ausrottung der Blattern.* Bückeberg, 1798.

Faust, Bernhard C. *An den Herrn Eduard Jenner, über einige Versuche zur weiteren Untersuchung der Wirkungen und zum Beweise der Unschädlichkeit der Kuhpocken-Materie.* Hanover: Hahn, 1802.

Faust, Bernhard C. "An den Kongreß zu Rastadt über die Ausrottung der Blattern." *Deutsches Magazin* 16 (1798): 373–90.

Faust, Bernhard C. *Gesundheits-Katechismus zum Gebrauche in den Schulen und beym häuslichen Unterricht.* Leipzig: Kummer, 1800.

Faust, Bernhard C. "Resultate der Kuhpocken-Einimpfung in Großbrittanien während des Jahrs 1799." *Reichs-Anzeiger* 2 (1800): 2401–411.

Faust, Bernhard C. "Versuch über die Pflicht der Menschen, jeden Blatternkranken der Gesunden abzusondern; und dadurch zugleich in Städten und Ländern und in Europa die Ausrottung der Blatternpest zu bewirken." *Philosophisches Journal* 4 (1794): 40–95. *Neue Montasschrift von und für Mecklenburg* 4 (1795): 89–97; 5 (1796): 345–50, 369–73.

"Fifty Articles of Literary and Philosophical Intelligence." *The Monthly Magazine* 7 (1799): 150–51.

Fischer, Gottlieb N. "Die Pocken können, und also sollen und müssen ausgerottet werden. Aufruf an seine Mitburger." *Halberstädtischen neuen gemeinnützigen Blättern,* no. 46 (1797): 8.

Fischer, Heinrich L. *Beiträge zur Beantwortung der Frage, ob Aufklärung schon weit genug gediehen oder vollendet sey? Als Anhang zu dem Buch vom Aberglauben.* Hanover: Rischer, 1794.

Fischer, Johann B. *Geschichte und ausführliche Beschreibung der markgräflich-Brandenburgischen Haupt-und Residenz-Stadt Anspach.* Ansbach: Fischer, 1786.

Formey, Ludwig. *Versuch einer medicinischen Topographie von Berlin.* Berlin: Felisch, 1796.

Frank, Johann P. *Abhandlung über eine gesunde Kindererziehung, besonders für Mütter, denen ihre und ihre Kinder Gesundheit am Herzen liegt.* Leipzig: Baumgärtner, 1794.

Fréron, Élie-Catherine. "Arrivée d'un de Mrs. Sutton & d'un de ses beaux-frères à Paris." In Vol. 3 of *L'année littéraire. Année 1771,* 188–98. Paris: Delalain, 1771.

Frewen, Thomas. *The Practice and Theory of Inoculation.* London: Austen, 1749.

Friebe, William C. *Physische, ökonomische und statistische Bemerkungen von Lief-und Ehstland, oder von den beiden Staathalterschaften Riga und Reval.* Riga: Hartnoch, 1794.

Friedrich II, King of Prussia. *Correspondance de Frédéric II, roi de Prusse,* edited by Johann D.E. Preuss and Adolph von Menzel. Vol. 9. Berlin: Decker, 1854.

Fritze, Johann G. "Eine Blatterimpfung." *Baldinger's neues Magazin für Aerzte* 9 (1787): 213–15.

Gatti, Angelo. *Nouvelles réflexions sur la practique de l'inoculation.* Brussels: Musier, 1767.

"Geheime Nachricht, von der wahre Ursache, warum der königliche Preussische Kalender des 1780sten Jahres wieder auf den alten Fuß gesetz worden." *Deutsches Museum* 1 (1781): 269–83.

Gellert, Christian F. "Lisette." In vol. 1 of *Christian F. Gellert: Fabeln und Erzählungen*, 119–21. Leipzig: Wendler, 1763.

George I, King of Great Britain, to his daughter Sophia Dorothea, Queen of Prussia, 26 May 1724. MS 9212/1, Box 229, Shelfmark PP/CRI/M/2/3. Wellcome Library, Archives and Manuscripts, London.

Gerstlacher, Carl F., ed. *Sammlung aller Baden-Durlachischen Anstalten und Verordnungen*. Vol. 1. Karlsruhe: Schmieder, 1773.

"Geschichte der Staaten. Aus Teutschland." *Berlinische priveligirte wöchentliche Relation der merkwürdigsten Sachen*, no. 10 (1756): 73–5.

"Geschichte von den Herrn Daniel Wilhelm Triller." In *Beyträge zur Historie der Gelartheit, worinnen die Geschichte der Gelehrten unserer Zeiten beschrieben worden*, 142–81. Hamburg, Geißler, 1748.

Girtanner, Christoph. *Historische Nachrichten und politische Betrachtungen über die Französische Revolution*. Berlin: Unger, 1792.

Girtanner, Christoph. *Krankheiten der Kinder und über die physische Erziehung derselben*. Berlin: Rottmann, 1794.

"Glücklicher Erfolg der Bemühungen eines Predigers, der seine Kirchkinder anzuweisen suchte, wie sie sich bei herrschenden Pocken in Ansehung ihrer kranken Kinder zu benehmen hätten." *Schlesische Provinzialblätter* 25 (1797): 147–51.

Goerres, Joseph. "Die teutschen Zeitungen." *Rheinische Merkur* 80 (1814): 1–4.

Goethe, Johann W. von. *Goethe's Werke*. Vol. 24, *Aus meinem Leben, Dichtung und Wahrheit*. Stuttgart and Tübingen: Cotta, 1839.

Goldstein, Augusta F. von. *Das Mädchen Wunderhold. Eine abendländische Romanesk in neuern Styl*. Leipzig, 1810.

Gretschel, Carl. *Geschichte des sächsischen Volkes und Staaten*. Vol. 3. Leipzig: Hinrichs, 1853.

Grot, Joachim C. "Kanzelrede von der Rechtmäßigkeit der Blatter-Einimpfung aus allgemeinen Gründen, am ersten Nov. 1769." *Journal für Prediger* 3 (1770): 349–50.

Gruner, Christian G. *Ein Paar Worte zur Belehrung, Beherzigung und Besserung an den Herrn Ex-Professor Fichte*. Jena, 1799.

Gruner Christian G. *Gedanken von der Arzneiwissenschaft und den Aerzten*. Breslau: Korn, 1772.

Gruner, Ernst von. *Leben MA von Thümmels*. Leipzig: Göschen, 1819.

Günther, Johann C. "An einen guten Freund," in *Sammlung von Johann Christian Günther's Gedichten*, 484–88. 2nd ed. Breslau and Leipzig: Hubert, 1739.

Günther, J.U. "Anleiting, gesund zu werden." *Verhandlungen und Schriften der hamburgischen Gesellschaft zur Beförderung der Künste und nützlichen Gewerbe* 4 (1797): 448–54.

Halle, Johann S. *Fortgesetzte Magie, oder die Zauberkräfte der Natur*. Berlin: Pauli, 1793.

Hamberger, Georg C. and Johann G. Meusel. *Das gelehrte Teutschland.* Lemgo: Meyer, 1776.

Hamberger, Georg C. and Johann G. Meusel. *Das gelehrte Teutschland.* Vol. 17. Lemgo: Meyer, 1778.

Hartenkeil, Johann J. "Nachricht für Nicht-Aerzte, die von der beyspiellosen Geschwätzigkeit und Zankzucht des Prof. Junckers in Halle such überzeugen wollen, da es die Aertze schon längstens sind." *Reichs Anzeiger* 1 (1799): 613–15.

Haygarth, John. *An Inquiry How to Prevent the Small-Pox and Proceedings of a Society for Promoting General Inoculation at Stated Periods and Preventing the Natural Small-Pox, in Chester*. Chester: Monk, 1784.

Hebenstreit, Ernst B.G. *Lehrsätze der medicinischen Policeywissenschaft.* Leipzig: Dyck, 1791.

Heim, Ernst L. "Ueber die Diagnostik der falschen Pokken mit Hinsicht auf die neuerlich behaupteten Fälle von echten Pokken nach vorhergegangener gelungener Vaccination." *Archiv für medizinische Erfahrung* 2 (1809): 183–219.

Helmershausen, Paul J.F. "Auszug eines Schreibens aus London in Betreff der Kuh-Pocken." *Reichs Anzeiger* 2 (1799): 1793–95.

Hennig, Friedrich W. *Abhandlung über das Selbstsäugen der Kinder*. Breslau: Korn, 1797.

Henschel, Elias. *Von den Blattern und deren Ausrottung.* Breslau and Leipzig: Korn, 1796.

Hermes, Johann T. *Sophiens Reise von Memel nach Sachsen.* Vol. 2. Leipzig: Junius, 1778.

Hess, Ludwig von. *Freymüthige Gedanken über Staatssachen.* Hamburg: J.J.C. Bode, 1775.

Hezel, William F. *Die Bibel mit vollständig-erklärenden Anmerkungen.* Part 4. Lemgo: Meyer, 1783.

Hinzberg, von. "An den Urheber der Kuhpockenimpfung, Doktor Jenner." *Der neue teutsche Merkur* 1 (1802): 5–6.

Hinze, August. *Lexicon aller Herzogl. Braunschweigischen Verordnungen, welche die medicinische Policey betreffen.* Stendal: Franzen und Grosse, 1793.

Hippel, Theodor G. von. *Über die bürgerliche Verbesserung der Weiber.* Berlin: Voß, 1792.

Hirschel, Leon E. "Gedanken über die Einimpfung der Pocken." *Mannigfaltigkeiten* 2 (1771): 654–61.

Hirschfeld, Christian C.L. Review of *Die Inoculation der Liebe. Eine Erzählung*, by Moritz A von Thümmel. *Allgemeine deutsche Bibliothek,* no. 2 (1771): 352–58.

Hirsching, Friedrich C.G. *Historisch-litterarisches Handbuch berühmter und denkwürdiger Personen welche im achtzehnten Jahrhundert gelebt haben.* Leipzig: Schwicker, 1810.

Hoffmann, Christoph L. *Pathologie der Pockenkrankheit.* Part 2, *Abhandlung von den Pocken.* Mainz, 1789.

Hoffmann, Christoph L. "Ueber die münsterschen Medizinalgesetze." *Deutsches Museum* 1 (1778): 28–47.

Holsche, August K. *Historisch-topographisch-statistische Beschreibung der Grafschaft Tecklenburg nebst einigen speciellen Landesverordnungen mit Anmerkungen als ein Beytrag zur vollständigen Beschreibung Westphalens.* Berlin and Frankfurt: Kunze, 1788.

Hübner, Johann. *Reales Staats-Zeitungs und Conversations-Lexicon.* Regensburg and Vienna: Baders, 1765.

Hufeland, Christoph W. *Bemerkungen über die natürlichen und geimpften Blattern, verschiedene Kinderkrankheiten und sowohl medizinische als diatetische Behandlung der Kinder.* 3rd ed. Berlin: Rottmann, 1798.

Hufeland, Christoph W. "Erklärung." *Intelligenzblatt der Allgemeine Literatur-Zeitung*, no. 71 (1795): 561–62.

Hufeland, Christoph W. *Gemeinnützige Aufsätze zur Beförderung der Gesundheit und das Wohlseyns.* Vienna: Schmidbauer and Kemp, 1797.

Hufeland, Christoph W. "Neue Aussicht zur Vertilgung der Blattern." *TM* 4 (1786): 167–81, 253–63.

Hufeland, Christoph W. "Neuer Vorschlag zur Verhüting der Blattern durch Inoculation der Kuhpocken." *Journal der practischen Arzneykunde und Wundarzneykunst* 6 (1798): 907–9.

"Ihre Kleider sind das schönste an ihr." In *Herrn von Hoffmannswaldau und anderer Deutschen auserlesener und bisher ungedruckter Gedichte*, 336–7. Part 2. Leipzig: Fritsch, 1697.

"Inoculation." *Journal Oeconomique, ou mémoires, notes et avis, Année 1770* (July 1770): 321–22.

Jani, Christian H. "Nachtrag zu meiner kleinen Schrift: Was müssen wir bey den jetzigen Bemuhungen deutscher Aerzte, die gänzliche Ausrottung der Blattern vorzubereiten, zur Mitwürkung thun?" *Reichs Anzeiger* 2 (1799): 1713–17.

Juncker, Johann C.W. "Antwort an den hrn Dr. Sponitzer auf die an mich gerichtete Erklärung im R-A d. J. Nr. 134." *Reichs Anzeiger* 1 (1798): 1711–13.

Juncker, Johann C.W. *Archiv der Aerzte und Seelsorger wider die Pockkenoth.* 7 Vols. Leipzig: Weygand, 1796–99.

Juncker, Johann C.W. "Celeberrimo Doctori G. Pearson." *Medical and Physical Journal* 4 (1800): 141–45.

Juncker, Johann C.W. "Einige Bemerkungen über die Ansatz des Dr. Sponitzer in *RA* nr. 67." *Reichs Anzeiger* 1 (1799): 1090–92.

Juncker, Johann C.W. *Gemeinnützige Vorschläge und Nachrichten über das beste verhalten der Menschen in Rücksicht der Pockenkrankheit. Erster Versuch, für die mittlern Stände, nebst einem Anhange für Aerzte.* Halle, 1792.

Juncker, Johann C.W. *Gemeinnützige Vorschläge wider die Pockenkrankheit. Dritter Versuch, für möglichst alle Aerzte, die der deutschen Sprache kundig sind; zur Sammlung ihrer Gutachten hierüber.* Halle and Leipzig: Hemmerde and Schwetschke, 1796.

Juncker, Johann C.W. *Mémoire addressée au Congrès de Rastadt concernant la petite vérole – affiche concernant la petite vérole à employer conformement aux ordres du gouvernement/ Pockentafel, auf Befehl der Regierung zu gebrauchen.* Halle, 1798.

Juncker, Johann C.W. “Nachricht die Pockennoth betreffend.” *Berlinische Monatsschrift* 28 (1796): 88–93.

Juncker, Johann C.W. “Nachricht für Aerzte von den neuesten und beyspiellosen Ungerechtigkeiten in der Hartenkeil’schen (Salzburger) Zeitung; in Betreff der Pockenangelegenheit.” *Reichs Anzeiger* 1 (1799): 285–89.

“Kalenderlegenden.” In *Almanach für Aerzte und Nichtärzte auf das Jahr 1782*, edited by Christian G. Gruner, 231–36. Jena: Cuno’s Erben, 1782.

Kilpatrick (Kirkpatrick), James. *Essay on Inoculation Occasioned by the Smallpox being brought into South-Carolina in the Year* 1738. London: Huggenson, 1743.

Kirkpatrick, James. *The Analysis of Inoculation.* London: Edward Brothers, 1754.

Kretschmar, Friedrich S. *Irrthumer, Warnungen, und Lehren.* Würzburg, Bamberg, Fulda: Stahel, 1770.

Krünitz, Johann G. *Oekonomisch-technologische Encylopädie.* Parts 32, 35, and 72. Berlin: Pauli, 1784, 1793, and 1799.

Krünitz, Johann G. *Verzeichniß der vornehmsten Schriften von der Kinderpocken und deren Einpfropfung.* Leipzig: Hilscher, 1768.

Krusen, Jürgen E. *Allgemeiner Hamburgischer Contorist.* Vol. 2. Hamburg: Krusen Erben, 1782–83.

Kühn, Johann G. *Medicinischer Briefwechsel eines Arztes mit einigen Frauenzimmern.* Breslau: Korn, 1796.

Kur-Badisches Regierungsblatt. Vol. 1, nos. 1–26 (1803).

Lenhardt, Joseph. *Arzneyen ohne Maske.* Leipzig, 1787.

Lentin, Leberecht F.B. *Beyträge zur ausübenden Arzneywissenschaft.* Leipzig: Crusius, 1789.

Lenz, Christian L. *Bemerkungen auf Reisen in Dänemark, Schweden und Frankreich.* Part 2. Gotha: Ettinger, 1801.

Lenz, Christian L. “Vertheidigung und Berichtigung.” *Reichs Anzeiger* 2 (1799): 2025–27.

“Letter to the editor.” *The Gentleman’s Magazine* 25 (1846): 592–93.

Lindemann, Christoph F.H. “Ueber die Ausrottung der Kinderblattern.” *Hannoverisches Magazin* 27 (1789): 561–90.

Livy. *The History of Rome.* Translated by D. Spillan and C. Edmonds. London: Bell, 1892.

Lüders, F.L. “Ueber die gefährlichen Folgen der Quacksalberei.” *Neues hannoverisches Magazin* 2 (1792): 1265–74.

Maitland, Charles. *Account of the Inoculation of the Small Pox.* London: Peele, 1723.

“Margrafschaft Baden, Kuhpocken.” *Schwäbische Chronik, Stuttgart* (July 31, 1801): 287.

Medicus, Friedrich C. *Send-Schreiben von der Ausrottung der Kinder-Blattern.* Frankfurt and Leipzig, 1763.

Meißner, August G. "Gustav Lindau, oder der Mann, der keinen Neid ertragen will. Fragment aus Branko's Reisejournal." In vol. 1 of *Meißner's Erzählungen und Dialogen*, 79–133. Karlsruhe: Schmieder, 1783.

Meißner, J.G. "Vorschlag, die Blattern zu vertilgen." *Neue bunzlauische Monatsschrift zum Nutzen und Vergnügen* 4 (1787): 358–361.

Mémoires pour l'histoire des sciences et beaux-arts. Vol. 1. Paris, 1766.

Mercy, Joseph A. "Freude des Patrioten. Ein Hymnus gesungen im Neujahr, 1790." *Deutsche Monatsschrift* 1 (1790): 105–6.

Merkel, Garlieb. *Die Letten in Liefland am Ende des philosophischen Jahrhunderts*. Leipzig: Graff, 1800.

Meyer, F.J.L. "Blatternausrottung, in der halbjährigen öffentlichen Versammlung der Gesellschaft, von 9 May 1795." *Verhandlungen und Schriften der hamburgischen Gesellschaft zur Beförderung der Künste und nützlichen Gewerbe* 4 (1797): 142.

M.L.R. *L'inoculation, poème en quatre chants*. Amsterdam: Lacombe, 1773.

Müller, Johann V. *Medizinisches praktisches Handbuch der Frauenzimmerkrankheiten zum Gebrauch der Aerzte und des schönen Geschlechts*. Frankfurt and Leipzig: Jäger, 1788.

"Nachrichten und Urtheile von den neuesten Predigten und andern dahin gehörigen Schriften." *Journal für Prediger* 8 (1777): 239–41.

"Nachricht von der Pockeninokulation zu Nennhausen bei Rathenow." In vol. 2 of *Jahrbücher der preussischen Monarchie unter der Regierung Friedrich Wilhelms des Dritten*, 97–100. Berlin: Unger, 1798.

"Nachricht von einem in Hummelshayn gefeierten Blatternfest." *Journal für Prediger* 22 (1790): 289–96.

"Nekrolog, Samuel Gottlieb Bürde." *Schlesische Provinzialblätter* 93 (1831): 445–46.

Nowak, Karl G. *Schlesisches Schriftsteller-Lexicon*. Part 5. Breslau: Korn, 1841.

Oeder, Georg C. "Ueber die Inokulation der Hornviehseuche." *Deutsches Museum* 1 (1776): 409–11.

Osiander, Friedrich B. *Lehrbuch der Hebammenkunst*. Göttingen: Rosenbusch, 1796.

Osiander, Friedrich B. "Urtheil über die vergebliche leichte Möglichkeit der Blatternausrottung in Europa, nebst einer Erinnerung an die Aerzte der gegenwärtigen Zeit, und der Uebersetzung eines französischen Briefes von Voltaire über diesen Gegenstand, zur Beherzigung der an Ausführbarkeit der Ausrottung Glaubenden und Nichtglaubenden." *Neues hannoverisches Magazin* 8 (1798): 1266–87.

Otto, Johann G. *Medicinische und chirurgische Bemerkungen*. Leipzig: Böhme, 1793.

Ovid. *Metamorphoses*. Translated by A.D Melville. Oxford: Oxford University Press, 1986.

Parabeln oder Gleichnißreden für Junge und Alte. Vienna: Deutschen Schulanstalt St. Anna, 1794.

Parhysius. "Ueber die mancherley Mißgriffe derer, welche aus Reformationssucht überall stürmend zu Werke gehen." *Patriotisches Archiv für Deutschland* 1 (1799): 290–331.

"Pastoralkorrespondenz." *Journal für Prediger* 8 (1777): 135–38.

Paulini, Kristian F. *Neu-Vermehrte heylsame Dreck-Apotheke.* Part 1. Frankfurt am Main: Köllner, 1714.

Ploucquet, Wilhelm G. *Initia Bibliothecae Medico-Practicae et Chirurgicae sive Repertorii Medicinae Practicae et Chirurgicae.* Vol. 8. Tübingen: Cotta, 1797.

Ploucquet, Wilhelm G. *Literatura Medica Digesta.* Vol. 4. Tübingen, Cotta, 1809.

Prussian Medical Board. "Kurze Anleitung wie der Landmann und diejenigen, die keinen Arzt erlangen können, bei der grassirenden Pocken sich zu verhalten haben." *Hannoverisches Magazin* 7 (1769): 561–76.

Prussian Medical Board. *Kurze Anweisung wie der Landmann bei grassierenden Pocken und Scharlachfieber sich zu verhalten habe, auf seiner Königlichen majestät Befehl vom Ober-collegium medicum zeitgemaß verändert und verbessert.* Berlin: Decker, 1796.

Pütter, Johann S. *Versuch einer academischen gelehrten-Geschichte von der Georg-Augustus Universität Göttingen.* Göttingen: Vandenhoek, 1765.

Pütter, Johann S. *Versuch einer academischen gelehrten-Geschichte von der Georg-Augustus Universität Göttingen.* Vol. 2, von 1766 bis 1788. Göttingen: Vandenhoek and Ruprecht, 1788.

Pufendorf, Friedrich L. von. *Ausführbare Vorschläge zur gänzlichen Vertilgung der Blattern. Regenten, Staatsmännern, und Menschenfreunden zu reiflicher Erwägung und Beherzigung empfohlen.* Brunswick: Schulbuchhandlung, 1792.

Pylarini, Jacob. "A New and safe Method of Communicating the Small-pox by Inoculation, lately invented and brought into use." *Philosophical Transactions of the Royal Society* 29 (1716): 207–10.

Rechberger, Anton J. *Vollständige Geschichte der Einimpfung der Blattern in Wien.* Vienna: Grässer, 1788.

Reich, Gottfried C. "Etwas über die Hornviehseuche." *Medicinisch-chirurgische Zeitung* 4 (1796): 365–84.

Reimarus, Johann A.H. "Ueber die Ausrottung der Blattern." *Sammlung auserlesener Abhandlungen zum Gebrauch praktischer Aerzte* 16 (1793): 517–19.

Reinecke, Johann C.M. "Epistel an den Congreß zu Rastadt." *Patriotisches Archiv für Deutschland* 1 (1799): 158–60.

Rengger, Albrecht. *Johann Georg Zimmerman's Briefe an einige seiner Freunde in der Schweiz.* Aarau: Sauerländer, 1830.

Review of *Archiv der Aerzte und Seelsorger wider die Pockkenoth,* Vols. 1–2, by Johann C.W. Juncker. *Medicinisch-chirurgische Zeitung* 3 (1797): 142–60.

Review of *Archiv der Aerzte und Seelsorger wider die Pockkenoth,* Vols. 3–6, by Johann C.W. Juncker. *Medicinisch-chirurgische Zeitung* 4 (1798): 369–83, 401–09. *Medicinisches Journal* 2, no. 4 (1797): 39–47.

Review of *Ausführbare Vorschläge zur gänzlichen Vertilgung der Blattern, Regenten, Staatsmännern, und Menschenfrunden zu reiflicher Erwägung und Beherzigung empfohlen*, by Friedrich L. von Pufendorf. *Medicinish-chirurgische Zeitung* 3 (1794): 212–18.

Review of *Darstellung der Gründe für und gegen die Blattereinimpfung für Leser aus allen Ständen*, by Gottlieb T. Ehrhart. *Allgemeine Literatur-Zeitung* 92 (1792): 470.

Review of *De divers ouvrages sur l'inoculation de la petite vérole*, by Carl C. Krause and Friedrich G. Beer. *Journal de médecin, chirurgie, pharmacie, etc.* 19 (1763): 387–410.

Review of *Essay on Inoculation Occasioned by the Smallpox being brought into South-Carolina in the Year 1738*, by James Kilpatrick. *Neuer Zeitungen von gelehrten Sachen, Leipzig* 1 (1744): 701–2.

Review of *Gemeinnützige Vorschläge wider die Pockenkrankheit. Dritter Versuch, für möglichst alle Aertzte, die der deutschen Sprache kündig sind*, by Johann C.W. Juncker. *Medicinisch-chirurgische Zeitung* 4 (1796): 190–92, 214–17.

Review of *Plan, nach welchem die Einimpfung der Pocken in einer ganzen Provinz allgemein eingeführt und die längst gewünschte Ausrottung der Seuche erreicht werden könnte*, by Abraham Zadig. *Medicinisch-chirurgische Zeitung* 1 (1799): 435–37. *Neue allegemeine deutsche Bibliothek* 36 (1798): 152–53.

Review of "On the most efficacious preservative against the contagion of the small-pox," by Christian A. Cothenius. *The Monthly Review, or Literary Journal* 43 (1771): 521–22.

Review of *Sendschreiben, Beantwortung der Frage: Was ist von den Impf-Predigern und von Empfehlung der Blatter-Einimpfung auf der Kanzel zu halten? Von zween Freunden der Wahrheit*, by Christian G. Hauck. *Allgemeime deutsche Bibliothek* 38, part 2 (1779): 445–46.

Review of *Send-Schreiben von der Ausrottung der Kinder-Blattern*, by Friedrich C. Medicus. *The Gentleman's Magazine and Historical Chronicle* 34 (1764): 290–91.

Review of *Ueber den nützen der Pocken-Inoculation in Vergleich des Schadens der natürlichen Pocken. Eltern und Menschen-freunden zur Beherzigung vorgestellt*, by Bernard J. Reyland. *Medicinisch-chirurgische Zeitung* 2 (1795): 463–64.

Review of *Von dem Ursprung und der Ursache der ansteckenden Krankheiten, insbesondere der Blattern, und deren leicht zu bewerkstelligenden Ausrottung*, by Francesco M. Scuderi. *Neues allgemeine deutsche Bibliothek* 2, Anhang (1797): 123–25.

Review of *Von der vorzüglichen Geschichtlichkeit des Herrn Georg Motherby, bey der Einpfropfung der Pocken, ertheilet aus eigner Erfahrung an seinem Kinde sichere Nachricht*, by Friedrich S. Bock. *Der teutsche Merkur*, no. 12 (1775): 283–92.

Review of *Vorschläge zur Ausrottung der Kinderblattern und andere ansteckenden Seuchen, nebst einer Vorrede von C.G. Salzmann*, by Francesco M. Scuderi. Translated by Christian L. Lenz. *Medicinisch-chirurgische Zeitung* 3 (1794): 218–20.

Rochow, Friedrich E. von. *Der Kinderfreund, ein Lesebuch zum Gebrauch in Landschulen*. Frankfurt: Eichenberg, 1779.

Rössler, Emil F. *Die Gründung der Universität Göttingen*. Göttingen: Vandenhoek and Ruprecht, 1855.

Rosenstein, Nils R. von. *Anweisung zur Kenntniß und Cur der Kinderkrankheiten*. Translated by Johann A. Murray. Göttingen and Gotha: Dieterich, 1768.

Rousseau, Jean-Jacques. *Julie, ou la nouvelle Héloïse*. Vol. 2. Amsterdam: Rey, 1772.

Rüling, Johann P. "Einige bey den Pocken zu beobachtende Vorschriften." *Hannoverisches Magazin* 16 (1778): 467–80.

Sachs, Johann J. *Christoph Wilhelm Hufeland: Ein Rückblick auf sein siebenzigjähriges Leben und Wirken*. Berlin: Hirschwald, 1832.

Salchow, Ulrich C. "Ein durch Versuch geprüftes und durch die Erfahrung bestätigtes vorbauungs-mittel wider die Pokken." *Berlinische Sammlungen zur Beförderung der Arzneywissenschaft* 9 (1777): 230–35.

Salzmann, Christian G. *Carl von Carlsberg, oder über das menschliche Elend*. Vol. 6. Leipzig: Crusius, 1788.

Schäffer, G.B. "Ueber medizinisches Aufklärung." *Neues hannoverisches Magazin* 2 (1792): 1393–1422.

Schäffer, Johann U.G. *Versuche aus der theoretischen Arzneykunde*. Nuremberg: Grattenauer, 1784.

Scherf, Johann C.F. *Archiv der medizinischen Polizey und die gemeinnützigen Arzneikunde*. Vols. 1–2. Leipzig: Weygand, 1783–84.

Schlegel, Johann A. "Auf die Schwester meines Freundes, Christiane Dorothee Gärtnern, nachmalige Ehegattin des Dichters Rost. 1746." In *Johann A. Schlegel: Vermischte Gedichte*, 291–94. Karlsruhe: Schmieder, 1788.

Schlichtegroll, Friedrich, ed. *Nekrolog auf das Jahr 1797*. Vol. 2. Gotha: Perthes, 1801.

Schlichtegroll, Friedrich, ed. *Nekrolog auf das Jahr 1799*. Vol. 2. Gotha: Perthes, 1805.

Schlichtegroll, Friedrich, ed. *Nekrolog der Teutschen für das neunzehnte Jahrhundert*. Vol. 3. Gotha: Perthes, 1805.

Schlözer, August L. von. *Von Russland's Bevolkerung überhaupt. Erster Theil. Von der Unschädlichkeit der Kindsblattern oder Pocken daselbst*. St. Petersburg: Royal Academie, 1768.

Schlözer, Christian von. *August Ludwig von Schlözer's öffentliches und Privatleben*. Leipzig: Hinrichs, 1828.

Schmidt, J.J. "Einige gemeinnützige Regeln über das beste Verhalten des Landmanns bei grassirenden Pokken und Scharlachfiebern." *Neue Monatsschrift von und für Mecklenburg* 6 (1797): 89–93.

"Schreiben eines Quacksalbers aufm Lande an seinen Herrn Gevatter in der Stadt." *Bunzlauische Monatsschrift zum Nutzen und Vergnügen* 3 (1776): 75–82.

"Schreiben eines Reisenden über die Blattern in Darmstadt." *Reichs Anzeiger* 2 (1800): 2859–62.

Schriften, die in die Sachen des ehemalige Grafen Johann Friedrich von Struensee, bey der königliche Inquisitions-Commission zu Copehagen übergeben sind (1772).

Schultz, David. *An Account of Inoculation.* London: A. Linde, 1758.

Schwabe, Ernst. *Anweisung zu den Pflichten und Geschäften eines Stadt- oder Land-Physikus.* 2 Vols. Erfurt: Keyser, 1786–87.

Schwager, Johann M. "Johann Moritz Schwager, Prediger zu Joellenbeck in der Grafschaft Ravensburg." *Niederrheinisch-westfälische Blätter* 1 (1801): 33–93.

Schwager, Johann M. "Ueber die Ravensburger Bauer." *Westphälisches Magazin zur Geographie, Historie und Statistik* 2 (1786): 49–74.

Schwager, Johann M. "Wie kann der Prediger sich das Zutrauen des gemeinen Mannes erwerben?" *Journal für Prediger* 2 (1789): 377–401.

Schweickhard, Christian L. *Ueber den Zustand des Wundarzneiwesens im Badischen.* Karlsruhe: Müller, 1787.

Seidel, Samuel. "Schlaf wohl! erblaßte Theodore, schlaf auserwählte Böttnerinn." In *Zeugnisse treuer Liebe nach dem Tode tugendhafter Frauen, von ihren Ehemännern,* 223–49. Hanover: Försters, 1743.

Selle, Christian Gottlieb. *Medicina Clinica oder Handbuch der medicinischen Praxis.* Berlin: Himburg, 1786.

Sharp, Samuel. *Treatise on the Operations of Surgery.* 4th ed. London, 1743.

"Sollte nicht gegen Orte, worin die Blattern-Epidemie herrscht, die Sperrung eingeführt worden?" *Reichs Anzeiger* 1 (1800): 104.

Sponitzer, Georg W. "Bemerkungen über das leidenschaftliche höchst unedle Benehmen des Prof. Juncker gegen die Dissenters seiner Meinungen." *Reichs Anzeiger* 1 (1799): 770–79.

Sponitzer, Georg W. "Freymüthige Erklärung an den herrn Professor Juncker und andere Gegner der artigen Bemerkungen zu den jetzigen Verhandlungen über die Blattern im XI Stück des J.d. Erfindung." *Reichs Anzeiger* 1 (1798): 1549–55.

Sprengel, Kurt. *Versuch einer pragmatischen Geschichte der Arzneikunde.* Part 5. Halle: Gebauer, 1803.

Stark, Johann C. *Auszüge aus dem Tagebuch des herzoglischen Jenaischen klinischen Instituts.* Jena: Cuno, 1789.

Stark, Johann C. "Widererklärung." *Intelligenzblatt der Allgemeine Literatur-Zeitung,* no. 89 (1795): 711–12.

Strobel, Leonis. *Geist der Wahrheit oder gesammelte Glaubens-und Sittenlehren.* Part 1. Freising: Mösmer, 1769.

Struve, Christian A. *Miscellaneen für Freunde der Heilkunde.* Breslau: Korn, 1796.

Struve, Christian A. *Neues Handbuch der Kinderkrankheiten, besonders zum Gebrauch für Eltern und Erzieher.* Breslau: Korn, 1797.

Süßmilch, Johann P. *Die göttliche Ordnung in den Veränderungen des menschlichen Geschlechts, aus der Geburt, dem Tode und der Fortpflanzung desselben erwiesen.* 2 Vols. 2nd ed. Berlin: Buchhandlung der Realschule, 1761–62.

Swieten, Gerhard van. *Erläuterungen der Boerhaavischen Lehrsätze von Erkentniss und Heilung der Krankheiten.* Frankfurt and Leipzig: Krauß, 1775.

Sydenham, Thomas. *The Whole Works of Dr. Thomas Sydenham*. Translated by John Pechey. 10th ed. London: Feales, 1734.

"The Opinion of his Majesty's Physicians and Surgeons, given Jan. 23, 1768, in regard to Messrs. Sutton's Practice of Inoculation, in Consequence of a Letter from Sir John Pringle." *Gentlemans Magazine* 38 (1768): 74–5.

Thilenius, Moritz G. "Lauterbach, am Vogelsberg, 5 December, 1783." *Politisches Journal* 2 (1783): 1226–27.

Thilenius, Moritz G. *Medicinische und chirurgische Bemerkungen*. 3 eds. Frankfurt am Main: Brönner, 1789; 1809; 1814.

Thümmel, Moritz A. von. *Die Inoculation der Liebe. Eine Erzählung*. Biel: Heilmann, 1773.

Tieftrunk, Johann H. *Philosophische Untersuchungen über die Tugendlehre*. Halle: Renger, 1797.

Timoni, Emanuele. "An Account, or History, of the Procuring the Small Pox by Incision, or Inoculation: as it has for Some Time Been Practiced at Constantinople." *Philosophical Transactions of the Royal Society* 29 (1714): 72–84.

Tissot, Samuel-Auguste D. *Anleitung für das Landvolk in Absicht auf seine Gesundheit*. Translated by H. C. Hirzel. Zürich: Heidegger, 1762.

Tissot, Samuel-Auguste D. *Avis au peuple sur sa santé*. Lausanne: Grasset, 1761.

Tissot, Samuel-Auguste D. *Leben des Ritters von Zimmermann, Hofrath und Leibarztes zu Hannover*. Hanover: Hahn, 1797.

Tissot, Samuel-Auguste D. *L'inoculation justifiée, ou dissertation pratique et apologétique sur cette méthode*. Lausanne, 1754.

Tode, Johann C. "Etwas von der medizinischen Aufklärung des Volks." *Der unterhaltende Arzt* 4 (1789): 141–7.

Triller, Daniel W. "Neujahrs-Gedicht, auf das Jahr 1743." In *Daniel W. Triller: Poetischer Betrachtungen über verschiedene Natur-und Sittenlehre*, 208–13. Hamburg: Herold, 1747.

"Ueber die Ausrottung der Blattern." *Münchner Intelligenzblatt*, no. 23 (1797): 280–83.

"Ueber die Pockeninoculation und die Pockenvertilgung. Ein Gespräch im Wirtshaus zu B…" *Deutsche Monatsschrift* 2 (1798): 180–92.

Uebersicht des politischen Zustandes Europens im Jahr 1786. Kempten: Kösel, 1787.

Ungnad, Christian S. "Nachricht von einer zahlreichen Blatter-impfung auf dem Land." In vol. 3 of *Jahrbücher der preussischen Monarchie unter der Regierung Friedrich Wilhelms des Dritten*, 303–8. Berlin: Unger, 1800.

Vater, Karl F.W.A. *Preussisch-Schlesische Civil Medicinal- and Sanitäts-Verfassung*. Part 2. Breslau: Korn, 1800.

"Vermischte Nachrichten." *Journal für Prediger* 3 (1773): 462–63.

"Vermischte Nachrichten." *Lausitzischen Magazin*, no. 3 (1771): 45.

Vogel, Samuel G. *Handbuch der practischen Arzneywissenschaft zum Gebrauche angehende Aerzte*. 1st ed. Vienna: Trattner, 1789. 3rd ed. Stendal: Franzen and Große, 1820.

Voltaire, *Collection Complette des Oeuvres de M. Voltaire*. Vol. 27, *Histoire du Parlement de Louis XV, Fragmens*. Geneva, 1776.

"Von den Calender-Prophezeihungen." *Hannoverisches Magazin* 5 (1767): 92–6.

Wagener, Samuel C. "Der Schulmeister vom Haina." *Patriotisches Archiv für Deutschland* 1 (1799): 156–60.

Wagener, Samuel C. "Staatsdiener! Schriftsteller! Leser jedes Standes!" *Patriotisches Archiv für Deutschland* 1 (1799): 1–15.

"Warnung gegen die medizinische Pfuscherey eines Geistlichen." *Journal von und für Deutschland* 7 (1790): 287–80.

"Warum man mit der Aufklärung der Bürger und Bauern noch so weit zurück, und wie weit man gleichwohl gekommen ist." *Beyträge zur vaterländischen Historie, Geographie, Statistik* 3 (1790): 352–70.

Wechsel. Untitled. *Schlesische Provinzialblätter* 30 (1799): 458.

Wehrs, G.F. "Vom Blatternkaufen unter den Landleuten, nebst einigen Anmerkungen über das Alter der Kinderpocken." *Hannoverisches Magazin* 27 (1789): 449–64.

Weinhold. "Schul Feierlichkeit." *Schlesische Provinzialblätter* 30 (1799): 456–58.

Weiße, Christian E. and Samuel G. Frisch. *Christian Felix Weißens Selbstbiographie*. Leipzig: Voß, 1806.

Weiße, Christian F. "Eitle Schönheit." In vol. 3 of *Christian F. Weiße: Kleine lyrische Gedichte*, 51–53. Leipzig: Weidmann's Erben und Reich, 1772.

Weiße, Christian F. *Komische Opern*. Leipzig: Dyck, 1773.

Weißmann, Immanuel. *Fata & imposturae variolosorum. Oder Muthmaßliche Gedanken und Ursachen, Wie? Und Warum? Manche Leute die sogenannte Urschlechten oder Kinds-Blattern als ein Göttliches Straff-Gericht nicht erkennen*. Ulm: Bartholomeo, 1713.

Wessely, Napthali H. *Dankfeyer auf die Genesung der Königlichen Kinder, nach glücklich erfolgter Blattern-Einimpfung: gehalten in der Synagoge der Judenschaft zu Berlin, am Sabat-Abend 18 Dezember, 1789*. Berlin, 1790.

Westenrieder, Lorenz von. *Beschreibung der Haupt-und Residenzstadt München (im gegenwärtigen Zustand)*. Munich: Strobel, 1782.

Wetsch, Ignaz J. *Das bestrittene Vorurtheil in zweyen Abhandlungen: die Einpfropfung der Kindspocken und die Beerdigung der Toten in den Kirchen und Städten betreffend*. Vienna: Krauß, 1764.

Willamov, Johann G. "Auf Ihro Russischkaiserlichen Majestät und des Durchlauigsten Großfürsten Wiedergenesung von Einimpfung der Blattern, im November 1768." In *Johann G. Willamov's Sämmtliche poetische Schriften*, 88–95. Leipzig: Schwickert, 1779.

"Wohlgemeinte Vorschläge zur Abschaffung der Quacksalberey in Schlesien." *Schlesische Provinzialblätter* 34 (1801): 219–24.

"Worms im Januar, 1791." *Intelligenzblatt der Allgemeine Literatur-Zeitung*, no. 81 (1791): 669–71.

Wreden, Johann E. *An Essay on the Inoculation of Smallpox. To which are Added, some Examples of Persons inoculated with Good Success at Hanover.* London, 1729.

Wrisberg, Heirich A. *Beytrag zur Pocken-Geschichte.* Göttingen: Vandenhoek, 1770.

Wrisberg, Heinrich A. *Dissertatio de insitione variolarum nonulla momenta recenset et simul ad sermonem academicum de physologia errores quosdam expurgante.* Göttingen, 1765.

Württemburgisches gelehrten Lexicon, so viel die jetztlebende Württemburgische Schriftensteller betrift. 1772.

Zaccharià, Justus F.W. "Die Seuche." In *Justus F.W. Zacharià: Scherzhafte epische Poesien, nebst einigen Oden und Liedern,* 385–86. Brunswick and Hildesheim: Schröder, 1754.

Zacchiroli, Francesco. "La Inoculazione." In *Francesco Zacchiroli: Versi,* 11–49. Lausanne, 1778.

Zadig, Abraham. *Plan, nach welchem die Einimpfung der Pocken in einer ganzen Provinz allgemein eingeführt und die längst gewünschte Ausrottung der Seuche erreicht werden könnte.* Breslau: Korn, 1797.

Secondary Materials

Albrecht, Peter."Wie hältst Du es mit der Blatterninokulation? Eine 'Gretchenfrage' im 18. Jahrhundert." *Praxis Geschichte* 5 (1999): 58–60.

Albrecht, Peter. "Von den vergeblichen Mühen, die Bevölkerung der Stadt Braunschweig von der Nützlichkeit des Impfens gegen Blattern zu überzeugen (1754–1787)." In *Gotts Verhengnis und seine Straffe – zur Geschichten der Seuche in der frühen Neuzeit,* edited by Petra Feuerstein-Herz, 127–37. Wolfenbüttel: Herzog August Bibliothek, 2005.

Alexander, John T. *Bubonic Plague in Early Modern Russia.* Oxford: Oxford University Press, 2003.

Baasner, Rainer. *Einführung in die Literatur der Aufklärung.* Darmstadt: Wissenschaftliche Buchgesellschaft, 2006.

Backhaus, Ursula. "Johann Heinrich Gottlob von Justi (1717–1771): Health as part of a State's Capital Endowment." In *The Beginnings of Political Economy,* edited by Jürgen G. Backhaus, 171–195. New York: Springer, 2009.

Bazin, Hervé. *Vaccination: a History. From Lady Montagu to Genetic Engineering.* Esher: John Libbey Eurotext, 2011.

Becker-Cantarino, Barbara. "The Scope of German Literature in the Eighteenth Century." In *German Literature of the Eighteenth Century: The Enlightenment and Sensibility,* edited by Barbara Becker-Cantarino, 1–31. Rochester: Camden House, 2005.

Behrend, Gustav. "Ueber Variolation." *Deutsche Medizinische Wochenschrift* 20 (1896): 307–11.

Bennett, Michael J. "Curing and Inoculating Smallpox: the Career of Simeon Worlock in Paris, Brittany, and Saint-Domingue in the 1770s." *French History and Civilization* 7 (2017): 27–38.

Bennett, Michael J. *War Against Smallpox. Edward Jenner and the Early Global Spread of Vaccination.* Cambridge: Cambridge University Press, 2020.

Bischoff, Cordula. "Aufklärung in Sachsen? Das höfische Familienporträt zwischen Staatsrepräsentation und Empfindsamkeit." *Das Achtzehnte Jahrhundert: Aufklärung und Hofkultur in Dresden* 37, part 2 (2013): 202–18.

Blanning, Tim C.W. *The Culture of Power and the Power of Culture; Old-Regime Europe, 1660–1789*. Oxford: Oxford University Press, 2002.

Blower, Sally. "Classic Paper: An Attempt at a New Analysis of the Mortality Caused by Smallpox and of the Advantages of Inoculation to Prevent it, by Daniel Bernoulli." *Reviews in Medical Virology* 14 (2004): 275–288.

Boerner, Peter. *Goethe*. Translated by Nancy Boerner. Haus: London, 2013.

Böning, Holger. "Johann Moritz Schwager als Volkskundler und Volksaufklärer." In *Er War ein Licht in Westfalen. Johann Moritz Schwager (1738–1804), ein Westfälische Aufklärer*, edited by Walter Gödden, Peter Hesselmann, and Frank Stückemann, 53–78. Bielefeld: Aisthesis, 2013.

Böth, Marieke. *Erzählweisen des Selbst. Körperpraktiken in den Briefen Liselottes von der Pfalz (1652–1722)*. Böhlau, Cologne, 2015.

Bohn, Heinrich. "Ueber Kant's Beziehungen zur Medizin." *Altpreussische Monatsschrift* 9 (1872): 609–26.

Boylston, Arthur. "The Origins of Inoculation." *Journal of the Royal Society of Medicine* 105 (2012): 309–13. https://doi:10.1258/jrsm.2012.12k044 (accessed 13 February 2021).

Brandes, Helga. "The Literary Marketplace and the Journal." In *German Literature of the Eighteenth Century: The Enlightenment and Sensibility*, edited by Barbara Becker-Cantarino, 70–102. Rochester: Camden House, 2005.

Brechka, Frank T. *Gerard van Swieten and His World 1700–177*. The Hague: Nijhoff, 1970.

Brockmann, Hartmut. *Der Deutsche Orden.* Munich: Beck, 1999.

Broman, Thomas. "Rethinking Professionalization: Theory, Practice, and Professional Ideology in Eighteenth-Century German Medicine." *The Journal of Modern History* 67 (1995): 835–72.

Broman, Thomas. *The Transformation of German Academic Medicine, 1750–1820*. Cambridge: Cambridge University Press, 1996.

Brügelmann, Jan. "Observations on the Process of Medicalization in Germany, 1770–1830, based on Medical Topographies." In *La Medicalisation de la Société Francaise 1770–1830,* edited by Jean-Pierre Goubert, 131–49. Waterloo, Ontario: Historical Reflections Press, 1982.

Brunschwig, Henri. *Enlightenment and Romanticism in Eighteenth-century Prussia.* Chicago and London: University of Chigaco Press, 1974.

Brunton, Deborah C. "Pox Britannica: Smallpox Inoculation in Britain, 1721–30." PhD thesis, University of Pennsylvania, 1990.

Brunton, Deborah C. "Smallpox Inoculation and Demographic Trends in Eighteenth-Century Scotland." *Medical History* 36 (1992): 403–29.

Campbell, Jill. "Lady Mary Wortley Montagu and the 'Glass Revers'd' of Female Old Age." In *Defects: Engendering the Modern Body,* edited by Helen Deutsch and Felicity Nussbaum, 213–51. Ann Arbor: University of Michigan Press, 2003.

Clark, Christopher. *Iron Kingdom. The Rise and Downfall of Prussia, 1600–1947.* London: Allen Lane, 2006.

Clausnitzer, Eduard. *Die Volksschulpädagogik Friedrichs des Grossen und der preussischen Unterrichtsverwaltung seiner Zeit.* Halle: Schroedel, 1902.

Clendinning, Philip H. "Dr. Thomas Dimsdale and Smallpox Inoculation in Russia." *Journal of the History of Medicine and Allied Sciences* 28 (1973): 109–25.

Cotoni, Marie-Hélène, ed. *Correspondance de Frédéric II avec Louise-Dorothée de Saxe-Gotha (1740–1767).* Oxford: Alden, 1999.

De Ford, Sara and Clarinda H. Lott. *Forms of Verse.* New York: Meredith, 1971.

Drews, Peter. "Johann Gottlieb Willamov – ein deutscher Dichter im Russland Katharinas II." *Germanoslavica* 3 (1996): 209–22.

Ebstein, William. "Georg und William Motherby und Ihren Beziehungen zur Variolation (Königsberg)." *Archiv für Geschichte der Medizin* 4 (1911): 31–42.

Emch-Dériaz, Antoinette S. "L' Inoculation Justifiée, or Was it?" *Eighteenth-Century Life* 7 (1982): 65–72.

Eriksen, Anne. "A Case of Exemplarity. C.F. Rotböll's History of Smallpox Inoculation in Denmark-Norway, 1766." *Scandinavian Journal of History* 35 (2010): 351–70.

Fenner, Frank, Donald A. Henderson, Isao Arita, Zdeněk Jezek, and Ivan D. Ladnyi. *Smallpox and its Eradication.* Geneva: World Health Organization, 1988.

Finckh, Ruth, ed. *Das Universitätsmamsellen-Lesebuch.* Göttingen: Göttingen University Press, 2015.

Frevert, Ute. *Krankheit als politisches Problem 1770–1880. Soziale Unterschichten in Preußen zwischen medizinischer Polizei und staatlicher Sozialversicherung.* Göttingen: Vandenhoek & Ruprecht, 1984.

Garland, Mary and Henry Garland. *The Oxford Companion to German Literature.* Oxford and New York: Oxford University Press, 1997.

Gehrmann, Rolf. *Bevölkerungsgeschichte Norddeutschlands zwischen Aufklärung und Vormärz.* Berlin: Spitz, 2000.

Gehrmann, Rolf. "The Impact of Smallpox and Vaccination in Northern Germany in the 18th and 19th Centuries." *Przeszlość Demograficzna Polski* 36 (2014): 39–54.

Gerber, Michael R. *Die Schlesische Provinzialblätter.* Sigmaringen: Thorbecke, 1995.

Gins, Heinrich A. *Krankheit wider den Tod.* Stuttgart: Fischer, 1963.

Glynn, Ian and Jennifer Glynn. *The Life and Death of Smallpox*. London: Profile, 2004.
Grant, Alicia. *Globalisation of Variolation: the Overlooked Origins of Immunity for Smallpox in the 18th Century*. New Jersey: World Scientific, 2018.
Gratton, Jacqueline. "Smallpox Prevention and the Dissemination of New Ideas in Spain 1725–1775." MA thesis, University of Tasmania, 2012.
Grundy, Isobel. *Lady Mary Wortley Montagu*. Oxford: Oxford University Press, 1999.
Halama, Udo, ed. *Ein + verbindet. 150 Jahre Marienkirche Jöllenbeck*. Bielefeld: Anzeigen & mehr, 2004.
Heinrich, Jörg. *Johann Theodor Eller. Ein bedeutender Arzt, Wissenschaftler und Medizinalbeamter in Brandenburg-Preussen in der ersten Hälfte des 18. Jahrhunderts*. Husum: Matthiesen, 2003.
Heller, Robert. "Johann Christian Reil's Training Scheme for Medical Auxiliaries." *Medical History* 19 (1975): 321–32.
Hellmuth, Eckhart and Wolfgang Piereth. "Germany, 1760–1815." In *Press, Politics, and the Public Sphere in Europe and North America, 1760–1820*, edited by Hannah Barker and Simon Burrows, 69–92. Cambridge: Cambridge University Press, 2002.
Henderson, Donald A. *Smallpox: the Death of a Disease*. New York: Prometheus, 2009.
Hess, Volker. "Vom Miasma zum Virus." In *Pocken zwischen Alltag, Medizin und Politik*, edited by Ragnhild Münch, 16–30. Berlin: Engel, 1994.
Hilliard, Kevin. "Religious and Secular Poetry and Epic (1700–1780)." In *German Literature of the Eighteenth Century: The Enlightenment and Sensibility*, edited by Barbara Becker-Cantarino, 105–128. Rochester: Camden House, 2005.
Hirsch, Erhard. "Naturwissenschaftlicher Unterricht am Dessauer Philanthropium." In *Johann Juncker (1679–1759) und seine Zeit*, edited by Wolfram Kaiser and Hans Hübner, 57–81. Halle-Wittenberg: Martin-Luther University, 1979.
Hochheim, Margot. *Der Pädagoge Salzmann*. Berlin: Springer, 1939.
Hölscher-Lohmeyer, Dorothea. *Johann Wolfgang von Goethe*. Munich: Beck, 2007.
Hopkins, Donald R. *The Greatest Killer: Smallpox in History*. Chicago: University of Chicago Press, 2002.
Hovorka, Oscar and Adolf Kronfeld. *Vergleichende Volksmedizin: eine Darstellung volksmedizinischer Sitten und Gebräuche, Anschauungen und Heilfaktoren, des Aberglaubens und der Zaubermedizin*. Stuttgart: Strecker and Schröder, 1909.
Huerkamp, Claudia. "The History of Smallpox Vaccination in Germany: a First Step in the Medicalization of the General Public." *Journal of Contemporary History* 20 (1985): 617–35.
Humphries, N.A. "English Vaccination and Small-Pox Statistics: with Special Reference to the Report of the Royal Commission, and to Recent Small-Pox Epidemics." *Journal of the Royal Statistical Society* 60 (1897): 503–51.
Im Hof, Ulrich. *Das Europa der Aufklärung*. Munich: Beck, 1993.

Ingen Housz, Jan Maarten, Norman Beale, and Elaine Beale. "The Life of Dr Jan Ingen Housz (1730–99), Private Counsellor and Personal Physician to Emperor Joseph II of Austria." *Journal of Medical Biography* 13 (2005): 15–21.

Israel, Jonathan I. *Democratic Enlightenment. Philosophy, Revolution and Human Rights 1750–1790*. Oxford: Oxford University Press, 2011.

Israel, Jonathan I. *Radical Enlightenment.* Oxford: Oxford University Press, 2002.

Jaeckel, Gerhard. *Die Charité. Die Geschichte eines Weltzentrums der Medizin von 1710 bis zur Gegenwart.* Berlin: Lehmanns Media, 2018.

Kaiser, Wolfram. "Impfärzte des 18. Jahrhunderts." *Zahn-, Mund, und Kieferheilkunde* 64 (1976): 385–96.

Kaiser, Wolfram and Kurt Werner. "Die Anfänge der Pockenschutzimpfung in Halle und Umgebung." *Zeitschrift für die gesamte Hygiene* 19 (1973): 806–12.

Klebs, Arnold C. *Die Variolation im achtzehnten Jahrhundert: ein historischer Beitrag zur Immunitätsforschung.* Gießen: Töpelmann, 1914.

Köpke, Rudolf. "Aus dem Leben des Johann Timotheus Hermes." *Zeitschrift für das Gymnasialwesen* 16 (1862): 657–68.

Konert, Jürgen. "S.A. Tissot und sein Einfluss auf den 'Dessau-Wörlitzer Kulturkreis.'" *Gesnerus* 49 (1992): 39–44.

Kopitzsch, Franklin. "Die Durchsetzung der Pockenimpfung. Zu Strategien und Mitteln aufgeklärter Reform in Hamburg und Schleswig-Holstein." In *Das Volk im Visier der Aufklärung*, eds. Anne Conrad, Arno Herzig, and Franklin Kopitzsch, 229–37. Hamburg: LIT, 1998.

Kübler, Peter. *Geschichte der Pocken und der Impfung.* Berlin: Hirschwald, 1901.

La Vopa, Anthony J. *Grace, Talent, and Merit. Poor Students, Clerical Careers, and Professional Ideology in Eighteenth-Century Germany.* Cambridge: Cambridge University Press, 1988.

Lindemann, Mary. "'*Aufklärung*' and the Health of the People; '*Volksschriften*' and Medical Advice in Braunschweig-Wolfenbüttel, 1756–1803." In *Das Volk als Objekt obrigkeitlichen Handelns,* edited by Rudolf Vierhaus, 101–20. Tübingen: Niemeyer, 1992.

Lindemann, Mary. *Health and Healing in Eighteenth-Century Germany.* Baltimore and London: Johns Hopkins University Press, 1996.

Lukitschev, Michail and Reimer Witt, eds. *Die Gottorfer auf dem Weg zum Zarenthron. Russisch-Gottorfische Verbindungen im 18. Jahrhundert.* Eine russisch-schleswig-holsteinische Archivausstellung in Landesarchiv Schleswig-Holstein. Schleswig, 1997.

McAlpin, Mary. *Female Sexuality and Cultural Degradation in Enlightenment France: Medicine and Literature.* Oxford and New York: Routledge, 2016.

MacGregor, Neil. *Germany. Memories of a Nation.* London: Allen Lane, 2014.

Maehle, Andreas-Holger. "Conflicting Attitudes Towards Inoculation in Enlightenment Germany." *Clio Medica* 29 (1995): 198–222.

Maehle, Andreas-Holger. "The Ethics of Prevention: German Philosophers of the Late Enlightenment on the Morality of Smallpox Inoculation." In *Coping with Sickness. Perspectives on Health-Care Past and Present,* edited by John Woodward and Robert Jütte, 91–114. Sheffield: E.A.H.M.H., 1996.

Mamlock, Gotthold L. "Friedrich der Grosse und die Einführung der Impfung in Berlin." *Aerztliche sachverständige Zeitung* 10 (1904): 38–41.

Mamlock, Gotthold L. *Friedrichs des Grossen Korrespondenz mit Aerzten.* Wiesbaden: Sändig, 1966.

Melton, James van Horn. *Absolutism and the Eighteenth-Century Origins of Compulsory Schooling in Prussia and Austria.* Cambridge: Cambridge University Press, 1988.

Messerli, Alfred. "'Der Pöbel aber bleibt versäumt' – Kalender als populäres Vehikel medizinischer Volksaufklärung." In *Gesundheit und Krankheit im 18.Jahrhundert,* edited by Helmut Holzhey and Urs Bosching, 89–105. Amsterdam and Atlanta: Rodopi, 1995.

Michalik, Kerstin. *Kindsmord. Soziale-und Rechtsgeschichte der Kindstötung im 18. und beginnenden 19. Jahrhundert, am Beispiel Preussen.* Pfaffenweiler: Centaurus, 1997.

Miller, Genevieve. *The Adoption of Inoculation for Smallpox in England and France.* Philadelphia: University of Pennsylvania Press, 1957.

Mörike, Klaus D. *Geschichte der Tübinger Anatomie.* Tübingen: Mohr, 1988.

Pischon, F.A. *Denkmäler der deutschen Sprache, von Haller bis jetzt.* Berlin, 1845.

Pistor, Moritz. "Geschichte der preussischen Medizinalverwaltung." *Deutsche Vierteljahrsschrift für öffentliche Gesundheitspflege* 40 (1908): 225–50, 500–554, 749–810.

Poeter, Elisabeth. "Gender, Religion, and Medicine in Enlightenment Germany: Dorothea Christiane Leporin's Treatise on the Education of Women." *NWSA Journal* 20 (2008): 99–119.

Powell, Barry. *Classical Myth.* Englewood Cliffs, NJ: Prentice Hall, 1995.

Razzell, Peter. *The Conquest of Smallpox: the Impact of Inoculation on Smallpox Mortality in Eighteenth-century Britain.* London: Caliban, 2003.

Rees, Joachim, Winfried Siebers and Hilmer Tilgner. "Reisen im Erfahrungsraum Europa. Forschungsperspektiven zur Reisetätigkeit politisch-sozialer Eliten des Alten Reichs (1750–1800)." *Das Achtzehnte Jahrhundert* 26, part 1 (2002): 35–62.

Rödel, Walter H. "Die Pocken in Mainz in Jahre 1766." *Medizinhistorisches Journal* 14 (1979): 53–80.

Rowbotham, Arnold H. "The 'Philosophes' and the Propaganda for Inoculation of Smallpox in France." *University of California Publications in Modern Philology* 18 (1935): 265–90.

Rusnock, Andrea A. *Vital Accounts. Quantifying Health and Population in Eighteenth-Century England and France.* Cambridge: Cambridge University Press, 2002.

Sander, Sabine. *Handwerkschirurgen: Sozialgeschichte einer verdrängten Berufsgruppe.* Göttingen: Vandenhoek & Ruprecht, 1989.

Schenda, Rudolf. *Volk ohne Buch; Studien zur Sozialgeschichte der populären Lesestoffe, 1770–1910*. Frankfurt am Main: Klostermann, 1970.

Schieder, Theodor. *Frederick the Great*. Translated and edited by Hamish M. Scott and Sabina Berkeley. London and New York: Longman, 2000.

Seitz, A. "Etwas vom Impfen aus dem Jahre 1768." *Archiv für Geschichte der Medizin* 2 (1909): 419–21.

Seth, Catriona. *Les rois aussi en mouraient. Les Lumières en lutte contre la petite vérole*. Paris: Desjonquères, 2008.

Shorter, Edward. "Die Grosse Umwalzung in der Mutter-Kind-Beziehung vom 18. bis zum 20. Jahrhundert." In *Zur Sozialgeschichte der Kindheit*, edited by Jochen Martin, August Nitschke, and Klaus Arnold, 503–24. Munich: K.A. Freiburg, 1986.

Siegert, Reinhart. "Aufklärung und Volkslektüre exemplarish dargestellt an Rudolph Zacharias Becker und seinem 'Not-und Hülfsbüchlein.'" In vol. 19 of *Archiv für Geschichte des Buchwesens*, edited by Berthold Hack, Reinhard Wittman, and Marietta Kleiss, 1025–1348. Frankfurt am Main: Buchhändler-Vereinigung, 1978.

Shuttleton, David E. *Smallpox and the Literary Imagination, 1660–1820*. Cambridge: Cambridge University Press, 2007.

Skold, Peter. "From Inoculation to Vaccination: Smallpox in Sweden in the Eighteenth and Nineteenth Centuries." *Population Studies* 50 (1996): 247–62.

Skold, Peter. "The Beauty and the Beast – Smallpox and Marriage in Eighteenth- and Nineteenth-Century Sweden." *Historical Social Research* 28 (2003): 141–61.

Skold, Peter. *The Two Faces of Smallpox. A Disease and its Prevention in Eighteenth and Nineteenth-Century Sweden*. Umea: Umea University Press, 1996.

Smith, John R. *The Speckled Monster*. Chelmsford: Essex Records Office, 1987.

Spalding, Almut. *Elise Reimarus (1735–1805): The Muse of Hamburg: A Woman of the German Enlightenment*. Würzburg: Königshausen and Neumann, 2005.

Starck, Christopher and Kurt Schönhammer. *Die Geschichte der Akademie der Wissenschaften*. Part 1. Berlin and Boston: de Gruyter, 2013.

Stricker, Wilhelm. "Pockenpoesie." *R. Virchow's Archiv für pathologische Anatomie und Physiologie und für klinische Medizin* 20 (1861): 394–99.

Stroup, Johann M. *The Struggle for Identity in the Clerical Estate*. Leiden: Brill, 1984.

Sumich, Christi. "'A Christian's Groans Under the Body of Sin': the Pox and the Pious Physician." *Clio Medica* 91 (2013): 135–72.

Szabo, Franz A.J. *The Seven Years War in Europe 1756–1763*. Harlow: Pearson Longman, 2008.

Tering, Arvo. "The Dissertations of Doctors of Medicine Active in Estland, Livland, and Courland defended at European Universities in the Eighteenth Century." *Ajalooline Ajakiri* 133–4 (2010): 367–402.

Tutzke, Dietrich. *Christian August Struve (1767–1807): Leben und Werke eines Görlitzer Arztes im Dienste des Humanismus der Aufklärungszeit*. Görlitz: Town Council, 1957.

Ulbricht, Otto. *Kindsmord und Aufklärung in Deutschland*. Munich: Oldenbourg, 1990.

Völker, Arina. "Einige Markierungspunkte aus der Geschichte der Pockenschutzimpfung." *Zeitschrift für die gesamte innere Medizin und ihre Grenzgebiete* 45 (1990): 392–96.

Völker, Arina. "Johann Christian Wilhelm Juncker (1761–1800) und die Dessauer Impfpropagisten." In *Johann Juncker (1679–1759) und seine Zeit*, edited by Wolfram Kaiser and Hans Hübner, 86–96. Halle-Wittenberg: Martin-Luther University, 1979.

Watson, Peter. *The German Genius*. London: Simon and Schuster, 2010.

Van Dulmen, Richard. *The Society of the Enlightenment, the Rise of the Middle Class and Enlightenment Culture in Germany*. Cambridge: Polity, 1992.

Van Zwanenberg, David. "The Suttons and the Business of Inoculation." *Medical History* 22 (1978): 71–82.

Wilson, W. Daniel. "Eighteenth-century Germany in its Historical Context." In *German Literature of the Eighteenth Century: The Enlightenment and Sensibility*, edited by Barbara Becker-Cantarino, 265–83. Rochester: Camden House, 2005.

Wimmer, Johannes. *Gesundheit, Krankheit, und Tod im Zeitalter der Aufklärung. Fallstudien aus den Habsburgischen Erbländern*. Vienna, Cologne: Böhlau, 1991.

Wittmann, Reinhard. *Buchmarkt und Lektüre im 18. und 19. Jahrhundert, Beiträge zum literarischen Leben, 1750–1880*. Tübingen: Niemeyer, 1982.

Wittmann, Reinhard. "Was there a Reading Revolution at the End of the Eighteenth Century?" In *A History of Reading*, edited by Gugliemo Cavallo and Roger Chartier, 284–312. Oxford: Blackwell, 1999.

Wolff, Eberhard. "Der 'willkommene Würgeengel,' Verstehende Innenperspektive und 'genaue' Quellen-interpretation – am Beispeil des erwünschten Kindertods in den Anfangen der Pockenschutzimpfung." In *Neue Wege in der Seuchengeschichte*, edited by Martin Dinges, 105–41. Stuttgart: Steiner, 1995.

Wolff, Eberhard. *Einschneidende Maßnahmen: Pockenschutzimpfung und traditionale Gesellschaft im Württemberg des frühen 19. Jahrhunderts*. Stuttgart: Steiner, 1998.

Ziolkowski, Theodore. *German Romanicism and its Institutions*. Princeton, NJ: Princeton University Press, 1990.

Index

www.ingramcontent.com/pod-product-compliance
Lightning Source LLC
Chambersburg PA
CBHW071253180926
51613CB00001B/24
* 9 7 8 9 0 0 4 4 6 5 1 3 8 *